Analog Methods for Computer-Aided Circuit Analysis and Diagnosis

ELECTRICAL ENGINEERING AND ELECTRONICS

A Series of Reference Books and Textbooks

1. Rational Fault Analysis, *edited by Richard Saeks and S. R. Liberty*
2. Nonparametric Methods in Communications, *edited by P. Papantoni-Kazakos and Dimitri Kazakos*
3. Interactive Pattern Recognition, *Yi-tzuu Chien*
4. Solid-State Electronics, *Lawrence E. Murr*
5. Electronic, Magnetic, and Thermal Properties of Solid Materials, *Klaus Schröder*
6. Magnetic-Bubble Memory Technology, *Hsu Chang*
7. Transformer and Inductor Design Handbook, *Colonel Wm. T. McLyman*
8. Electromagnetics: Classical and Modern Theory and Applications, *Samuel Seely and Alexander D. Poularikas*
9. One-Dimensional Digital Signal Processing, *Chi-Tsong Chen*
10. Interconnected Dynamical Systems, *Raymond A. DeCarlo and Richard Saeks*
11. Modern Digital Control Systems, *Raymond G. Jacquot*
12. Hybrid Circuit Design and Manufacture, *Roydn D. Jones*
13. Magnetic Core Selection for Transformers and Inductors: A User's Guide to Practice and Specification, *Colonel Wm. T. McLyman*
14. Static and Rotating Electromagnetic Devices, *Richard H. Engelmann*
15. Energy-Efficient Electric Motors: Selection and Application, *John C. Andreas*
16. Electromagnetic Compossibility, *Heinz M. Schlicke*
17. Electronics: Models, Analysis, and Systems, *James G. Gottling*
18. Digital Filter Design Handbook, *Fred J. Taylor*
19. Multivariable Control: An Introduction, *P. K. Sinha*
20. Flexible Circuits: Design and Applications, *Steve Gurley, with contributions by Carl A. Edstrom, Jr., Ray D. Greenway, and William P. Kelly*
21. Circuit Interruption: Theory and Techniques, *Thomas E. Browne, Jr.*
22. Switch Mode Power Conversion: Basic Theory and Design, *K. Kit Sum*
23. Pattern Recognition: Applications to Large Data-Set Problems, *Sing-Tze Bow*
24. Custom-Specific Integrated Circuits: Design and Fabrication, *Stanley L. Hurst*
25. Digital Circuits: Logic and Design, *Ronald C. Emery*
26. Large-Scale Control Systems: Theories and Techniques, *Magdi S. Mahmoud, Mohamed F. Hassan, and Mohamed G. Darwish*
27. Microprocessor Software Project Management, *Eli T. Fathi and Cedric V. W. Armstrong* (*Sponsored by Ontario Centre for Microelectronics*)
28. Low Frequency Electromagnetic Design, *Michael P. Perry*
29. Multidimensional Systems: Techniques and Applications, *edited by Spyros G. Tzafestas*
30. AC Motors for High-Performance Applications: Analysis and Control, *Sakae Yamamura*

31. Ceramic Materials for Electronics: Processing, Properties, and Applications, *edited by Relva C. Buchanan*
32. Microcomputer Bus Structures and Bus Interface Design, *Arthur L. Dexter*
33. End User's Guide to Innovative Flexible Circuit Packaging, *Jay J. Miniet*
34. Reliability Engineering for Electronic Design, *Norman B. Fuqua*
35. Design Fundamentals for Low-Voltage Distribution and Control, *Frank W. Kussy and Jack L. Warren*
36. Encapsulation of Electronic Devices and Components, *Edward R. Salmon*
37. Protective Relaying: Principles and Applications, *J. Lewis Blackburn*
38. Testing Active and Passive Electronic Components, *Richard F. Powell*
39. Adaptive Control Systems: Techniques and Applications, *V. V. Chalam*
40. Computer-Aided Analysis of Power Electronic Systems, *Venkatachari Rajagopalan*
41. Integrated Circuit Quality and Reliability, *Eugene R. Hnatek*
42. Systolic Signal Processing Systems, *edited by Earl E. Swartzlander, Jr.*
43. Adaptive Digital Filters and Signal Analysis, *Maurice G. Bellanger*
44. Electronic Ceramics: Properties, Configuration, and Applications, *edited by Lionel M. Levinson*
45. Computer Systems Engineering Management, *Robert S. Alford*
46. Systems Modeling and Computer Simulation, *edited by Naim A. Kheir*
47. Rigid-Flex Printed Wiring Design for Production Readiness, *Walter S. Rigling*
48. Analog Methods for Computer-Aided Circuit Analysis and Diagnosis, *edited by Takao Ozawa*
49. Transformer and Inductor Design Handbook, Second Edition, Revised and Expanded, *Colonel Wm. T. McLyman*

Additional Volumes in Preparation

Signal Processing Handbook, *edited by C. H. Chen*

Electrical Engineering-Electronics Software

1. Transformer and Inductor Design Software for the IBM PC, *Colonel Wm. T. McLyman*
2. Transformer and Inductor Design Software for the Macintosh, *Colonel Wm. T. McLyman*
3. Digital Filter Design Software for the IBM PC, *Fred J. Taylor and Thanos Stouraitis*

Analog Methods for Computer-Aided Circuit Analysis and Diagnosis

edited by

Takao Ozawa

Kyoto University
Kyoto, Japan

MARCEL DEKKER, INC. New York and Basel

Library of Congress Cataloging-in-Publication Data

Analog methods for computer-aided circuit analysis and
diagnosis.

(Electrical engineering and electronics ; 48)
Includes bibliographies and index.
1. Electric circuit analysis--Data processing.
2. Analog electronic systems. I. Ozawa, Takao
1934 II. Series.
TK454.A475 1988 621.319'1'1287 87-37983
ISBN: 0-8247-7843-0

MARCEL DEKKER, INC.
270 Madison Avenue, New York, New York 10016

Current printing (last digit):
10 9 8 7 6 5 4 3 2 1

PRINTED IN THE UNITED STATES OF AMERICA

Preface

Both the scale and the complexity of electronic circuits are now growing rapidly as the demand for electronic circuits and devices used in various systems increases. This continuously creates needs for new and more efficient analog methods for circuit analysis. For example, all large-scale analog circuits require careful setting of operating points. Because of the nonlinear characteristics of transistors and diodes, computationally efficient modeling of elements and algorithms for solving nonlinear equations are essential in DC circuit analysis. Even for digital circuits accurate waveform calculation is necessary in order to attain desirable circuit performance, especially fast switching speed. Parasitic capacitances and resistances must be taken into consideration, and thus the transient analysis must deal with stiff equations describing both very fast and very slow behavior of circuits. For lightly damped nonlinear circuits, computational efficiency is of special importance to obtain the periodic steady-state response. Switched-capacitor circuits and circuits containing time-varying elements require special AC analysis techniques.

Although testing and fault diagnosis of analog circuits has a long history, significant contributions to this problem with general theoretical foundations and computational algorithms have been made quite recently. This is perhaps because the formulation of fault diagnosis is not as straightforward as that of analysis. In the case of analysis, equations for the circuit response can be obtained from the circuit tolopogy and the characteristics of elements, whereas in diagnosis, these differ at least in part from the nominal ones because of faults. Besides, the location of faults is generally not known.

Whether or not faults can be located under given measurement conditions, how diagnostic equations are derived and how they can be solved efficiently, where measurements should be made, and how the tolerances of element values affect the diagnosis are a few examples of the problems encountered in circuit diagnosis.

Of course, circuit analysis, diagnosis, and design techniques are closely related to one another. Circuit simulation, which consists of repeated circuit analysis, is a most popular method for checking circuit designs. Circuit simulation used for fault diagnosis may have features different from those of simulation for design, but they have many numerical techniques in common. Methods for element value calculation to detect faults can also be used to determine element values in circuit design. Optimization techniques for circuits can be used for both design and diagnosis.

This book consists of chapters on circuit analysis and diagnosis covering important aspects of this field such as modeling, DC, AC, transient, and symbolic analyses, diagnosability, element value calculation, fault dictionary construction, fault verification, and optimization techniques. Emphasis is put on computational approaches so that the techniques presented here can be used in practice. As can be seen from the short descriptions given in the Introduction, the chapters present some advanced methodology and techniques for problems that cannot be handled by standard and well-established methods. Because of space limitations, papers appearing in conference proceedings or technical journals often lack preparatory descriptions and details of the methods used, or papers on the same subject appear separately. This book is intended to provide consistent and comprehensible descriptions of the subject matter for clear understanding. Whenever possible, fundamental concepts as well as analysis and diagnosis algorithms are illustrated by examples. It is hoped that engineers, researchers, and graduate students who want to study recent advances in this field or develop their own computer programs will use this book as a guide or a reference volume. It is assumed that the readers are familiar with the basic techniques of circuit analysis.

Although existing standard circuit simulators such as SPICE and ASTAP adopt a number of techniques for handling large-scale circuits, it has been found that they are not always efficient enough, taking too much CPU time and too much storage if they are run in conventional computers. Progress in manufacturing very large-scale integrated circuits, on the other hand, is now making new ways of computation possible. Analysis algorithms taking full advantage of vector or array processors or multiprocessor data processing systems will be able to handle far larger circuits. Theories, algorithms, and techniques presented in this book will provide the foundation for further developments in circuit analysis and diagnosis.

Takao Ozawa

Contents

Preface iii

Contributors vii

Introduction ix

1 Computationally Efficient Modeling of Transistors 1
Ryo Dang

2 LU Decomposition Algorithms for Parallel and Vector Computation 37
Martin Vlach

3 Piecewise Linear Analysis 65
Jos T. J. van Eijndhoven

4 Decomposition Techniques in Circuit Simulation 93
Martin Vlach

5 Waveform Relaxation Algorithms 117
Sadatoshi Kumagai

6 Computer Methods for Analysis of Switched-Capacitor Networks 139
Jiri Vlach

7 Techniques for Finding the Periodic Steady-State Response of Circuits 169
Kenneth S. Kundert, Alberto Sangiovanni-Vincentelli and Tsutomu Sugawara

8 Symbolic Network Analysis 205
Tadashi Matsumoto

9 Diagnosability of Analog Circuits 241
Takao Ozawa

10 Fault Location by Nodal Equations 265
Janusz A. Starzyk and Mohamed El-Gamal

11 Tableau Approach to Fault Diagnosis 299
Lawrence A. Rapisarda and Raymond A. DeCarlo

12 Computational Approaches to Fault Dictionary 325
Pen-Min Lin and Y. S. Elcherif

13 Decomposition Approaches to Fault Location 365
Takao Ozawa

14 Optimization Techniques for Modeling, Diagnosis, and Tuning 381
John W. Bandler and Qi-Jun Zhang

Index

Contributors

John W. Bandler Department of Electrical and Computer Engineering, McMaster University, Hamilton, Ontario, Canada

Ryo Dang Electrical Engineering Department, Hosei University, Koganei, Tokyo, Japan

Raymond A. DeCarlo School of Electrical Engineering, Purdue University, West Lafayette, Indiana

Jos T. J. Eijndhoven Department of Electrical Engineering, Eindhoven University of Technology, Eindhoven, The Netherlands

Y. S. Elcherif Department of Electrical and Communication Engineering, Cairo University, Giza, Egypt

Mohamed A. El-Gamal Department of Electrical and Computer Engineering, Ohio University, Athens, Ohio

Sadatoshi Kumagai Department of Electronic Engineering, Osaka University, Suita, Osaka, Japan

Kenneth S. Kundert Department of Electrical Engineering, University of California at Berkeley, Berkeley, California

Pen-Min Lin School of Electrical Engineering, Purdue University, West Lafayette, Indiana

Tadashi Matsumoto Department of Electrical Engineering, Fukui University, Fukui, Japan

Takao Ozawa, Department of Electrical Engineering, Kyoto University, Kyoto, Japan

Lawrence A. Rapisarda Department of Electrical Engineering, United States Military Academy, West Point, New York

Alberto Sangiovanni-Vincentelli Department of Electrical Engineering and Computer Sciences, University of California at Berkeley, Berkeley, California

Janusz A. Starzyk Department of Electrical and Computer Engineering, Ohio University, Athens, Ohio

Tsutomu Sugawara Research and Development Center, Toshiba Corporation, Kawasaki, Japan

Jiri Vlach Department of Electrical Engineering, University of Waterloo, Waterloo, Ontario, Canada

Martin Vlach Analogy, Inc., Beaverton, Oregon

Qi-Jun Zhang Department of Electrical and Computer Engineering, McMaster University, Hamilton, Ontario, Canada

Introduction

Device modeling is an essential step in circuit analysis. At present, it seems that no single model can represent all types of metal-oxide-semiconductor field effect transistors (MOSFET), and many MOSFET models are in use. The Ebers-Moll model has been the basis of all bipolar transistor models and some sophisticated extensions have been developed. For large-scale circuit simulation it is very important to choose proper device models, computationally efficient and yet accurate enough to express the physical effects that are to be taken into consideration. Trade-offs between efficiency and accuracy may have to be made. Therefore it is important to know how these models are derived. Starting from the basic fluid model of carriers, Chapter 1 presents analytical modeling of MOSFET and bipolar transistors and also numerical modeling of MOSFET. Analytical models are developed from the basic models by including various second-order effects, such as the short-channel and narrow-channel effects for MOSFET and space-charge region recombination and the Early effect for bipolar transistors. Normalization, linearization, and discretization of the basic equations to obtain numerical models are explained.

Very often DC and transient circuit analyses involve solving nonlinear equations by the Newton-Raphson method, which in turn is reduced to solving linear simultaneous equations repeatedly. Small-signal AC analysis, of course, consists of solving linear equations. A standard way to solve such linear simultaneous equations is by LU decomposition of the coefficient matrix. Since the number of times the equations are solved is very large, efficient algorithms for LU decomposition are very useful for all kinds of circuit analysis. Chapter 2 gives LU decomposition algorithms where the circuit to be analyzed has a hierarchical structure. The coefficient matrix, which has a nested (recursive) bordered-block-diagonal form, can be derived from the circuit, and the LU decomposition of a block is obtained from the decompositions of smaller subblocks contained in it. This gives rise to the possibility of using parallel processors to obtain the overall solution.

When the circuit to be simulated contains components with strongly nonlinear characteristics, the Newton-Raphson iteration often consumes a large amount of computation time and sometimes does not even converge. Piecewise linear methods have very attractive features such as strong global convergence properties, flexibility for choosing coarse or fine models depending on the desired accuracy, and the possibility of constructing models directly from measured data. Chapter 3 presents the basic principles of piecewise linear modeling and analysis for both static and dynamic circuit systems. A matrix notation is used for compact definition and manipulation of piecewise linear models, and the problem is solved as a linear complementarity problem, for which powerful algorithms are known.

Another powerful approach to piecewise linear analysis of large-scale circuits is presented in Chapter 4. This approach is based on the Katzenelson algorithm and decomposition techniques are used to speed up the algorithm. Two decomposition approaches—structural decomposition and relaxation decomposition, which is also known as temporal decomposition—are dealt with.

Recently, very efficient algorithms, called waveform relaxation algorithms, for the transient analysis of large-scale circuits were introduced. They are essentially iterative methods; the circuit is decomposed into subcircuits and then the subcircuits are analyzed in turn over the specified time interval repeatedly until the convergence of waveforms is attained. In Chapter 5 important problems inherent in waveform relaxation algorithms, such as the convergence conditions and the partitioning of circuits, are discussed. The algorithms are well suited to parallel computation, and a report on a parallel circuit simulator based on waveform relaxation algorithms is included.

Chapter 6 summarizes basic steps of switched-capacitor network analysis. With the assumption that the characteristics of switches, capacitors, and voltage sources are ideal, a simple and systematic method for deriving a system of equations describing the network behavior is given. Two-graphs, that is, a V-graph (voltage graph) for Kirchhoff's voltage law and an I-graph (current graph) for Kirchhoff's current law, are used so that a mininum system of equations is obtained. Formulas are derived for time domain solutions, frequency domain solutions, sensitivities in the frequency domain, and the group delay. They are numerically efficient, since most of the operations are transferred into the preprocessing, which must be done only once.

Three basic methods for computing periodic steady-state responses of nonlinear circuits are discussed in Chapter 7. The first is the shooting method, which essentially tries to find an initial state that eliminates any transient behavior and immediately results in periodicity. The second is the finite-difference method for solving finite-difference equations on mesh points that cover one period. The third is the expansion method, typically represented by the harmonic balance method, where the response is expressed as a linear combination of trigonometric functions whose coefficients are determined by balancing harmonics in the expression. These three methods are contrasted in a unified mathematical framework.

In designing a circuit, the dependence of circuit responses or network functions on some variables may be wanted in symbolic form. Since the number of variables (the exciting frequency, element values, etc.) associated with a circuit is, in general, very large, it is practical to express circuit responses or network functions in terms of the exciting frequency and/or a small number of variables in symbols while the remaining variables are given numerical values. Again, computationally efficient methods for deriving symbolic expressions are desired. Chapter 8 gives an overview of symbolic analysis followed by descriptions of important symbolic analysis methods including numerical interpolation algorithms using Fast Fourier Transform (FFT) and signal flow graph methods.

At present, approaches to analog circuit diagnosis can be classified in two main categories: fault-simulation-before-test methods and diagnosis-after-test methods. The former methods consist of two major steps. The first step is construction of a fault dictionary by analysis of the circuit under test for various fault situations, and the second is comparison of the simulated results in this dictionary with measurement data to locate faults. The latter methods try to locate faults directly from measurement data by calculating element or parameter values or by verifying fault assumptions.

Diagnosability is a far more important problem in circuit diagnosis than the solvability problem in analysis, since data available to diagnose a circuit are in general very limited. Equations derived under the given diagnostic conditions may or may not be solvable in the first place, and their intrinsic instability must be distinguished from that due to numerical methods used to solve them. Also, very often there exists fault ambiguity. Since the measurements can, in general, be performed at limited points in the circuit, two or more faults may give the same measurement data. Then they cannot be separated and are said to constitute an ambiguity set. The diagnosability problem is considered in Chapter 9 based on the principle partition of two-graphs (the voltage graph and the current graph). Diagnosable faults can be determined by graph algorithms.

Node equations, which are most commonly used in circuit analysis, can also be a basis for circuit diagnosis. Diagnosability of node faults (a node is said to be faulty if any of the elements connected to it is faulty) and algorithms to locate them are given in Chapter 10 utilizing node equations. First, algebraic conditions are derived for diagnosability and are given topological interpretations using the Coates flow graph and also the two-graph representation. Then an algorithm for locating faults in subnetworks is given. In the third and fourth parts methods are presented for evaluating faulty elements. Multiple circuit excitations and multifrequency measurements are assumed.

In general, equations for determining element values from measurement data such as input and output voltages become nonlinear. One numerically efficient approach to solving this problem of element value calculation is to formulate equations for element values in such a way that at most quadratic nonlinear equations appear. It follows then that a solution technique for fast convergence of the Newton-Raphson iteration becomes applicable by taking advantage of this special formulation. Chapter 11 presents this novel approach, which is called the tableau approach. The component connection model is used to derive network equations, and sparse tableau techniques are utilized in handling the equations.

The previous three chapters dealt with so-called soft faults or faults caused by element value or parameter value deviations outside the tolerance bounds. For diagnosing hard faults or faults caused by open circuits and/or short circuits the fault dictionary approach is well suited. Although the amount of computation required to simulate faults is very large, this has to be done only once. Chapter 12 presents a review of an existing fault dictionary approach and some new techniques to be used in fault dictionary construction. Open circuits and short circuits are represented by switches. In DC fault dictionary, construction nonlinear resistive networks containing switches are dealt with. Then a numerically efficient way to solve the problem is to use piecewise-linear models for nonlinear elements and apply the complementary pivot algorithm. A systematic fault isolation technique based on the ambiguity set concept is presented. Heuristic algorithms for selecting test or measurement points in the network to attain good separation of faults are also included.

If the given circuit can be decomposed into smaller subcircuits in such a way that the terminal voltages of each subcircuit can be measured and the terminal currents can be calculated from the terminal voltages, then the decomposition approach presented in Chapter 13 is applicable. The terminal currents are calculated individually for each subcircuit using nominal element values and measured terminal voltages. Then the calculated values are tested if they satisfy Kirchhoff's current law at terminals in the original circuit. A very simple and efficient algorithm is given for locating, from the test results, the faulty region that is the minimum-ambiguity subcircuit set containing faults. The effect of element value deviations within tolerance bounds is investigated, and an algorithm for determing the most likely faulty subcircuit in the sense of Hamming distance between two vectors is presented.

If the measurement is not enough to calculate actual element values, it is reasonable to find elements that are most likely to be faulty. One approach is to determine element values so that they minimize a certain measure and then to isolate as faulty the elements that exhibit large changes from their nominal values. Then the fault location problem is reduced to an optimization problem. Closely related to diagnosis problems are modeling and turning problems. Chapter 14 shows how these problems can be formulated as various optimization problems, what properties the formulated problems have, and how they can be solved efficiently. Among the methods and techniques discussed are the least-squares methods and the quadratic programming method for diagnosis, the reduction of model parameters and the multicircuit approach for modeling, and the functional approach and the deterministic approach for postproduction tuning.

Analog Methods for Computer-Aided Circuit Analysis and Diagnosis

1

Computationally Efficient Modeling of Transistors

Ryo Dang

Hosei University
Koganei, Tokyo, Japan

1 INTRODUCTION

Modeling, as considered in this chapter, is aimed at the construction of models to describe various device characteristics. In the early days of semiconductor electronics, models were usually developed in parallel with or sometimes even before the device itself. This is no longer true since the advent of very large scale integration (VLSI). In only about a decade we have witnessed a several hundredfold change in integration scale. This implies shrinking of basic devices—transistors, especially metal-oxide-semiconductor field effect transistors (MOSFETs)—by more than an order of magnitude in each of their three dimensions. This shrinking of basic devices is so drastic that many physical effects of a two- or three-dimensional nature have become conspicuous (the short-channel effect [1], narrow-channel effect [2], inverse narrow-channel effect [3], and so on), but none of them has yet been modeled in a completely satisfactory way.

The fact that some of the latest circuit simulators, especially commercially available ones such as SPICE [4], include more than a dozen models for the MOSFET shows, on the one hand, that many "equivalent" efforts [5–12] have been carried out to develop a good circuit model for this device and, on the other hand, that a "decisive" model is yet to be found.

For the bipolar transistor, the number of models is limited. However, the most widely used circuit model, the Gummel-Poon model [13], an extension of the basic Ebers-Moll model [14], has become so sophisticated that it sometimes proves to be cumbersome. Moreover, it seems difficult for an average circuit engineer to have a thorough knowledge of every detail of this model.

A recent trend is to develop numerical models [15–18] not only for accurate simulation of device terminal characteristics but also for probing the inside of the device to investigate physical phenomena that could not be observed with a "conventional" measuring instrument. This greatly aids understanding of the physics of transistors. Numerical models have also made their way into circuit simulators, either as a built-in model [19] or as a table-model generator [20].

With the above in mind, it can be seen that a full account of transistor modeling would exceed the framework of the present text. Therefore, it is not our intention here to make a survey or a comparative study of all available models. Rather, we will limit ourselves to providing a guide on how device models, analytical as well as numerical, are being developed. For details of specific models, if needed, readers are referred to the original work, to more comprehensive treatises and guidebooks, or to the manuals which are usually provided with circuit simulators. Nevertheless, to be consistent, only simplified versions of numerical and analytical models, of moderate accuracy but easy to handle computationally, will be presented here.

2 BASIC EQUATIONS—FLUID MODEL

Let us first derive the basic equations describing the movement of carriers in a semiconductor device. In these equations, electrons and holes are treated as if they form a flow of fluid that is distributed continuously in time and space. This view of the carriers constitutes what is usually called the "fluid model." By contrast, there is another view in which electrons and holes are considered as particles, and device characteristics are analyzed on the basis of their individual movements. This latter view, termed the "particle model," has attracted much attention of late. In this chapter, however, we will limit ourselves to the fluid model because it is the mainstream model at present.

The basic equations for the fluid model can be derived from the classical Maxwell equations where the current vector is given by the Boltzmann transport equation.

The Maxwell equations, which form the foundation of electromagnetics, are written as follows:

$$\operatorname{div} D = \rho \tag{2.1}$$

$$\operatorname{div} B = 0 \tag{2.2}$$

$$\operatorname{rot} E = -\frac{\delta B}{\delta t} \tag{2.3}$$

$$\operatorname{rot} H = J + \frac{\delta D}{\delta t} \tag{2.4}$$

$$D = \varepsilon E \tag{2.5}$$

$$B = \mu H \tag{2.6}$$

where all the symbols have their conventional meaning.

If the magnetic field is negligible small, that is, $B = H = 0$, then from (2.3) we have $\operatorname{rot} E = 0$, which implies that there exists in the vector field E a potential ψ that satisfies $\operatorname{grad}\psi = -E$. In addition, if we now take the divergence of both sides of (2.4) we have

$$\operatorname{div} J + \frac{\delta(\operatorname{div} D)}{\delta t} = \operatorname{div} J + \frac{\delta\rho}{\delta t} = 0 \tag{2.7}$$

Thus, for the case of no magnetic field, the Maxwell equations reduce to

Current continuity equation:

$$\operatorname{div} J + \frac{\delta\rho}{\delta t} = 0 \tag{2.7a}$$

Poisson equation:

$$\operatorname{div}(-\varepsilon \operatorname{grad}\psi) = \rho \tag{2.8}$$

where

$$E = -\operatorname{grad}\psi \tag{2.9}$$

Since charge in a semiconductor consists of components due to electrons (n), holes (p), ionized donors (N_D), and acceptors (N_A), we have

Poisson equation:

$$\operatorname{div}(-\varepsilon \operatorname{grad}\psi) = q(p - n + N_D - N_A) \tag{2.10}$$

where q is the elementary electronic charge.

It can be seen that the Maxwell equations also serve as the basis for the fluid model. For the current vector J, the derivation is not as simple as that above and will not be attempted here. However, the result, given below, is quite familiar.

Transport equation for electrons:

$$\begin{aligned} J_n &= q \cdot V_{\text{drift}} \cdot n + q \cdot D_n \cdot \operatorname{grad} n \\ &= -q(\mu_n \cdot n \cdot \operatorname{grad}\psi - \mathrm{D}_n \cdot \operatorname{grad} n) \end{aligned} \tag{2.11}$$

Transport equation for holes:

$$J_p = -q(\mu_p \cdot \operatorname{grad} \psi + D_p \cdot \operatorname{grad} p) \tag{2.12}$$

The above equations postulate that the current density consists of two components, namely a drift component proportional to the carrier velocity, v_{drift}, and a diffusion component proportional to the carrier density gradient.

Substituting the total current $J = J_n + J_p$ into (2.7) and taking account of the fact that $-qn$ and qp are the only time-varying components among the terms on the right-hand side of (2.10), we have

$$\operatorname{div} J_n - q\frac{\delta n}{\delta t} + \operatorname{div} J_p + p\frac{\delta p}{\delta t} = 0$$

or

$$\operatorname{div}\left(-\frac{J_n}{q}\right) + \frac{\delta n}{\delta t} = \operatorname{div}\left(\frac{J_p}{q}\right) + \frac{\delta p}{\delta t} = G' \tag{2.13}$$

If we consider a system that has reached a steady state, then $\delta/\delta t = 0$, and G' must represent the total number of electrons and holes that emerge from the region of interest through the process of generation (G) and recombination (R).

In summary, the basis for the fluid model of a semiconductor device consists of the following set of equations.

$$\operatorname{div}(-\varepsilon \operatorname{grad} \psi) = q(p - n + C) \tag{2.10}$$

$$\operatorname{div} J_n = -q(G - R) \tag{2.13}$$

$$\operatorname{div} J_p = q(G - R) \tag{2.13a}$$

$$J_n = -q(\mu_n n \operatorname{grad} \psi - D_n \operatorname{grad} n) \tag{2.11}$$

$$J_p = -q(\mu_p p \operatorname{grad} \psi + D_p \operatorname{grad} p) \tag{2.12}$$

where we have put $C \equiv N_D - N_A$ and $G - R \equiv G'$.

Now, for simplicity, assuming a Boltzmann distribution (in a strict sense, a Fermi distribution must be applied) for electrons and holes, we have

$$n = n_i \exp[\beta(\psi - \phi_n)] \tag{2.14}$$

$$p = n_i \exp[\beta(\phi_p - \psi)] \tag{2.14a}$$

with

$$\beta = \frac{q}{kT} \tag{2.15}$$

where ϕ_n and ϕ_p are quasi-Fermi levels for electrons and holes, respectively, n_i

is the intrinsic carrier density, k is the Boltzmann constant, and T is the absolute temperature.

Using (2.14) and (2.15), we can rewrite (2.11) and (2.12) as follows.

$$J_n = q\mu_n n \,\mathrm{grad}\,\psi + q(\beta D_n)n_i \exp[\beta(\psi - \phi_n)] \times \{\mathrm{grad}\,\psi - \mathrm{grad}\,\phi_n\}$$

$$= -q\mu_n n \,\mathrm{grad}\,\phi_n \tag{2.11a}$$

$$J_p = -q\mu_p p \,\mathrm{grad}\,\psi - q(\beta D_p)n_i \exp[\beta(\phi_p - \psi)] \times \{\mathrm{grad}\,\phi_p - \mathrm{grad}\,\psi\}$$

$$= q\mu_p p \,\mathrm{grad}\,\phi_p \tag{2.12a}$$

Thus, in the case of a semiconductor device at steady state, we have three equations [(2.10), (2.13) and (2.13a)] for three unknowns (either ψ, n, and p or ψ, ϕ_n, and ϕ_p) with J_n and J_p given by either (2.11) and (2.12) or (2.11a) and (2.12a). In other words, any problem related to semiconductor device characteristics that originate from the movement of electrons and holes can be solved at least formally. In actuality, however, since the basic equations are highly nonlinear, they can be solved analytically only in some special cases, such as those presented in the following sections for analytical models. For the general case one has to resort to a numerical solution, which will be mentioned briefly in Section 5.

3 MOSFET MODELING

The prototype MOSFET analytical model was established in the mid-1960s [5]. This basic model, however, has been extensively revised to cope with the various two- and three-dimensional effects that have shown up along with the microminiaturization of the devices.

Here, we will first present the simplest MOSFET model. Then we will briefly introduce the inclusion of various second-order effects, such as short-channel effect [1] and the narrow-channel effect [2].

3.1 Threshold Voltage

Figure 1.1 shows a cross-sectional view of a typical MOSFET. When the channel length L and channel width W are larger than the depletion layer thicknesses Y_{DS}, Y_{DD}, Y_{DB} in the source, drain, and channel regions, respectively, then the electric field can be considered one-dimensional for most of the channel. This condition is usually known as the "gradual-case approximation" [21]. In this case, one has only to consider the field in the vertical (transverse) direction, where Gauss's theorem is applied to obtain the following charge conservation law:

$$Q_G + G_{ss} + Q_B + Q_C = 0 \tag{3.1}$$

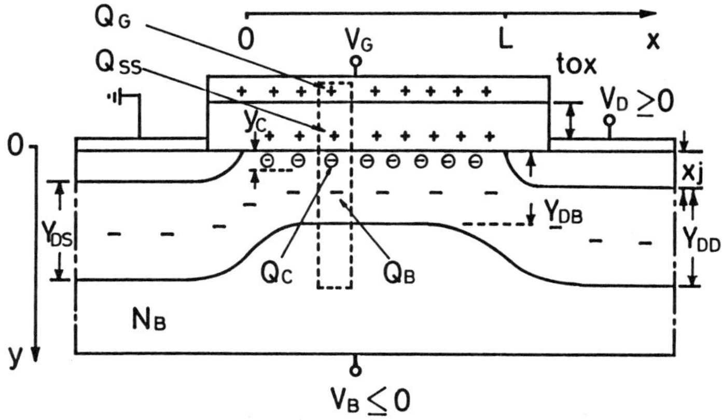

Figure 1.1 Cross-sectional view (along the channel length) of a MOSFET. See text for definitions of the various quantities shown.

where Q_C is the channel mobile charge; the other terms are shown in the figure.

If ϕ_{MS} is the work function difference between the gate and the substrate, then the gate charge Q_G will be given by

$$Q_G = (V_G - \phi_{MS} - \psi_s)C_{ox} \tag{3.2}$$

where $C_{ox} = \varepsilon_{ox}/t_{ox}$ is the gate capacitance per unit area and ψ_s is the channel surface potential. Using the depletion layer approximation, Q_B can be obtained as follows:

$$Q_B = -\gamma C_{ox}\sqrt{(\psi_s - V_B)} \tag{3.3}$$

where $\gamma = \sqrt{(2\varepsilon_s q N_B)}/C_{ox}$ is termed the "body factor."

The potential ψ_s will increase with increasing V_G, but when it has reached a value of about $2\phi_F$ the carrier density close to the source will become so large that, due to its shielding effect, ψ_s will increase so slowly that it can be considered virtually locked at $2\phi_F$. This situation is referred to as the "strong inversion state" and the threshold voltage V_T, defined as the gate voltage to produce this state, is given by

$$V_T = 2\phi_F + V_{FB} - \frac{Q_B}{C_{ox}} \tag{3.4}$$

where $V_{FB} = \phi_{MS} - Q_{ss}/C_{ox}$ (Q_{ss} being the charge due to surface states) is called the "flat-band voltage."

In circuit simulations, for simplicity, the MOSFET is considered to be in a conducting state (ON state) when $V_G > V_T$ and in a nonconducting state (OFF state) when $V_G < V_T$.

3.2 Drain Current

In deriving the model formula for the MOSFET drain current, it is usually assumed, in addition to the gradual-case condition, that

1. Carrier generation and recombination are negligible ($G = R = 0$).

2. Minority carrier current is negligible.

Then when considering an n-channel, the drain current I_D, using (2.11), is given by

$$I_D = -W \int_0^{y_C} \left[q\mu_n n \left(\frac{\delta \phi_n}{\delta x} \right) \right] dy \,(=\text{constant}) \tag{3.5}$$

where y_C is the channel depth.

In addition, if the carrier mobility μ_n is considered constant and the quasi-Fermi potential is considered almost constant in the transverse direction ($\delta\phi_n/\delta y \doteqdot 0$), then (3.5) simplifies to

$$I_D = W\mu_n Q_C(\psi_s) \frac{d\psi_s}{dx} \tag{3.6}$$

where $\psi_s = \psi_s(x) = \phi_n(X) - \phi_n(0)$. The channel mobile charge Q_C is now given by

$$Q_C = -C_{ox}(V_G - \psi_s - V_T) \tag{3.7}$$

if one considers that the channel does not conduct when $V_G < V_T$, as mentioned above.

Substituting (3.7) into (3.6) and integrating from source to drain, one has

$$I_D \int_0^L dx = -W\mu_n C_{ox} \int_{\psi_s(0)=V_S=0}^{\psi_s(L)=V_D} [(V_G - V_T) - \psi_s] \, d\psi_s$$

or

$$I_D = -\left(\frac{W}{L} \right) \mu_n C_{ox} \left[(V_G - V_T)V_D - \frac{V_{D^2}}{2} \right] \tag{3.8}$$

The above formula represents the simplest model formulation for the drain current of a MOSFET. It can readily be seen that, in addition to not giving the drain current at $V_G < V_T$ (subthreshold conduction), as mentioned above, this formula does not apply in the case $V_D > (V_G - V_T)$ (saturation region). In the latter case, the current is taken as the value at $V_D = (V_G - V_T)$ as follows:

$$I_D = -\left(\frac{W}{L} \right) \left(\frac{\mu_n C_{ox}}{2} \right) (V_G - V_T)^2 \tag{3.9}$$

More elaborate analytical models applicable for all voltage ranges are described briefly in the Appendix.

In the following, however, we will retain the fundamental form of (3.8) and show how second-order effects, such as field-dependent mobility and short-channel and narrow-channel effects, are taken into account.

Field-Dependent Mobility

The field dependence of carrier mobility is considered in two directions. In the transverse direction, the following model is widely used [22]:

$$\mu = \frac{\mu_0}{1 + \theta(V_G - V_T)} \tag{3.10}$$

where μ_0, the low-field mobility, and θ, a fitting parameter, are to be obtained by measurements. On the other hand, a number of models have been proposed for the field dependence of the mobility in the longitudinal direction. The one given below is assumed here because it is easy to handle analytically:

$$\mu = \frac{\mu_0}{1 + E_x/E_c} = \frac{\mu_0}{1 + \mu_0 E_x/v_s} \tag{3.11}$$

where E_x is the electric field strength in the channel direction, E_c is the E_x value at which carriers reach the saturation velocity v_s ($\equiv \mu_0 E_c$).

Using (3.10) and (3.11), the drain current becomes [23]

$$I_{D'} = \left[\frac{\mu_0}{1 + \theta(V_G - V_T)}\right]\left[1 + \left(\frac{\mu_0}{v_s}\right)\left(\frac{V_D}{L}\right)\right]^{-1} I_D \tag{3.12}$$

where I_D is given by (3.8).

Short-Channel Effect

When the channel length L of a MOSFET is shortened, its threshold voltage V_T drops. This phenomenon is called the short-channel effect. Because of its two-dimensional nature, a thorough analysis of this effect requires the use of a two-dimensional numerical simulator (see Section 5). Here we will present only a simple but reasonably accurate model that has been implemented in the all-purpose circuit simulator SPICE [4].

Essentially, this simple model for the short-channel effect is expressed in terms of what is called a correction factor for the short-channel effect, K, whose definition will become clear very soon. In Figure 1.2 the depletion charge right below the gate corresponds to Q_B in (3.1). One can see in this figure that the two extreme parts of Q_B are overlapped by the depletion layers of the source and the drain. It is conceivable that the charge contained in these overlapped regions is controlled by both the gate voltage and the

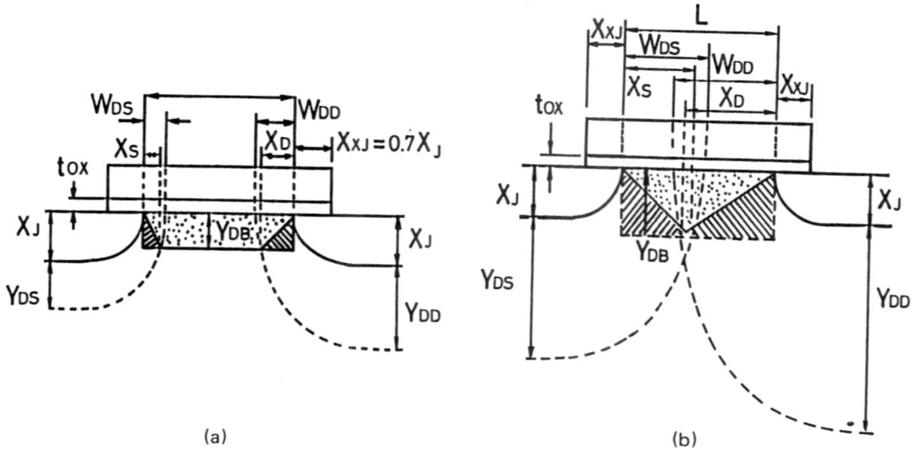

Figure 1.2 Model for the short-channel effect in a MOSFET. The shaded area [trapezoid in (a), triangle in (b)] represents bulk depletion charge (Q_B) in the formula for $V_{T,\text{short}}$. The total area of hatched regions corresponds to the difference between two threshold voltages, $V_{T,\text{long}}$ and $V_{T,\text{short}}$.

source/drain voltage. Therefore, it is reasonable to assume equal sharing between these two voltages, and this will result in a Q_B as represented by the shaded trapezoidal area. Note that when the channel is very short and/or the biases are very high, the trapezoid reduces to a triangle as shown in Figure 1.2b. For simplicity, the charge represented by either the shaded trapezoid of Figure 1.2a or the shaded triangle of Figure 1.2b will be denoted by $Q_{B,\text{trapezoid}}$ in the following. In other words, the threshold voltage of a short-channel MOSFET becomes

$$V_{T,\text{short}} = 2\phi_F + V_{FB} - \frac{Q_{B,\text{trapezoid}}}{C_{ox}} \tag{3.13}$$

For convenience of comparison, the threshold voltage of a long channel, given by (3.4) is rewritten below:

$$V_{T,\text{long}} = 2\phi_F + V_{FB} - \frac{Q_{B,\text{rectangle}}}{C_{ox}} \tag{3.4a}$$

The difference between $V_{T,\text{long}}$ and $V_{T,\text{short}}$ can be expressed in terms of the correction factor K, defined as

$$K = \frac{Q_{B,\text{trapezoid}}}{Q_{B,\text{rectangle}}} = \frac{V_{T,\text{short}} - 2\phi_F - V_{FB}}{V_{T,\text{long}} - 2\phi_F - V_{FB}} \tag{3.14}$$

$V_{T,\text{short}}$ can now be rewritten as follows.

$$V_{T,\text{short}} = 2\phi_F + V_{FB} - \frac{KQ_{B,\text{rectangle}}}{C_{ox}} \tag{3.15}$$

For the simple case of constant bulk impurity K reduces to the ratio between the areas of the trapezoid and the rectangle. Assuming that the edge of the depletion layer across the curved parts of the source/drain junctions takes the form of an ellipse, K becomes [23]

$$K = 1 - \frac{X_s + X_D}{2L} \qquad \text{for } X_S + X_D \leqq L \tag{3.16}$$

and

$$K = \frac{0.5L}{X_S + X_D} \qquad \text{for } X_S + X_D \geqq L \tag{3.16a}$$

where

$$X_S = (W_{DS} + 0.7x_j)\sqrt{\left[1 - \frac{Y_{DB^2}}{(Y_{DS} + x_j)^2}\right]} - 0.7x_j \tag{3.17}$$

$$X_D = (W_{DD} + 0.7x_j)\sqrt{\left[1 - \frac{Y_{DB^2}}{(Y_{DD} + x_j)^2}\right]} - 0.7x_j \tag{3.18}$$

$$Y_{DB} = \gamma C_{ox}\sqrt{(2\phi_F - V_B)} \tag{3.19}$$

$$Y_{DS} = \gamma C_{ox}\sqrt{(V_{BI} + V_S - V_B)} \tag{3.20}$$

$$Y_{DD} = \gamma C_{ox}\sqrt{(V_{BI} + V_D - V_B)} \tag{3.21}$$

$$2\phi_F + V_S - V_B = \left(\frac{qN_B}{2\varepsilon_s}\right)x_j^2\left(1 + \frac{W_{DS}}{x_j}\right)^2 \times \left\{\ln\left(1 + \frac{W_{DS}}{x_j}\right) - 0.5 + \left.\frac{0.5}{1 + W_{DS}/x_j}\right)^2\right\} \tag{3.22}$$

$$2\phi_F + V_D - V_B = \left(\frac{qN_B}{2\varepsilon_s}\right)x_j^2\left(1 + \frac{W_{DD}}{x_j}\right)^2 \times \left\{\ln\left(1 + \frac{W_{DD}}{x_j}\right) - 0.5 + \frac{0.5}{1 + W_{DD}/x_j)^2}\right\} \tag{3.23}$$

where V_{BI} is the built-in voltage of the junctions.

The logarithmic function in the last two equations can be approximated by a polynomial to reduce the computer time in a drastic manner [23].

Narrow-Channel Effects

Depending on the shape of the field oxide, two kinds of narrow-channel effects have been observed. One, found in LOCOS and other nonrecessed oxide structures, is expressed in terms of the threshold voltage, which increases with decreasing channel width [2]. The other, found in fully recessed oxide structures [24], has the opposite dependence on the channel width. In other words, a MOSFET with a fully recessed field oxide exhibits a threshold voltage that decreases with decreasing channel width. The former narrow-width effect is termed the "(conventional) narrow-channel effect" and the latter is the "inverse narrow-channel effect" [3]. These two effects are three-dimensional and therefore very difficult to treat analytically. A numerical approach, which is briefly described in a later section, can serve to clarify the mechanism that underlies these narrow-width effects [3]. Here, for simplicity, we will only show how, in practice, the conventional narrow-channel effect is taken into account in a formula for threshold voltage. The inverse narrow-channel effect, on the other hand, is ignored.

Figure 1.3 shows a cross section along the channel width of a conventional MOSFET structure. The hatched areas represent excess charges that are induced under the thick field oxide due to the gate parts that overlap the two

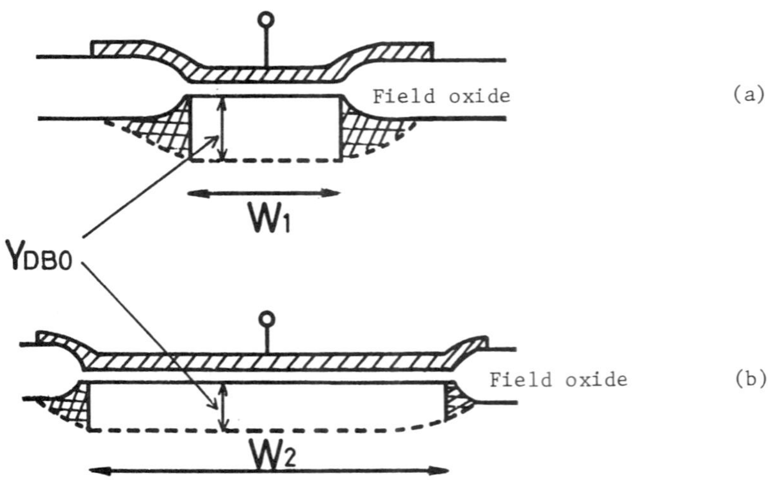

Figure 1.3 Cross-sectional view (along the channel width) of a MOSFET. The induced charge under the thick field oxide corresponds to an increase of threshold voltage in a narrow-width MOSFET. The area ratio between the crosshatched regions and total depletion region is large in the narrow channel W_1 (a) and small in the wide channel W_2 (b). This results in an increase of threshold voltage in narrow-width MOSFETs.

field regions on both sides (flanks) of the channel. The excess charges add up to the bulk charge Q_B in (3.4) to produce a voltage shift ΔV_T that can be expressed as follows:

$$\Delta V_T = \frac{\eta q N_B Y_{DBO}}{C_{ox} W} \tag{3.24}$$

where Y_{DBO} is the depletion layer depth corresponding to $V_B = 0$ and η is a fitting parameter that depends mostly on the shape of the field oxide.

3.3 MOSFET Equivalent Circuit

The total equivalent circuit of an MOSFET can now be drawn as shown in Figure 1.4a. Compared to a variety of drain current (analytical) models that agree fairly well with measurements, capacitance models have not been given adequate attention. One reason is that MOSFET capacitances do not vary much with bias conditions and in many cases it is difficult to isolate them from other parasitic capacitances, which are often larger. Here, we will not attempt to develop a complete model for the capacitances. Interested readers can find a more detailed and critical discussion of various capacitance models in Ref. [25]. Instead we will point out that the numerical simulation

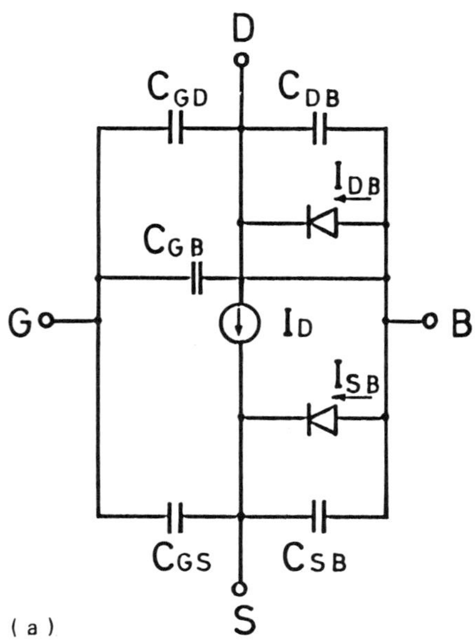

Figure 1.4 Equivalent circuit of a MOSFET (a) and capacitance variations with bias conditions (b).

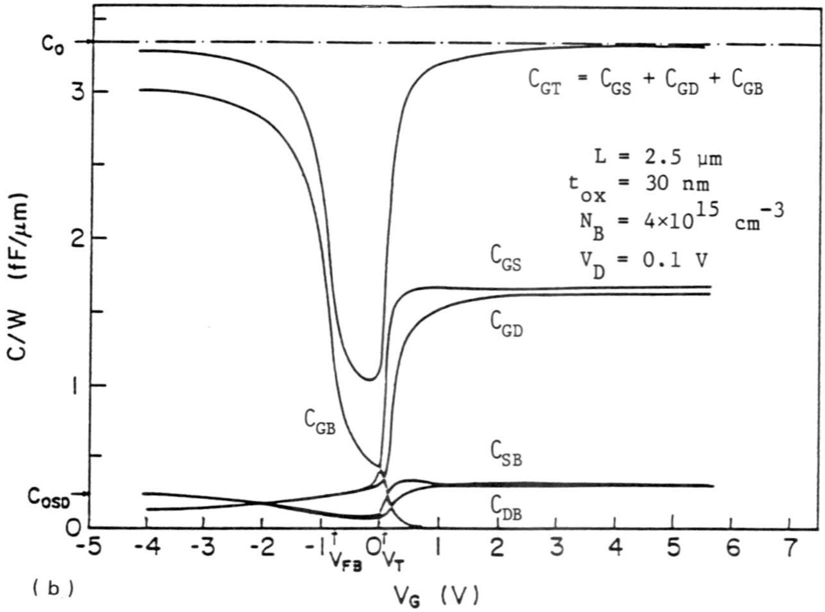

Figure 1.4 (b)

approach, described later can be used to obtain a variation of the capacitances with bias conditions, as shown in Figure 1.4b [26]. Note that the two capacitances due to the gate overlaps on the source and the drain, C_{GSO} and C_{GDO}, are included in C_{GS} and C_{GD}.

It can be seen that the total gate capacitance C_{GT} looks very similar to the familiar MOS capacitance. The gate-bulk capacitance C_{GB} shows the same gate voltage dependence as C_{GT} in the subthreshold region, but it drops quickly to zero above threshold as the substrate is shielded from the gate by the inversion layer that forms at the channel surface at this bias condition. One can also see that C_{SB} and C_{DB} are essentially capacitances due to the source and drain junctions and that they do not vary much with gate bias.

4 BIPOLAR TRANSISTOR MODELING

The basic circuit model for a bipolar transistor, the Ebers-Moll model, was established more than 30 years ago [14]. The most widely used model for computer simulation at present, the Gummel-Poon model [13], is an extension of the Ebers-Moll model.

4.1 Basic Ebers-Moll Model

The derivation of the basic current model for a bipolar transistor starts with the transport equations (2.11) and (2.12), which are rewritten in one-dimensional form as follows:

$$J_n = q\mu_n n E_x + qD_n \frac{dn}{dx} \tag{4.1}$$

$$J_p = q\mu_p p E_x - qD_p \frac{dp}{dx} \tag{4.2}$$

Consider a one-dimensional *npn* bipolar transistor of unit cross-sectional area (Figure 1.5) where the current in the base is dominated by injected electrons from the emitter ($J_p \doteqdot 0$). One has from (4.2)

$$E_x = \left(\frac{D_p}{\mu_p}\right)\left(\frac{1}{p}\right)\left(\frac{dp}{dx}\right) = \left(\frac{kT}{q}\right)\left(\frac{1}{p}\right)\left(\frac{dp}{dx}\right) \tag{4.3}$$

taking account of the Einstein relation.

Equation (4.3) is now substituted into (4.1) to yield the total current:

$$I_n = A \cdot J_n = kT\mu_n\left(\frac{n}{p}\right)\left(\frac{dp}{dx}\right) + qD_n\left(\frac{dn}{dx}\right) = \left(\frac{qD_n}{p}\right)\frac{d(pn)}{dx} \tag{4.4}$$

where A is the cross-sectional area, which has been taken as unity here.

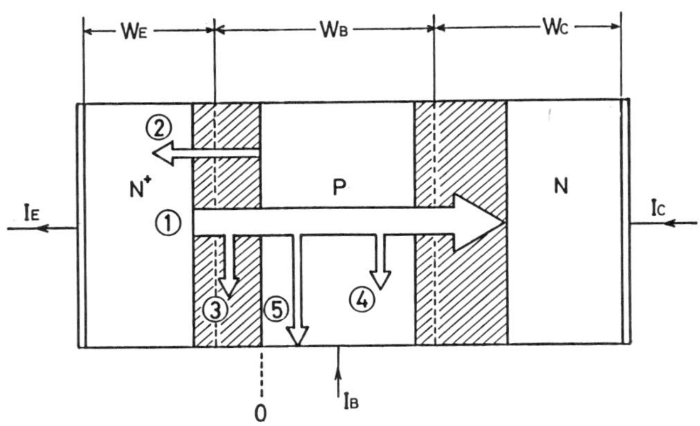

Figure 1.5 Cross-sectional view of a one-dimensional bipolar transistor. Various current components are shown by arrows whose widths represent their comparative magnitudes. 1, Injected electrons; 2, injected holes; 3, recombination in emitter depletion layer; 4, recombination in base region; 5, recombination at device surface.

Equation (4.4) is now integrated across the base (0 to W_B) to yield

$$\int_0^{W_B} \left(\frac{I_n}{D_n}\right)\left(\frac{p}{q}\right) dx = \left(\frac{I_n}{D_n}\right)\left(\frac{1}{q}\right) \int_0^{W_B} p\, dx = \int_0^{W_B} d(pn) = p(W_B)n(W_B) - p(0)n(0) \tag{4.5}$$

where D_n has been assumed constant and recombination in the base neglected so that I_n becomes constant throughout the base.

Using the Boltzmann distribution approximation for carrier densities [2.14) and (2.14a)], we have

$$\begin{aligned} pn &= n_i \exp[\beta(\psi - \phi_n)] n_i \exp[\beta(\phi_p - \psi)] = n_i^2 \exp[\beta(\phi_p - \phi_n)] \\ &= n_i^2 \exp(\beta V_a) \end{aligned} \tag{4.6}$$

where V_a is the applied voltage.

Substitution of (4.6) in (4.5), keeping in mind that the voltages across emitter and collector junctions are V_{BE} and V_{BC}, respectively, we obtain

$$I_n = \frac{q n_i{}^2 D_n [\exp(\beta V_{BC}) - \exp(\beta V_{BE})]}{\int_0^{W_B} p\, dx} \tag{4.7}$$

The integral in the denominator of (4.7) is the total major-carrier density in the base. Let Q_B denote the charge associated with it, namely

$$Q_B = q \int_0^{W_B} p\, dx \tag{4.8}$$

then (4.7) becomes

$$I_n = I_s[\exp(\beta B_{BC}) - \exp(\beta V_{BE})] \tag{4.9}$$

where

$$I_s = \frac{q^2 n_i^2 D_n}{Q_B} \tag{4.10}$$

I_n represents the current flowing between the emitter and the collector and therefore is called the "linking current."

Let us now consider the base current. Let I_{DE} be the saturation current of the base-emitter *pn* junction (ideal) diode; then we have the current component flowing between the base and the emitter I_{BE} as follows, using the (ideal) diode equation:

$$I_{BE} = I_{DE}[\exp(\beta V_{BE}) - 1] \tag{4.11}$$

where

$$I_{DE} = q n_i^2 \left(\frac{D_p}{N_{DE} L_p} + \frac{D_n}{N_{AB} L_n}\right) \tag{4.12}$$

Since the current in the emitter is the difference between the linking current and the emitter-base diode current, we have

$$\begin{aligned} I_E &= I_s[\exp(\beta V_{BC}) - \exp(\beta V_{BE})] - I_{OE}[\exp(\beta V_{BE}) - 1] \\ &= -(I_s + I_{OE})[\exp(\beta V_{BE}) - 1] + I_s[\exp(\beta V_{BE}) - 1] \end{aligned} \tag{4.13}$$

Similarly, we have the collector current as follows:

$$\begin{aligned} I_C &= I_s[\exp(\beta V_{BE}) - \exp(\beta V_{BC})] - I_{DC}[\exp(\beta V_{BC}) - 1] \\ &= -(I_s + I_{OC})[\exp(\beta V_{BC}) - 1] + I_s[\exp(\beta V_{BE}) - 1] \end{aligned} \tag{4.14}$$

using the following collector-base diode current

$$I_{BC} = I_{OC}[\exp(\beta V_{BC}) - 1] \tag{4.15}$$

with

$$I_{OC} = qn_i^2\left(\frac{D_n}{N_{DC}L_n} + \frac{D_p}{N_{AB}L_p}\right) \tag{4.16}$$

Let us now define

$$I_{Es} = I_s + I_{OE} \qquad I_{Cs} = I_s + I_{OC} \qquad \alpha_F = \frac{I_s}{I_{Es}} \qquad \alpha_R = \frac{I_s}{I_{Cs}} \tag{4.17}$$

Then (4.13) and (4.14) become

$$I_E = -I_{Es}[\exp(\beta V_{BE}) - 1] + \alpha_R I_{Cs}[\exp(\beta V_{BC}) - 1] \tag{4.18}$$

$$I_C = -I_{Cs}[\exp(\beta V_{BC}) - 1] + \alpha_F I_{Es}[\exp(\beta V_{BE}) - 1] \tag{4.19}$$

The equation pair (4.18) and (4.19) form the well-known Ebers-Moll relations for an *npn* bipolar transistor. For a *pnp* transistor, the current directions are to be changed suitably to account for the polarity of the emitter-base and collector-base junctions.

Among the four parameters of the Ebers-Moll model given above, only three are independent, since from the last two equalities of (4.17) we have

$$\alpha_F I_{Es} = \alpha_R I_{Cs} = I_s \tag{4.20}$$

which is usually referred to as the "reciprocity relationship" of the bipolar transistor.

If we again define

$$I_F = I_{Es}[\exp(\beta V_{BC}) - 1] \tag{4.21}$$

$$I_R = I_{Cs}[\exp(\beta V_{BE}) - 1] \tag{4.22}$$

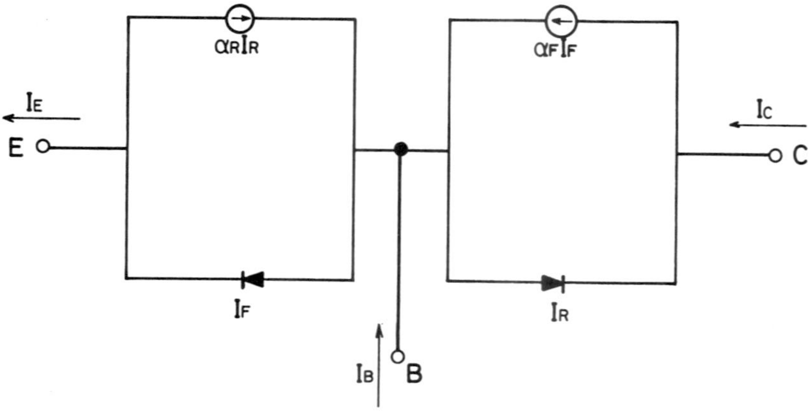

Figure 1.6 Simplest equivalent circuit of a bipolar transistor.

then the Ebers-Moll equations become

$$I_E = -I_F + \alpha_R I_R \tag{4.23}$$

$$I_C = -I_R + \alpha_F I_F \tag{4.24}$$

and the base current can now be expressed by

$$I_B = -(I_E + I_C) = I_F(1 - \alpha_F) + I_R(1 - \alpha_R) \tag{4.25}$$

Equations (4.23)–(4.125) can be represented by the equivalent circuit shown in Figure 1.6.

It can be seen from the above that only four parameters, namely α_F, α_R, I_{Es} and I_{Cs}, are needed to describe the current-voltage characteristics of the bipolar transistor. These parameters are related to device geometry and other parameters through (4.17) and related expressions for I_s [(4.11)], I_{OE} [(4.12)], and I_{OC} [(4.15)].

The Ebers-Moll model is valid for all ranges of bias but cannot serve as a current model for computer simulation. The reason is that it does not take into account the various second-order effects of the "actual" bipolar transistor. A more elaborate model, the Gummel-Poon model, presented below, is based on the Ebers-Moll model and is widely used for this purpose, especially since many general-purpose circuit simulators have been available.

4.2 Gummel-Poon Model

The construction of the Gummel-Poon model begins with (4.13) and (4.14) (which are sometimes referred to as the transport version of the Ebers-Moll model). Using the linking current, (4.10), and (4.18) and (4.19), it is possible to rewrite the Ebers-Moll equations as follows:

$$I_E = -\left(\frac{I_s}{\beta_F}\right)[\exp(\beta V_{BE}) - 1] + I_s[\exp(\beta V_{BC}) - 1]$$
$$= I_s[\exp(\beta V_{BC}) - \exp(\beta V_{BE})] - \left(\frac{I_s}{\beta_F}\right)[\exp(\beta V_{BE}) - 1]$$
$$= I_n - \left(\frac{I_s}{\beta_F}\right)[\exp(\beta V_{BE}) - 1] \tag{4.26}$$

$$I_C = -I_n - \left(\frac{I_s}{\beta_R}\right)[\exp(\beta V_{BE}) - 1] \tag{4.27}$$

$$I_B = \left(\frac{I_s}{\beta_F}\right)[\exp(\beta V_{BE}) - 1] + \left(\frac{I_s}{\beta_R}\right)[\exp(\beta V_{BC}) - 1] \tag{4.28}$$

where

$$\beta_{F,R} = \frac{(1 - \alpha_{F,R})}{\alpha_{F,R}} \tag{4.29}$$

In the form of (4.26)–(4.28), one sees that the Ebers-Moll model can now be described by the three parameters I_s, β_F, and β_R. The Gummel-Poon model using (4.26)–(4.28) is completed by including additional terms to account for various second-order effects as follows.

Space-Charge Region Recombination

First, the ideal diode relationships, (4.12) and (4.16), are replaced by more realistic ones where recombination in the space-charge region is accounted for. This modification is effected by superimposing two nonideal components on the ideal base current given by (4.28)

$$I_B = \left(\frac{I_s}{\beta_F}\right)[\exp(\beta V_{BE}) - 1] + I_1\left[\exp\left(\frac{\beta V_{BE}}{n_E}\right) - 1\right]$$
$$+ \left(\frac{I_s}{\beta_R}\right)[\exp(\beta V_{BC}) - 1] + I_2\left[\exp\left(\frac{\beta V_{BC}}{n_C}\right) - 1\right] \tag{4.30}$$

(I_1, n_E) and (I_2, n_C) are related to the emitter junction and the collector junction, respectively.

High-Injection and Base-Width Modulation (Early Effect)

The effect of high-current operation and the Early effect can be included simultaneously in (4.26)–(4.28) through I_s, where the charge Q_B is now

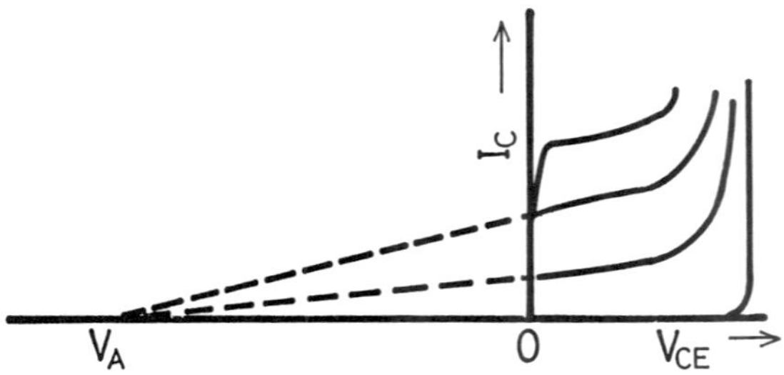

Figure 1.7 Determination of Early voltage for forward operation.

expressed as follows:

$$
\begin{aligned}
Q_{BT} = A_E Q_B &= A_E q \int_0^{W_B} N_{AB}(x)\,dx + Q_{E1} + Q_{E2} + Q_{C1} + Q_{C2} \\
&= Q_{B0} + C_{jE} V_{BE} + \left(\frac{Q_{B0}}{Q_{BT}}\right) \tau_F I_s[\exp(\beta V_{BE}) - 1] \\
&\quad + \left(\frac{A_E}{A_C}\right) C_{jC} V_{BC} + \left(\frac{Q_{B0}}{Q_{BT}}\right) \tau_R I_s[\exp(\beta V_{BC}) - 1]
\end{aligned}
\tag{4.31}
$$

where Q_{E1}, Q_{E2} represent charges due to the emitter storage and forward injection of minority carriers from the emitter to the base; Q_{C1}, Q_{C2} are charges related to the collector storage and reverse injection of minority carriers from the collector into the base; A_E and A_C denote the emitter and collector areas, respectively, which are usually different in an actual transistor as shown in Figure 1.8.

For computational ease, both sides of (4.31) are now normalized by Q_{B0} to yield

$$
\begin{aligned}
q_{bT} = \frac{Q_{BT}}{Q_{B0}} &= 1 + \left(\frac{C_{jE} V_{BE}}{Q_{B0}}\right) + \left(\frac{C_{jC} V_{BC}}{Q_{B0}}\right)\left(\frac{A_E}{A_C}\right) \\
&\quad + \left(\frac{1}{q_{bT}}\right)\left\{\left(\frac{\tau_F I_s}{Q_{B0}}\right)[\exp(\beta V_{BE}) - 1] \right. \\
&\quad \left. + \left(\frac{\tau_R I_s}{Q_{B0}}\right)[\exp(\beta V_{BC}) - 1]\right\}
\end{aligned}
\tag{4.32}
$$

$$
= q_1 + \frac{q_2}{q_{bT}} \tag{4.32a}
$$

or

$$
q_{bT} = \frac{q_1}{2} + \left[\left(\frac{q_1}{2}\right)^2 + q_2\right]^{1/2} \tag{4.32b}
$$

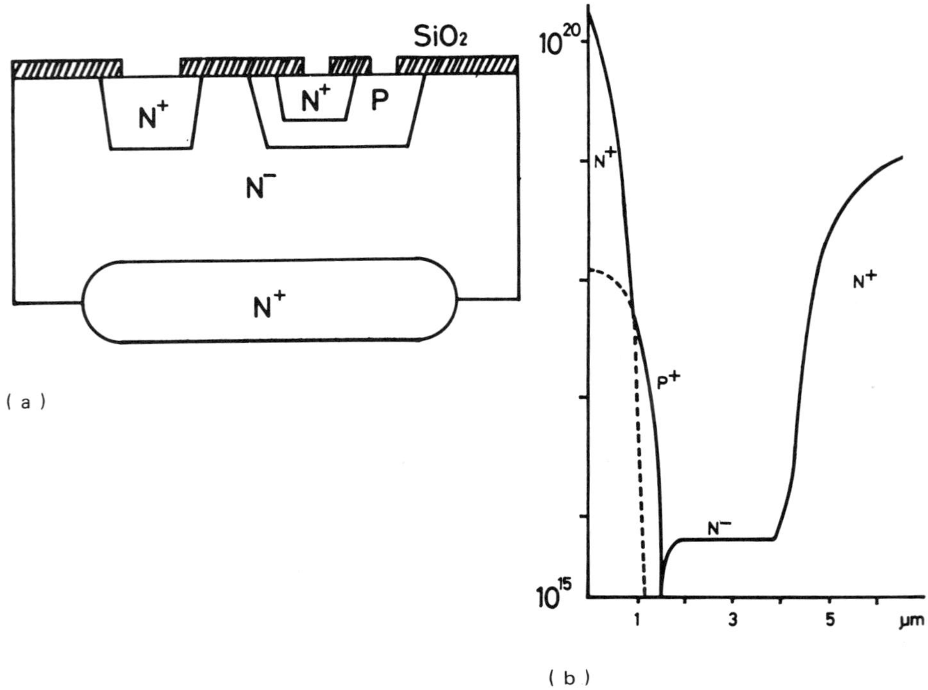

Figure 1.8 Cross-sectional view of an actual bipolar transistor (a) and the impurity profile in its various regions (b).

where

$$q_1 = 1 + \frac{V_{BE}}{|V_B|} + \frac{V_{BC}}{|V_A|} \tag{4.33}$$

$$q_2 = \left(\frac{I_s}{I_{KF}}\right)[\exp(\beta V_{BE}) - 1] + \left(\frac{I_s}{I_{KR}}\right)[\exp(\beta V_{BC}) - 1] \tag{4.34}$$

with

$$V_A \equiv \left(\frac{Q_{BO}}{C_{jC}}\right)\left(\frac{A_C}{A_E}\right) \qquad V_B \equiv \frac{Q_{BO}}{C_{jE}} \qquad I_{KF} \equiv \frac{Q_{BO}}{\tau_F} \qquad I_{KR} \equiv \frac{Q_{BO}}{\tau_R} \tag{4.35}$$

V_A and I_{KF} are the Early voltage and knee current for forward operation, respectively, and, as shown in Figure 1.9, are easily obtained by measurements. Also shown in the same figure are I_1 and n_E, mentioned above. The terms V_B, I_{KR}, I_2, n_C are the reverse-operation duals of V_A, I_{KF}, I_1, n_E and therefore can be obtained similarly from reverse-operation measurements.

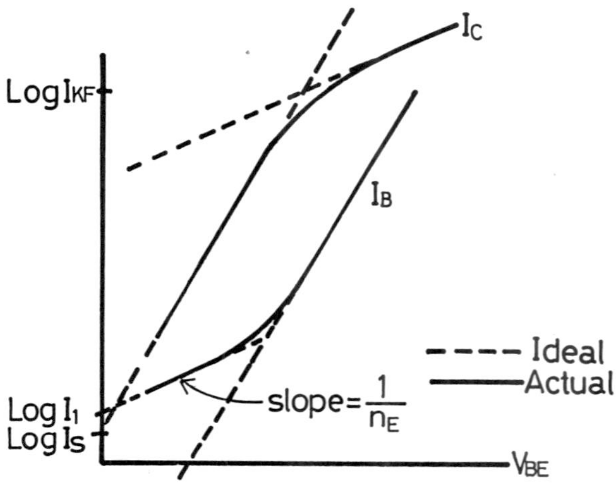

Figure 1.9 Determination of I_{KF}, I_S, I_1, and n_E (forward operation).

C_{jE} and C_{jC} are capacitances associated with emitter and collector junctions, respectively. τ_F and τ_R are time constants related to forward and reverse operations, respectively. τ_F and β_F are related to each other by the expression

$$\beta_F = \frac{I_C}{I_B} = \frac{\tau_{BF}}{\tau_F} \tag{4.36}$$

where

$$\tau_{BF} = \frac{Q_F}{I_B} \tag{4.37}$$

with Q_F being the sum of the charges associated with injection of electrons from the emitter to the base and injection of holes from the base to the emitter. If the emitter efficiency γ,* which represents the share of electron current in the total emitter current, is almost unity (implying that hole injection from the base into the emitter is negligible), Q_F reduces to the total injected electron charge in the base (Q_{nB}) and thus τ_F reduces to τ_B ($\equiv Q_{nB}/I_C$), which is the base transit time. Note that τ_B is related to the base width by the

---

*For the ideal one-dimensional transistor of Figure 1.5, γ is given by

$$\gamma = \frac{I_{nE}}{(I_{nE} + I_{pE})} = \left(1 + \frac{W_B N_{AB} D_{pE}}{W_E N_{DE} D_{nB}}\right)^{-1} \tag{4.40}$$

where subscripts B and E refer to the base region and the emitter region, respectively.

equation

$$\tau_B = \frac{W_B{}^2}{2D_n} \tag{4.38}$$

C_{jC} is the capacitance related to the collector-base junction:

$$C_{jC} = \left|\frac{dQ_B}{dV_{BC}}\right| \tag{4.39}$$

A similar expression can be obtained for C_{jE} (for reverse operation).

In general, a junction capacitance (C_j) is related to the junction voltage by a function of the form

$$C_j = C_0\left(1 - \frac{V_j}{V_0}\right)^{-m} \tag{4.41}$$

where m is a parameter that depends mostly on the impurity profile across the junction. For a step junction $m = 1/2$ and for a linearly graded junction $m = 1/3$. For an actual junction, however, m should be fitted to measurements.

The use of (4.41) for a junction capacitance, however, gives rise to an unrealistic situation at $V_j = V_0$, where C_j tends to infinity. This is avoided in computer simulation by various methods that essentially consist of replacing the above function by one that yields a finite value at $V_j = V_0$. A fairly detailed account of this problem can be found in the literature [27].

Using (4.32) for the total base charge, the collector and emitter currents given by (4.26) and (4.27) become as follows:

$$I_C = \left(\frac{I_s}{q_{bT}}\right)\left[\exp(\beta V_{BE}) - \exp(\beta V_{BC})\right] - \left(\frac{I_s}{\beta_R}\right)\left[\exp(\beta V_{BC}) - 1\right] - I_2\left[\exp\left(\frac{\beta V_{BC}}{n_C}\right) - 1\right] \tag{4.42}$$

$$I_E = \left(\frac{I_s}{q_{bT}}\right)\left[\exp(\beta V_{BE}) - \exp(\beta B_{BC})\right] - \left(\frac{I_s}{\beta_F}\right)\left[\exp(\beta V_{BE}) - 1\right] - I_1\left[\exp\left(\frac{\beta V_{BE}}{n_E}\right) - 1\right] \tag{4.43}$$

In summary, the Gummel-Poon model consists of the above two relations plus one for the base current, (4.30), with related parameters given by (4.32)–(4.41).

Base Widening

In the version of the Gummel-Poon model presented above, the so-called base push-out or base-widening effect is not accounted for. This effect becomes important, however, in an integrated transistor, where the collector includes a comparatively thick low-doped epitaxial region (Figure 1.8). This low-doped region is useful in several ways, such as enhancing the collector-base breakdown voltage, lowering the collector capacitance, and reducing the base-width modulation effect. The existence of this epitaxial region, however, gives rise to a considerable voltage drop between the collector electrode ("outer collector") and the collector-base junction. Therefore, even when the outer collector is reverse-biased (that is, positively biased for an *npn* structure), the collector-base junction may still become forward-biased. This state of operation is termed quasi-saturation, and the hole charge piled up in the epitaxial layer space-charge region, Q_{epi} $(=q\int p\,dx)$, for compensating electrons that result from the Kirk effect, will add to the original base charge in such a manner as to widen the base by a factor B, defined as follows [13]:

$$B = \left\{1 + \left(\frac{W_{\text{epi}}}{4W_B}\right)\frac{\{\sqrt{[(I_C + I_{C1})^2 + I_{C2}^2]} - (I_C + I_{C1})\}^2}{(I_C^2 + I_{C1}^2)}\right\}^{n_{\text{epi}}} \tag{4.44}$$

where

$$I_{C1} = \frac{A_E(V_{OC} - V_{CB})}{\rho W_{\text{epi}}} \tag{4.45}$$

with W_{epi} being the epitaxial layer thickness and ρ its resistivity. Other quantities in (4.44) are fitting parameters.

It can be seen that the application of B to cover the quasi-saturation is quite subtle since it requires considerable fitting, and therefore it is open for more refinement.

Kull et al. [28] proposed a straightforward treatment that essentially consists of solving the transport equation (4.1) for the epitaxial layer, assuming the following field dependence for the majority carrier:

$$\mu_n = \frac{\mu_{n0}}{1 + (\mu_{n0}/v_s)|d\phi_n/dx|} \tag{4.46}$$

which is identical to (3.11) considered in the case of MOSFET modeling.

The current in the epitaxial layer becomes

$$I_{\text{epi}} = \frac{\kappa_1(V_{CBO}) - \kappa_1(V_{CBW}) - \ln\{[1 + \kappa_1(V_{CBO})]/[1 + \kappa_1(V_{CBW})]\} + \beta(V_{CBO} - V_{CBW})}{\beta R_{co}(1 + |V_{CBO} - V_{CBW}|/V_0)} \tag{4.47}$$

where

$$R_{c0} = \frac{W_{\text{epi}}}{q\mu_{n0}N_{\text{epi}}A_E}$$

$$\eta = \frac{2n_i}{N_{\text{epi}}}$$

$$\kappa_1(V) = \sqrt{1 + \eta \exp(\beta V)} \tag{4.48}$$

$$V_0 = \frac{W_{\text{epi}}v_s}{\mu_{n0}}$$

V_{CBW} = outer collector-base voltage

V_{CB0} = inner collector-base voltage

Kull et al. [28] showed that this current model agrees with numerical (physical) simulation.

5 NUMERICAL MODELING

In this section, we will show very briefly how the basic equations given in Section 2 are solved numerically to obtain various characteristics of a semiconductor device. For convenience, we will take the MOSFET as the example device. The method presented, however, applies well to a bipolar or other transistor.

Generally speaking, there exist two basic methods for solving the basic equations: the finite-difference method (FDM) and the finite-element method (FEM). In this chapter, the FDM is employed.

5.1 Normalization

For computational convenience, the various physical quantities frequently encountered in numerical analysis of semiconductor devices are customarily normalized as summarized in Table 1.1.

Using Table 1.1, the basic equations in Section 2 now take the following form.

Basic Equations

Poisson equation:

$$\nabla \cdot (-\varepsilon \nabla \psi) = \exp(\phi_p - \psi) - \exp(\psi - \phi_n) + \Gamma \tag{5.1}$$

Electron continuity equation:

$$\frac{d[\exp(\psi - \phi_n)]}{\delta t} + \nabla \cdot [\mu_n \exp(\psi - \phi_n) \nabla \phi_n] = -\left(\frac{\varepsilon_0 \varepsilon_s R_0}{n_i^2 \mu q}\right)(R_n - G_n) \tag{5.2}$$

Table 1.1 Unit Transformation for Numerical Analysis (NA)[a]

Physical quantity	NA notation	Normalizing factor
Coordinates x, y, z	λ_x, λ_y, λ_z	$\lambda = \sqrt{(\varepsilon_0 \varepsilon_s kT/n_i q^2)}$
Time t	τ_t	$\tau = \varepsilon_0 \varepsilon_s / \mu_0 q n_i$
Mobilities μ_n, μ_p	$\mu_0 \mu_n$, $\mu_0 \mu_p$	μ_0
Particle densities n, p, C	$n_i n$, $n_i p$, $n_i \Gamma$	n_i
Potentials ψ, ϕ_n, ϕ_p	ψ/β, ϕ_n/β, ϕ_p/β	$1/\beta = kT/q$
Generation/recombination G, R	$R_0 G$, $R_0 R$	R_0
Current densities J_n, J_p	$J_0 J_n$, $J_0 J_p$	$J_0 = \mu_0 n_i / \lambda$

[a]Notes: (1) $\nabla \equiv (\delta/\delta x,\ \delta/\delta y,\ \delta/\delta z) \equiv (1/\lambda)\nabla_{\text{NA}}$, (2) grad $\psi = \nabla\psi$, $\operatorname{div} J = \nabla \cdot J$, $\operatorname{rot} E = \nabla \times E$.

Hole continuity equation:

$$\frac{\delta[\exp(\phi_p - \psi)]}{\delta t} + \nabla \cdot [\mu_p \exp(\phi_p - \psi)\nabla\phi_p] = -\left(\frac{\varepsilon_0 \varepsilon_s R_0}{n_i^2 \mu_q}\right)(R_p - G_p) \tag{5.2a}$$

Electron transport equation:

$$J_n = J_0 \mu_n \exp(\psi - \phi_n)\nabla\phi_n \tag{5.3}$$

Hole transport equation:

$$J_p = J_0 \mu_p \exp(\phi_p - \psi)\nabla\phi_p \tag{5.3a}$$

Electron density:

$$n = \exp(\psi - \phi_n) \tag{5.4}$$

Hole density:

$$p = \exp(\phi_p - \psi) \tag{5.4a}$$

In practice, it is rarely necessary to solve all the above equations at the same time. On the contrary, it is usually possible to neglect a few of them, depending on the nature of the problem in question. For example, if one is considering a steady-state problem, then the time-varying terms in (5.2) and (5.2a) become zero. Again, if an n-channel device is being considered, one may assume a dominant electron current J_n and neglect the hole current ($J_p \doteqdot 0$) altogether. Then, from (5.3a) one has ϕ_p = constant. Finally, if the device is operating under normal bias voltages, one may also neglect R_n and G_n. Under these conditions, it is necessary to consider only two basic equations:

$$\nabla\cdot(-\varepsilon\nabla\psi) = \exp(\phi_p - \psi) - \exp(\psi - \phi_n) + \Gamma \tag{5.1}$$

$$\nabla\cdot[\mu_n \exp(\psi - \phi_n)\nabla\phi_n] = 0 \tag{5.5}$$

5.2 Linearization (Gummel Algorithm)

The Gummel algorithm [29] is a typical and successful method for solving basic semiconductor equations. The essentials of this method can be understood through the following example. Let us take the case where we have to solve the following system of three equations:

$$\nabla\cdot(-\varepsilon\nabla\psi) = \exp(\phi_p - \psi) - \exp(\psi - \phi_n) + \Gamma \tag{5.1}$$

$$\nabla\cdot[\mu_n \exp(\psi - \phi_n)\nabla\phi_n] = 0 \tag{5.5}$$

$$\nabla\cdot[\mu_p \exp(\phi_p - \psi)\nabla\phi_p] = 0 \tag{5.6}$$

One can see very well that these equations are nonlinear in terms of the unknowns ψ, ϕ_n, ϕ_p. Therefore, if we discretize them using a lattice of about a few thousand mesh points, which is usually necessary for a typical semiconductor device, we will have to face the desperate problem of solving a system of thousands of nonlinear equations!

The Gummel algorithm consists of following steps used to solve the above problem.

First, the zeroth solution $\psi^{(0)}$, which differs from the true solution ψ by only a small amount $\Delta\psi$, is assumed.

$$\psi = \psi^{(0)} + \Delta\psi \tag{5.7}$$

If $\Delta\psi$ is sufficiently small, then by expanding the exponential function and taking only the first term, we have

$$\exp(\psi) = \exp(\psi^{(0)} + \Delta\psi) \doteqdot [\exp(\psi^{(0)})](1 + \Delta\psi) \tag{5.8}$$

Using this, we can rewrite (3.1) as follows:

$$\begin{aligned}\nabla\cdot(-\varepsilon\nabla\Delta\psi) + [\exp(\psi^{(0)} - \phi_n) - \exp(\phi_p - \psi^{(0)})\Delta\psi \\ = \nabla\cdot(\varepsilon\nabla\psi^{(0)}) - \exp(\psi^{(0)} - \phi_n) + \exp(\phi_p - \psi^{(0)}) + \Gamma\end{aligned} \tag{5.9}$$

which is now linearized in terms of $\Delta\psi$.

On the other hand, since

$$\exp(\psi - \phi_n)\nabla\phi_n = -\exp(\psi)\nabla[\exp(-\phi_n)] \tag{5.10}$$

one has

$$\nabla\cdot\{\mu_n \exp(\psi)\nabla[\exp(-\phi_n)]\} = \nabla\cdot\{\mu_n \exp(\psi)\nabla\zeta_n\} = 0 \tag{5.11}$$

which is also linearized in terms of $\zeta_n = \exp(-\phi_n)$.

Similarly, (5.6) becomes

$$\nabla \cdot [\mu_p \exp(\psi) \nabla \zeta_p] = 0 \tag{5.11a}$$

where $\zeta_p = \exp(\phi_p)$.

Thus, the Gummel algorithm can be summarized in the following steps.

1. Determine the $(i-1)$st approximate solution $\psi^{(i-1)}$, $\phi_n{}^{(i-1)}$, $(\phi_p{}^{(i-1)})$ of $\psi^{(i)}(\phi_p{}^{(i)})$.
2. Solve (5.9) to obtain $\Delta\psi^{(i-1)}$, then perform the substitution $\psi^{(i)} \leftarrow \psi^{(i-1)} + \Delta\psi^{(i-1)}$.
3. Solve (5.11) [5.11a)] to obtain $\exp(-\phi_n^{(i)})$ $[\exp(\phi_p^{(i)})]$.
4. Return to step 2.

The iteration is continued until a sufficiently small $\Delta\psi$ is obtained for all mesh points.

5.3 Discretization (Poisson Equation)

In deriving finite-difference equations for the basic equations described in Section 5.1, the following method (box integration [30]) is mostly used. Here, only its application to the Poisson equation will be shown. Application to the current continuity equation is similar and will be omitted.

First, the Poisson equation is rewritten in the following form, where $\varepsilon(r)$ is used to account for the variation of the dielectric constant with position in the MOSFET:

$$\nabla \cdot \{\varepsilon(r) \cdot \nabla \psi(r)\} = -\rho(r) \tag{5.12}$$

For the two-dimensional case shown in Figure 1.10, if we apply Gauss's theorem in the integration of (5.12), we obtain the finite-difference approximation for the Poisson equation as follows.

$$\begin{aligned}\iint_S \varepsilon(r) \cdot \nabla \psi(r)\, dS &= \int_\Sigma \varepsilon(r) \left[\frac{\delta \psi(r)}{\delta v}\right] d\xi \\ &\doteqdot \left(\frac{\varepsilon_1 dx_i}{2} + \frac{\varepsilon_8 dx_{i+1}}{2}\right) \frac{(\psi_N - \psi_P)}{dy_j} \\ &\quad + \left(\frac{\varepsilon_7 dy_j}{2} + \frac{\varepsilon_6 dy_{j+1}}{2}\right) \frac{(\psi_W - \psi_P)}{dx_i} \\ &\quad + \left(\frac{\varepsilon_5 dx_i}{2} + \frac{\varepsilon_4 dx_{i+1}}{2}\right) \frac{(\psi_S - \psi_P)}{dy_{j+1}} \\ &\quad + \left(\frac{\varepsilon_2 dy_j}{2} + \frac{\varepsilon_3 dy_{j+1}}{2}\right) \frac{(\psi_E - \psi_P)}{dx_{i+1}}\end{aligned} \tag{5.13}$$

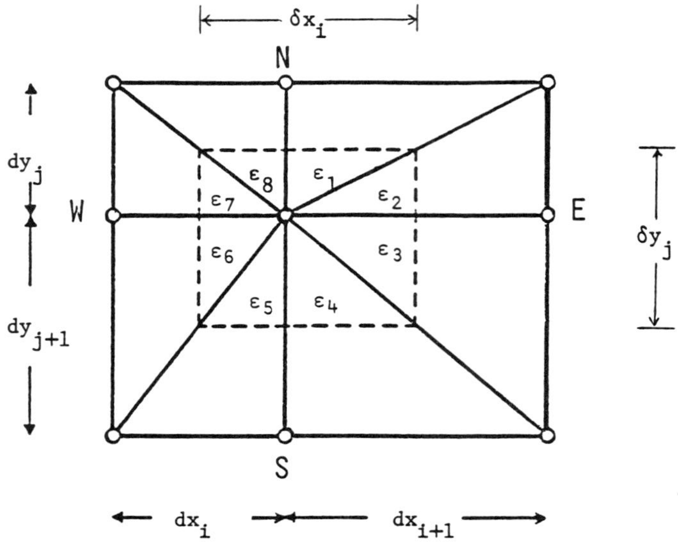

Figure 1.10 Discretization of the Poisson equation.

$$\iint_S -\rho(r)\,dS \fallingdotseq \rho(P)\cdot\delta x_i\cdot\delta y_j \tag{5.13a}$$

5.4 Numerical Simulation Examples

Figure 1.11a shows a MOSFET structure where the impurity profile is assumed to have the form shown in Figure 1.11b. As seen, an implantation is performed to make the impurity concentration at the channel surface somewhat higher than that of the bulk. Figures 1.11c–1.11e and Figures 1.11c′–1.11e′ represent potential, electron, and hole distributions for the cases where the gate is at 0 and 1 volt, respectively. Other conditions are identical and are given in the figure legend. Comparing the two electron distributions, one finds that the channel surface is strongly inverted at the gate bias of 1 volt. On the other hand, the two hole distributions show that while a thick depletion layer can be seen around the drain junction in the case of zero gate bias, the hole concentration in the vicinity of the drain is almost as high as in the bulk when the gate bias is raised to 1 volt. Thus, for a short-channel device, the hole current should always be considered if the device terminal characteristics are to be simulated correctly. Note that in the calculation leading to the results shown in Figures 1.11b–1.11e′, generation due to impact ionization was also taken into account. Details of the program with which these simulations were obtained can be found in Ref. [18].

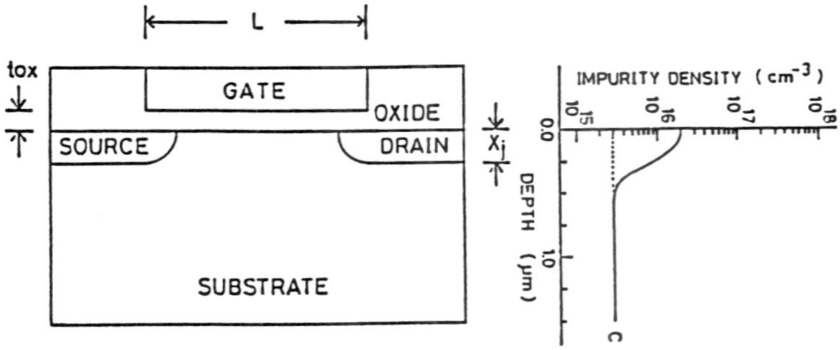

Figure 1.11 (a) structure under consideration

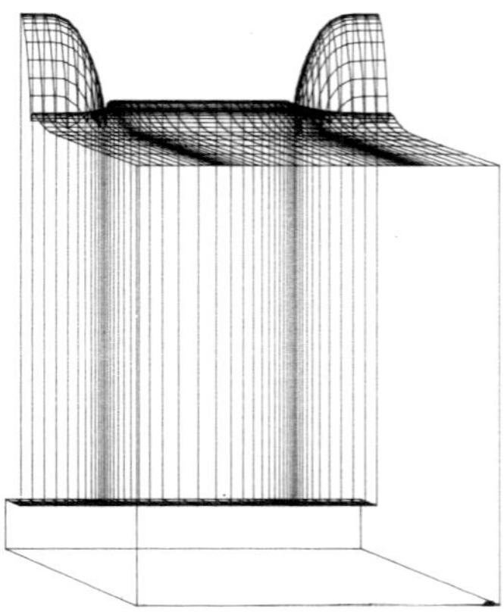

Figure 1.11 (b) impurity profile

Figure 1.11 (a) Two-dimensional simulation results based on a MOSFET structure with impurity profile at channel center shown at the right. (b) Overall impurity profile also shown by stereo plot. Potential, electron, and hole distributions are shown, also in stereo plots, for two gate biases: (c, d, e) $V_G = 0$ [V]; (c′, d′, e′) $V_G = 1$ [V]. Other parameters are $L = 1\,\mu$m, $t_{ox} = 35$ nm, $x_j = 0.25\,\mu$m.

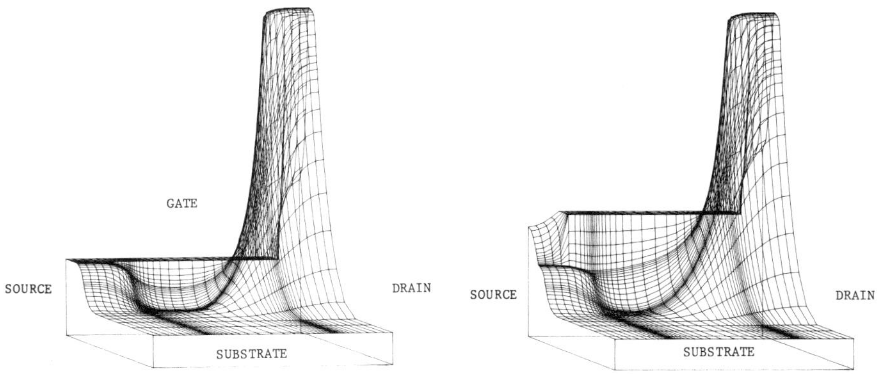

Figure 1.11 (c), (c)′ potential distributions

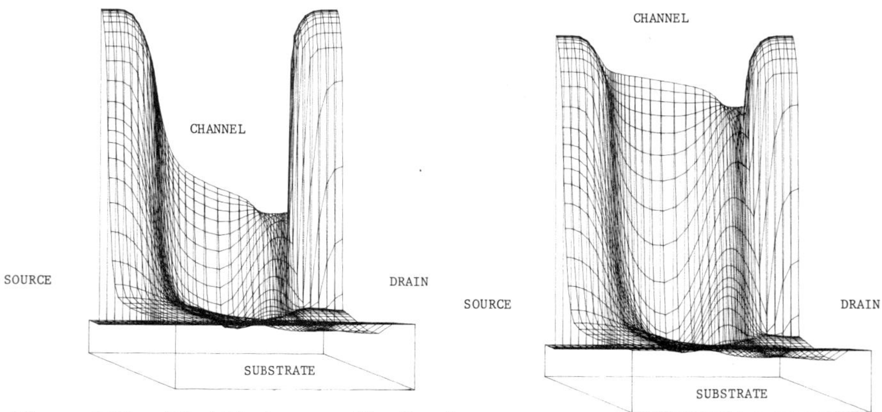

Figure 1.11 (d), (d)′ electron distributions

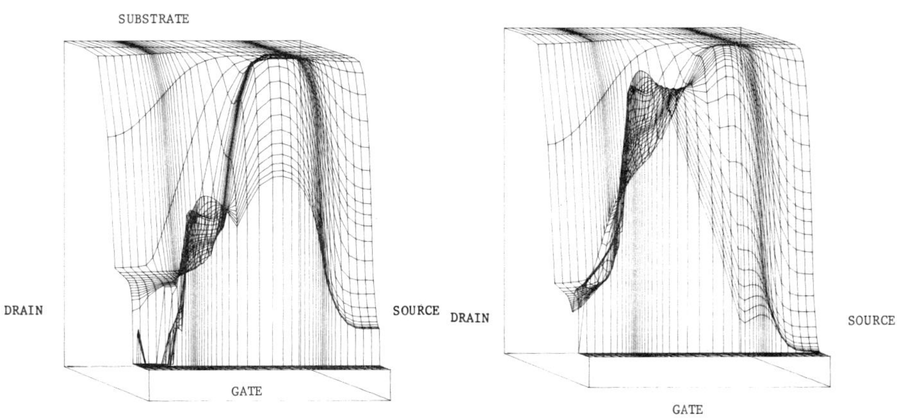

Figure 1.11 (e), (e)′ hole distributions

APPENDIX: ELABORATE MODELS FOR MOSFET DRAIN CURRENT (DANG MODEL AND PAO-SAH MODEL)

In Section 3.2, when proceeding from (3.5) to (3.6), it is assumed that $\delta\phi_n/\delta x \fallingdotseq 0$. Comparison of (2.11) and (2.11a) reveals that this is equivalent to neglecting the diffusion current component $qD_n \operatorname{grad} n$. In the following, however, we will present two formulas where the diffusion current component is also taken into account. The first formula was derived by Dang [7] under the assumption that the drain current flows only at the channel surface ("sheet current"). The second, called Pao-Sah model, is (3.5) itself given in the form of a double integral [6]. We will see that the calculated currents based on the two models are practically identical.

Dang Model

Under the sheet current assumption, it is possible to consider the drain current as being one-dimensional. Thus, in the case of an n-channel, the drain current per unit channel width will be given as follows:

$$J_D = \frac{I_D}{W} = \mu_n E_x Q_i + D_n \frac{dQ_i}{dx} \tag{A.1}$$

where Q_i is the total mobile charge per unit channel width at point x.

Substitution of $E_x = -dV_x/dx$, $D_n = \mu_n(kT/q) = \mu_n/\beta$ and integration from source to drain yields

$$I_D \int_0^L dx = I_D L = \mu_n W \left\{ -\int_{V_x(0)}^{V_x(L)} Q_i \, dV_x + \left(\frac{1}{\beta}\right) \int_{Q_i(0)}^{Q_i(L)} dQ_i \right\} \tag{A.2}$$

Let V_G denote the gate voltage. Then by virtue of charge conservation, we have

$$V_G - V_x = \frac{Q_i + Q_d}{C_{ox}} \tag{A.3}$$

where Q_d is the depletion charge per unit channel width at point x.

Using the one-sided junction formula to calculate this depletion charge, we have

$$Q_d = \sqrt{(2\varepsilon_s q N_B V_x)} \tag{A.4}$$

and therefore

$$Q_i = \frac{V_G - Q_d^2/(2\varepsilon_s q N_B)}{C_{ox} - Q_d} \tag{A.5}$$

Use of (A.4) and (A.5) in the above integral yields the following formula [7]:

$$I_D = \left(\frac{\mu_n W C_{ox}}{L}\right)\left\{\left(\frac{1}{2}\right)[V_s^2(L) - V_s^2(0)]\left(\frac{2\gamma}{3}\right)[\sqrt{V_s^3(L)} - \sqrt{V_s^3(0)}]\right.$$

$$\left. - \left(V_G + \frac{1}{\beta}\right)(V_s(L) - V_s(0))\left(\frac{1}{\beta}\right)\gamma(\sqrt{V_s(L)} - \sqrt{V_s(0)})\right\} \tag{A.6}$$

where

$$V_s(0) = \psi_s(0) + V_S - V_B \tag{A.7}$$

$$V_s(L) = \psi_s(L) + V_D - V_B \tag{A.7a}$$

A relation between ψ_s and V_G is derived as follows.

The one-dimensional Poisson equation in the vertical direction is written as

$$\frac{d^2\psi_s(x)}{dy^2} = \left(\frac{-q}{\varepsilon_s}\right)(-N_B + p - n)$$

$$= \left(\frac{-qN_B}{\varepsilon_s}\right)\left\{-1 + \exp(-\beta\psi_s(x) - V_B)\right.$$

$$\left. + \left(\frac{n_i}{N_B}\right)^2 \exp(\beta\psi_s(x) - V_x(x))\right\} \tag{A.8}$$

where $\chi_s(x) = V_x(x) - V_B$ is the difference between the quasi-Fermi levels for holes and electrons.

When (A.8) is multiplied by $2d\psi_s(x)/dy$ and integrated, we obtain $[d\psi_s(x)/dy]^2$, whose square root times ε_s will give the total charge Q_s in the semiconductor, by virtue of Gauss's theorem, as follows:

$$Q_s = C_{ox}(V_G - V_{FB} - \psi_s(x)) = \sqrt{(2\varepsilon_s q N_B)}$$

$$\times \left\{\psi_s(x) - V_B + \left(\frac{1}{\beta}\right)[\exp(-\beta\psi_s(x) - V_B) - 1\right.$$

$$\left. + \exp(\beta\psi_s(x) - 2\phi_F - V_x(x)) - \exp(V_B - 2\phi_F - V_x(x))\right\}^{1/2} \tag{A.9}$$

Again putting $V_G - V_{FB} - V_B = V_G$, $\psi_s(x) - V_B = \psi_s(x)$, we have, after arranging terms,

$$\frac{\beta(V_G - \psi_s(x))^2}{\gamma^2} - \beta\psi_s(x) + 1 - \exp(-\beta\psi_s(x))$$

$$-\exp(-\beta[2\phi_F + \chi_s(x)])\{\exp(\beta\psi_s(x)) - 1\} = 0 \tag{A.10}$$

Pao-Sah Model

As mentioned above, the Pao-Sah model also starts from the basic equation (2.11a). But, in this case, the latter equation is merely integrated across the inversion layer and from source to drain to yield [6]

$$I_D = \left(\frac{W}{L}\right)\left(\frac{\lambda}{\sqrt{2}}\right)\mu_n q n_i \int_{\chi_s(0)}^{\chi_s(L)} \int_{\psi_s(x)}^{\phi_F} \frac{\exp \beta(\psi_s - \chi_s + \phi_F)}{F} d\psi_s \, d\chi_s \tag{A.11}$$

where

$$[F(\psi_s(x), \chi_s(x))]^2 = \beta\psi_s(x) - 1 + \exp(-\beta\psi_s(x)) + \exp(-\beta[2\phi_F + \chi_s(x)])\{\exp(\beta\psi_s(x)) - 1\} \tag{A.12}$$

It can be seen that in the calculation of the drain current based on the Dang model, one has to compute (A.10) only twice—once at the source and once at the drain. But in the Pao-Sah model it is also necessary to compute (A.12) twice in each of the subintervals during the numerical integration of (A.11). Therefore, the computer time for the Pao-Sah model is many tens of

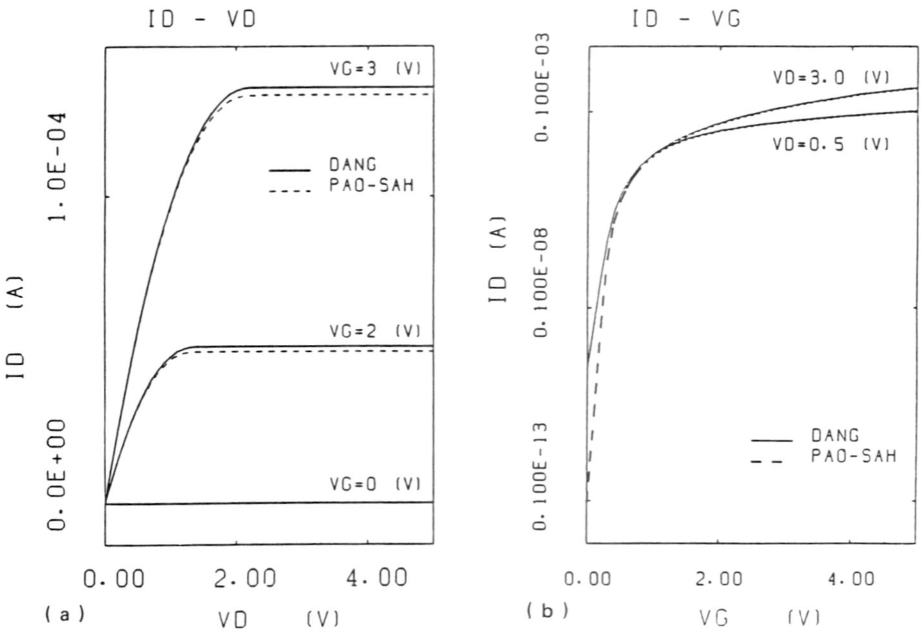

Figure 1.12 Comparison of the Pao-Sah model and the Dang model in terms of (a) $I_D - V_D$ characteristics and (b) $I_D - V_G$ characteristics. Other parameters are $L = 5\,\mu$m, $W = 5\,\mu$m, $t_{ox} = 50$ nm, $N_B = 5 \times 10^{15}$ cm^{-3}.

times that for the Dang model. In terms of the final calculated results, however, a comparison of the two models presented in Figure 1.12 shows that the calculated current values based on the two models are virtually identical for all voltage ranges, either subthreshold or superthreshold.

ACKNOWLEDGMENTS

The author wishes to thank his graduate students, M. Nakamura and T. Kojima, for the preparation of Figures 1.11 and 1.12. The VLSI Research Center, Toshiba Research and Development Center, is acknowledged for providing a copy of the two-dimensional numerical simulator MOS2C, which was developed under the supervision of the author when he was associated with Toshiba Corporation.

REFERENCES

1. L. D. Yau, A simple theory to predict the threshold voltage of short-channel IGFET's, *Solid-State Electron.*, vol. 17, pp. 1059–1063, 1974.
2. K. E. Kroell and G. K. Ackermann, Threshold voltage of narrow-channel transistors, *Solid-State Electron.*, vol. 19, pp. 77–81, 1976; K. O. Jeppson, Influence of the channel width on the threshold voltage modulation in MOSFET's, *Electron. Lett.*, vol. 11, pp. 297–298, 1975.
3. N. Shigyo, M. Konaka, and R. L. M. Dang, Three-dimensional simulation of inverse narrow-channel effect, *Electron. Lett.*, vol. 18, pp. 274–2751, 1982.
4. L. W. Nagel, SPICE2: A computer program to simulate semiconductor circuits, Memo. No. ERL-M520, Univ. of California, Berkeley, 1975.
5. H. K. J. Ihantola and J. L. Moll, Design theory of a surface field-effect transistor, *Solid-State Electron.*, vol. 7, pp. 423–430, 1964.
6. H. C. Pao and C. T. Sah, Effects of diffusion current on characteristics of metal-oxide (insulator)-semiconductor transistors, *Solid-State Electron.*, vol. 11, pp. 927–937, 1966.
7. L. M. Dang, A one-dimensional theory on the effect of diffusion current and carrier velocity saturation on E-type IGFET current-voltage characteristics, *Solid-State Electron.*, vol. 20, pp. 781–788, 1977.
8. J. R. Brews, A charge-sheet model of the MOSFET. *Solid-State Electron.*, vol. 21, pp. 345–355, 1978.
9. G. Baccarani et al., Analytical i.g.f.e.t. model including drift and diffusion, *Solid-State Electron Devices*, vol. 2, pp. 62–67, 1978.
10. F. Van de Wiele, A long-channel MOSFET model, *Solid-State Electron.*, vol. 22, pp. 991–997, 1979.

11. L. L. Lewyn and J. D. Meindl, An IGFET inversion charge model for VLSI systems, *IEEE Trans. Electron Devices*, vol. ED-32, pp. 434–440, 1985.
12. G. T. Wright, A simple and continuous MOSFET model, *IEEE Trans. Electron Devices*, vol. ED-32, pp. 1259–1263, 1985.
13. H. K. Gummel and H. C. Poon, An integral charge control model of bipolar transistors, *BSTJ*, vol. 49, pp. 827–852, 1970.
14. J. J. Ebers and J. L. Moll, Large signal behaviour of junction transistors, *Proc. IRE*, vol. 42, pp. 1761–1772, 1954.
15. D. P. Kennedy and R. R. O'Brien, Computer aided two-dimensional analysis of the junction field-effect transistor, *IBM J. Res. Dev.*, vol. 14, pp. 95–116, 1970.
16. M. S. Mock, A two-dimensional mathematical model of the insulated-gate field-effect transistor, *Solid-State Electron.*, vol. 16, pp. 601–609, 1973.
17. S. Selberherr, A. Schutz, and H. W. Potzl, MINIMOS—a two-dimensional MOS transistor analyzer, *IEEE Trans. Electron Devices*, vol. ED-27, pp. 1540–1550, 1980.
18. T. Wada and R. Dang, Development and application of a high-speed two-dimensional time dependent device simulator (MOS2C), in *NASECODE-IV* (Proc. 4th Int. Conf. Numerical Analysis of Semiconductor Devices and Integrated Circuits, June 19–21, 1985, Trinity College, Dublin), J. J. H. Miller, ed., pp. 108–119, Boole Press; 1985.
19. W. L. Engl, R. Laur, and H. K. Dirks, MEDUSA—a simulator for modular circuits, *IEEE Trans. Computer-Aided Design of Integrated Circuits and Systems*, vol. CAD-1, pp. 85–93, 1982.
20. T. Shima, H. Yamada, and R. L. M. Dang, Table look-up MOSFET modeling system using a 2-D device simulator and monotonic piecewise cubic interpolation, *IEEE Trans. Computer-Aided Design of Integrated Circuits and Systems*, vol. CAD-2, pp. 121–126, 1983.
21. W. Shockley, A unipolar field-effect transistor, *Proc. IRE*, vol. 41, pp. 1365–1381, 1952.
22. R. H. Crawford, *MOSFET in Circuit Design*, pp. 66–69, McGraw-Hill, New York, 1967.
23. L. M. Dang, A simple current model for short-channel IGFET and its application to circuit simulation, *IEEE J. Solid-State Circuits*, vol. SC-14, pp. 358–369, 1979.
24. K. Kurosawa, T. Shibata, and H. Iizuka, A new bird's-beak free field isolation technology for VLSI devices, *IEDM Tech. Digest*: pp. 384–387, 1981.

25. F. M. Klaassen, Compact MOSFET modeling, in *Process and Device Modeling*, W. L. Engl, ed., pp. 402–404, North-Holland, 1986.
26. N. Shigyo and R. Dang, Three-dimensional device simulation using a mixed process/device simulation, in *Process and Device Modeling*, W. L. Engl, ed., pp. 301–327, North-Holland, 1986.
27. H. C. De Graaff, Compact bipolar transistor modeling, in *Process and Device Modeling*, W. L. Engl, ed., pp. 416–418, North-Holland, 1986.
28. G. M. Kull, L. W. Nagel, S. W. Lee, P. Lloyd, E. J. Prendergast, and H. Dirks, A unified circuit model for bipolar transistors including quasi-saturation effects, *IEEE Trans. Electron Devices*, vol. ED-32, pp. 1103–1113, 1985.
29. H. K. Gummel, A self-consistent iterative scheme for one-dimensional steady state transistor calculations, *IEEE Trans. Electron Devices*, vol. ED-11, pp. 455–465, 1964.
30. J. A. Greenfield and R. W. Dutton, Nonplanar VLSI device analysis using the solution of Poisson's equation, *IEEE Trans. Electron Devices*, vol. ED-27, pp. 1520–1532, 1980.

2

LU Decomposition Algorithms for Parallel and Vector Computation

Martin Vlach

Analogy, Inc.
Beaverton, Oregon

Tearing methods for large systems have been widely studied and applied over the last decade. Most of the applications used single-level partitioning of a system into subsystems. In this chapter, tearing is applied to hierarchically described systems, where each subsystem is itself composed of subsystems, and so on to arbitrary depth. This structure gives rise naturally to "recursive" bordered block diagonal (BBD) matrices, where each diagonal block is itself in the BBD form. Algorithms for LU decomposition and forward and back substitution of such matrices are described.

1 INTRODUCTION

A method of solving large systems of equations, called tearing, has been investigated in a number of applications. In tearing, the system is decomposed or "torn" into smaller units, and each subsystem is solved separately. This approach, also called piecewise analysis or diakoptics, was first used by Kron [1]. Although the original method involved dense matrix inverses, sparse matrix techniques and LU decomposition have been applied to diakoptics [2–4].

From an algebraic point of view, tearing can be considered as a partitioning of the equations in a special way, and applying block matrix manipulations to the resulting form [5, 6].

Tearing does not necessarily save computations as compared to direct sparse matrix methods [3], but the subnetworks are handled independently and parallel processing can also be exploited. In the case of identical subnetworks, tearing may lead to savings in storage as well as in computation time [2]. It also becomes important in applications where the system must be solved repeatedly while only a small proportion of the subnetworks change. This may come about either from the properties of the external algorithm, such as the multilevel Newton iteration [7] or a block relaxation algorithm (see Chapter 4), or from the dynamic properties of the circuit itself, i.e., the latency concept [7, 8].

Two major interdependent areas of research in solving systems of equations by tearing or partitioning can be identified. One area is concerned with finding a good partitioning for a given system of equations. A major stumbling block is the lack of definition of what constitutes a good partitioning. An algorithm useful in "node tearing nodal analysis" [9] was presented in Ref. [10]. Several references to other papers dealing with this problem can be found there, and also in a review paper by Duff [11].

The other area under investigation is finding the best method for solving a partitioned system of equations assuming that the partitioning is known *a priori*. Hajj [5] gives a number of block algorithms, their operation counts, and comparisons. Questions of stability of block methods are addressed in Ref. [12].

In all of the works cited, the tearing/partitioning was applied on a single level only, although several authors mentioned the possibility of or briefly described recursive partitioning and decomposition [2, 13–15]. In Ref. [16] a multilevel decomposition approach based on tearing is described, using circuit-theoretical arguments and connecting two subnetworks at a time. In a recent publication [17], an approach similar to that described here is discussed.

With hierarchical design, the subnetworks to be torn will be known *a priori*. Algebraically, the matrix to be solved will have a BBD structure. Since each subnetwork is composed of lower-level networks, each of the diagonal blocks will itself be in the BBD form, and so on. We say that such a matrix is in the recursively bordered block diagonal form.

In this chapter we will describe an efficient implementation of a decomposition algorithm for such matrices. The approach taken (similar to that used in [18]) leads to a hierarchical decomposition and solution from considerations of the structure of the system matrix.

2 STRUCTURE OF THE SYSTEM MATRIX

In this section we will develop ideas related to and representations of hierarchical systems.

Consider a subnetwork with some internal structure and terminals where other networks may be connected. The subnetwork can be described by a (possibly nonlinear) function

$$\mathbf{g}(\mathbf{x}) = 0 \tag{1}$$

where the independent variables x_i may represent voltages and/or currents. Let us partition the vector $\mathbf{x}$ into internal variables (those which do not interact with the external world), and external variables—those associated with the terminals of the subnetwork:

$$\mathbf{x} = \begin{bmatrix} \mathbf{x}^I \\ \mathbf{x}^E \end{bmatrix} \tag{2}$$

We will assume that the description (1) of the subnetwork is such that, for each terminal, there exists an explicit function which determines the terminal current or terminal voltage in terms of the other variables. In other words, $\mathbf{g}$ will include a function of *one* of the following forms:

$$i - f(\mathbf{x}_{(-i)}) = 0 \tag{3a}$$

$$v - f(\mathbf{x}_{(-v)}) = 0 \tag{3b}$$

for each terminal. Here $\mathbf{x}_{-i}$ $(\mathbf{x}_{-v})$ is the vector $\mathbf{x}$ excluding the current (voltage) under consideration. We can therefore partition $\mathbf{g}$ into the internal and external parts

$$\mathbf{g} = \begin{bmatrix} \mathbf{g}^I \\ \mathbf{g}^E \end{bmatrix} = \begin{bmatrix} \mathbf{g}^I(\mathbf{x}^I, \mathbf{x}^E) \\ \mathbf{g}^E(\mathbf{x}^I, \mathbf{x}^E) \end{bmatrix} \tag{4}$$

If nodal formulation is used, $\mathbf{g}^I$ consists of Kirchhoff's current law equations for each internal node, and $\mathbf{g}^E$ gives the terminal currents of the subnetwork. The Jacobian (or its approximation) of the function (1), which will be needed in a solution algorithm, may be partitioned from (2) and (4) as

$$\frac{\partial \mathbf{g}}{\partial \mathbf{x}} = \begin{bmatrix} \dfrac{\partial \mathbf{g}^I}{\partial \mathbf{x}^I} & \dfrac{\partial \mathbf{g}^I}{\partial \mathbf{x}^E} \\[2ex] \dfrac{\partial \mathbf{g}^E}{\partial \mathbf{x}^I} & \dfrac{\partial \mathbf{g}^E}{\partial \mathbf{x}^E} \end{bmatrix} = \begin{bmatrix} \mathbf{D} & \mathbf{C} \\ \mathbf{R} & \mathbf{E} \end{bmatrix} \tag{5}$$

When the terminals of several subnetworks are connected at a single node, we are forcing those terminals to be at the same voltage and the sum of the terminal currents to be zero:

$$v_{k_1}{}^1 = v_{k_2}{}^2 = \cdots = v_{k_n}{}^n \tag{6a}$$

$$i_{k_1}{}^1 + i_{k_2}{}^2 + \cdots + i_{k_n}{}^n = 0 \tag{6b}$$

(Here the superscripts indicate different subnetworks and subscripts different terminals.) Let us now consider the two possible "constitutive equations" for the terminal variables indicated in (3a) and (3b). We will also assume that all terminals connected at a node are described by a function of the same type.

Consider first (3a):

$$i_{k_j}{}^{j} = g_{k_j}{}^{j}(\mathbf{x}_{(-i)k_j}{}^{j}) \qquad (j = 1, \ldots, n) \tag{7}$$

From (6a) we see that the n terminal voltages of the subnetworks are *merged* into a single voltage (an independent variable) of the connection network

$$v = v_{k_j}{}^{j} \qquad j = 1, \ldots, n \tag{8}$$

The number of independent variables in the combined network is reduced by $n - 1$. The n functions (7) can then be combined into a single function according to (6b):

$$\sum_{j=1}^{n} g_{k_j}{}^{j}(\mathbf{x}^{j}) = 0 \tag{9}$$

reducing the number of equations by $n - 1$.

This operation is performed for each node of the connection network where subnetwork terminals are attached. The external variables of all the subnetworks are thus relabeled [by (8)] to be some variable of the connection network. The independent variables of the interconnected system will be the internal variables of all the subnetworks plus the variables of the connection network. If the variables of the subnetworks are

$$\begin{bmatrix} \mathbf{x}^{I_1} \\ \mathbf{x}^{E_1} \end{bmatrix}, \begin{bmatrix} \mathbf{x}^{I_2} \\ \mathbf{x}^{E_2} \end{bmatrix}, \ldots, \begin{bmatrix} \mathbf{x}^{I_n} \\ \mathbf{x}^{E_n} \end{bmatrix}$$

then the independent variables of the interconnected system will be

$$\mathbf{x} = \begin{bmatrix} \mathbf{x}^{I_1} \\ \cdots \\ \mathbf{x}^{I_n} \\ \mathbf{x}^{C} \end{bmatrix} \tag{10}$$

where $\mathbf{x}^C$ are the variables of the interconnection network and the external variables of each subnetwork are selected entries of $\mathbf{x}^C$,

$$\mathbf{x}^{E_j} = \mathbf{S}^{j}\mathbf{x}^{C} \tag{11}$$

The "gather" operator $\mathbf{S}^j$ is a matrix whose rows are elementary unit vectors (e.g., row i of $\mathbf{S}^j$ is $\mathbf{e}_k$, corresponding to the selection $x_i{}^{E_j} = \mathbf{x}_k{}^{C}$).

The formation of the vector of independent variables $\mathbf{x}$ is illustrated graphically in Figure 2.1. Notice that there is no restriction on the columns of $\mathbf{S}^j$; the terminals of a subnetwork may be connected by the connection network.

If the connection network forms the overall system, the variables $\mathbf{x}^C$ can be considered as the internal variables of the connection network, and the entire vector of independent variables can be considered as a series of internal variables of all the subsystems involved:

$$\mathbf{x} = \begin{bmatrix} \mathbf{x}^{I_1} \\ \cdots \\ \mathbf{x}^{I_n} \\ \mathbf{x}^{I_c} \end{bmatrix} \tag{12}$$

Note that in our terminology, "internal" variables of a network do *not* include the internal variables of any of its subnetworks; for example, $\mathbf{x}^{Ic}$ are the only "internal" variables of the connection network, and $\mathbf{x}^{I_1}, \mathbf{x}^{I_2}, \ldots$ are "internal" variables of the subnetworks.

Let us now turn to consideration of the structure of the system matrix of the connected network. Using the gather matrices $\mathbf{S}^j$, we can write equation

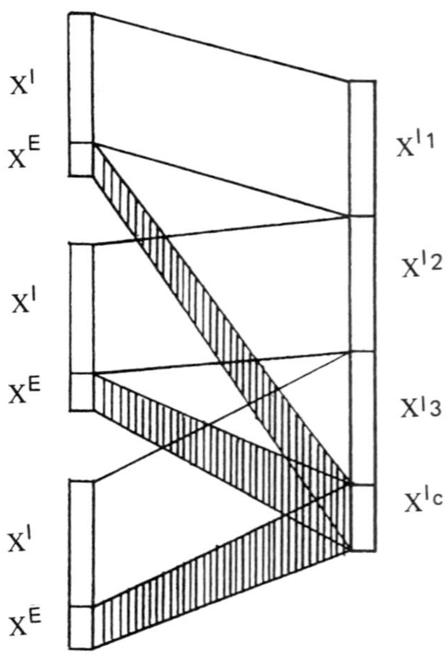

Figure 2.1 Merging external variables.

(9) for the entire interconnection network as

$$\sum_{j=1}^{n} \mathbf{S}^{jT}\mathbf{g}^{E_j} = 0 \tag{13}$$

since the operation $\mathbf{S}^{jT}\mathbf{g}^{Ej}$ scatters the entries of the vector $\mathbf{g}$ to the rows corresponding to the $\mathbf{x}^C$ entries where the terminals are connected. Combining (10), (11), and (13), the system of equations will be

$$\mathbf{g}(\mathbf{x}) = \begin{bmatrix} \mathbf{g}^{I_1}(\mathbf{x}^{I_1}, \mathbf{S}^1\mathbf{x}^C) \\ \cdots \\ \mathbf{g}^{I_n}(\mathbf{x}^{I_n}, \mathbf{S}^n\mathbf{x}^C) \\ \sum_{j=1}^{n} \mathbf{S}^{jT}\mathbf{g}^{E_j}(\mathbf{x}^{I_j}, \mathbf{S}^j\mathbf{x}^C) \end{bmatrix} = 0 \tag{14}$$

and, since from (11)

$$\frac{\partial \mathbf{g}^{I_i}}{\partial \mathbf{x}^C} = \frac{\partial \mathbf{g}^{I_i}}{\partial \mathbf{x}^{E_i}} \frac{\partial \mathbf{x}^{E_i}}{\partial \mathbf{x}^C} = \frac{\partial \mathbf{g}^{I_i}}{\partial \mathbf{x}^{E_i}} \mathbf{S}^i$$

the Jacobian becomes

$$\mathbf{J} = \frac{\partial \mathbf{g}}{\partial \mathbf{x}} = \begin{bmatrix} \frac{\partial \mathbf{G}^{I_1}}{\partial \mathbf{x}^{I_1}} & \cdots & & \frac{\partial \mathbf{g}^{I_1}}{\partial \mathbf{x}^{E_1}}\mathbf{S}^1 \\ \cdots & \ddots & & \cdots \\ & & \frac{\partial \mathbf{G}^{I_n}}{\partial \mathbf{x}^{I_n}} & \frac{\partial \mathbf{g}^{I_n}}{\partial \mathbf{x}^{E_n}}\mathbf{S}^n \\ \mathbf{S}^{1T}\frac{\partial \mathbf{g}^{E_1}}{\partial \mathbf{x}^{I_1}} & \cdots & \mathbf{S}^{nT}\frac{\partial \mathbf{g}^{E_n}}{\partial \mathbf{x}^{I_n}} & \sum_{j=1}^{n} \mathbf{S}^{jT}\frac{\partial \mathbf{g}^{E_j}}{\partial \mathbf{x}^{E_j}}\mathbf{S}^j \end{bmatrix}$$

$$= \begin{bmatrix} \mathbf{D}_1 & & & & \tilde{\mathbf{C}}_1 \\ & \mathbf{D}_2 & & & \tilde{\mathbf{C}}_2 \\ & & \cdots & & \cdots \\ & & & \mathbf{D}_n & \tilde{\mathbf{C}}_n \\ \tilde{\mathbf{R}}_1 & \tilde{\mathbf{R}}_2 & \cdots & \tilde{\mathbf{R}}_n & \sum_{j=1}^{n} \tilde{\mathbf{E}}_j \end{bmatrix} \tag{15}$$

where

$$\begin{aligned} \tilde{\mathbf{C}}_i &= \mathbf{C}_i\mathbf{S}^i \\ \tilde{\mathbf{R}}_i &= \mathbf{S}^{iT}\mathbf{R}_i \\ \tilde{\mathbf{E}}_i &= \mathbf{S}^{iT}\mathbf{E}_i\mathbf{S}^i \end{aligned} \tag{16}$$

and $\mathbf{D}_i$, $\mathbf{C}_i$, $\mathbf{R}_i$, and $\mathbf{E}_i$ correspond to the subdivision of the Jacobian in (5) in each subnetwork. It should be noted that no new nonzeros are created by the interconnection process. (If subnetwork terminals are connected by an outer network, some rows and columns are superimposed.) Graphically, the structure of the interconnected system with a single level of subcircuits is illustrated in Fig. 2.3.

This structure of the matrix relies on the assumption that the terminal variables (voltages and currents) are related as in (3a). The partitioning just described is called node-tearing analysis in network theory [5, 9].

If the impedance description (3b) were used as the starting point, we would obtain the "branch tearing" formulation. Since it leads to systems which are larger than in node tearing, [5] we will assume that the interaction between subnetworks can be described as in (3a). This assumption is reasonable, since this is the prevalent method of interconnections of electrical networks.

So far, we have shown the structure of an interconnected sytem on a single level. Often, the connected system will form a subnetwork of a larger system. The variables of a connection network can be again subdivided into internal and external variables

$$\mathbf{x}^C = \begin{bmatrix} \mathbf{x}^I \\ \mathbf{x}^E \end{bmatrix}$$

and the description (14) can be similarly partitioned. Graphically, the Jacobian of Figure 2.2 can be split as in Figure 2.3. Performing the interconnection on a higher level network, we will arrive at the recursive bordered block diagonal form of Figure 2.4.

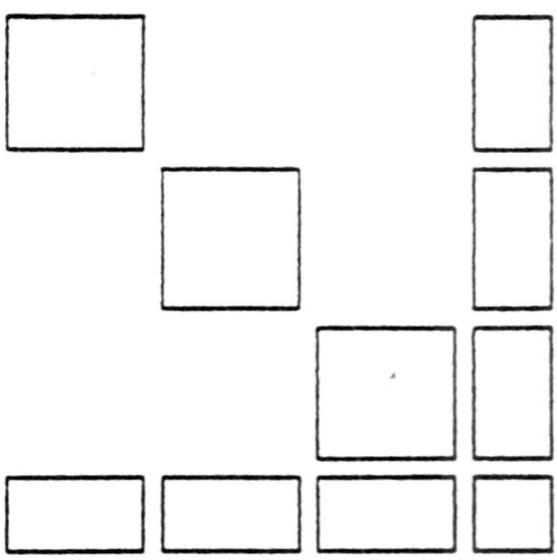

Figure 2.2 Bordered block diagonal structure of single-level interconnection.

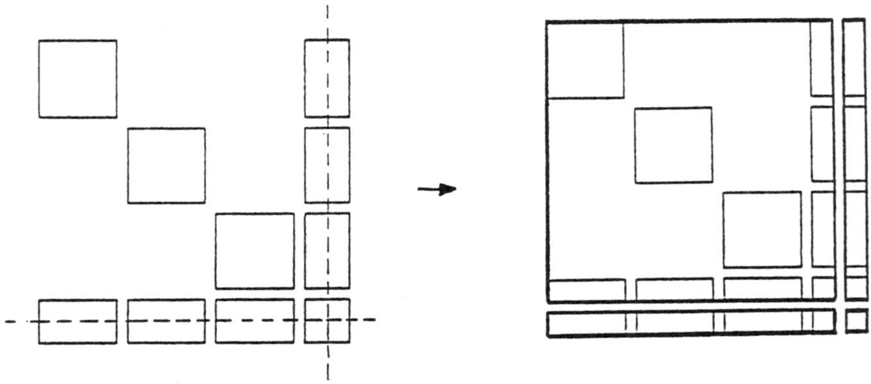

Figure 2.3 Interconnected system as a subnetwork.

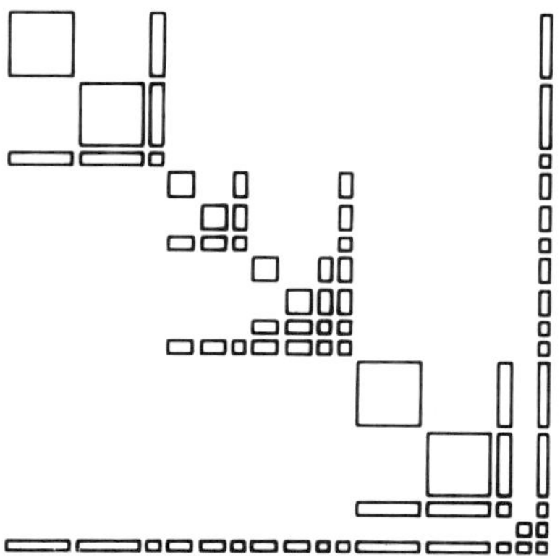

Figure 2.4 Recursive BBD form of a multilevel interconnected system.

As in the single-level case, the unknowns of the entire system will be a series of the internal variables of the various subsystems involved. No new nonzero rows or columns are generated by the multilevel interconnection.

Although we have constructed the matrix by a bottom-up process, connecting subnetworks into higher-level networks, we could just as well have proceeded top-down, splitting a system into subnetworks and then splitting the subnetworks further. In fact, both concepts will be found useful in the description of the various algorithms to follow.

3 REPRESENTATION OF THE INTERCONNECTED SYSTEM

In the description of the connected system, it was assumed that all interactions of a subnetwork with other subnetworks are described strictly by interconnections in an outer or higher-level network. Such a relationship can be represented graphically as a tree (Figure 2.5). Often many identical subnetworks are connected to form an overall system. A relationship between the *types* of subcircuits may be conveniently represented by a directed graph (Figure 2.6). Notice that as far as the circuit types are concerned, we do not require a tree structure.

This representation of the system allows certain invariant information, such as equation renumbering and sparse LU pointers, to be shared among circuits of the same type. It is also useful for checking purposes—for example, a circuit must not be described in terms of itself; that is, the "type graph" must not contain directed loops.

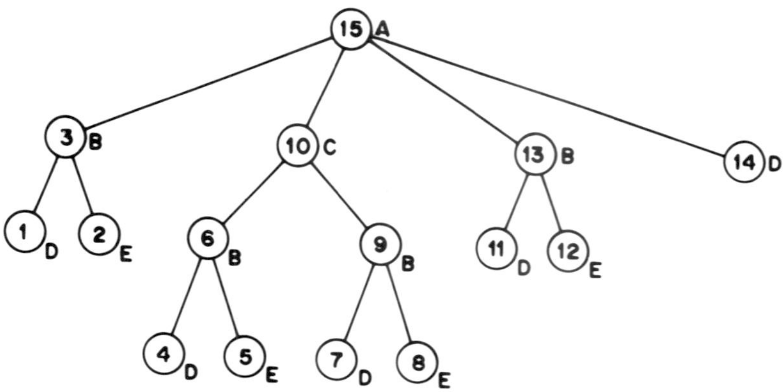

Figure 2.5 Representation of the subnetwork relationships.

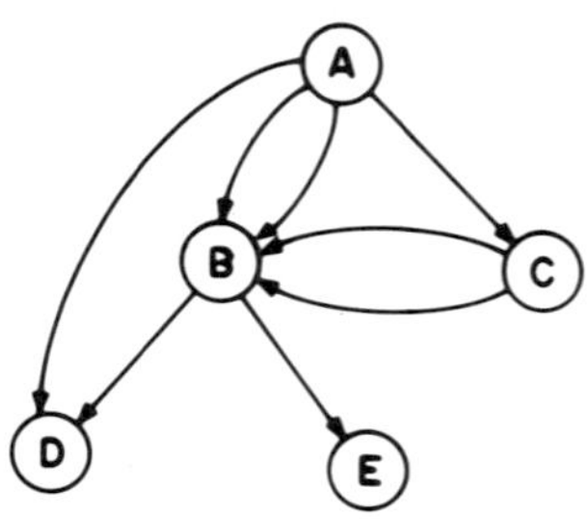

Figure 2.6 Relationship between circuit types—the type graph.

4 LU DECOMPOSITION

Let us recall the algorithm for the LU decomposition of a matrix:

Algorithm 1: The Crout algorithm for LU decomposition

For $k = 1, n$

$$u_{kk} = u_{kk} - \sum_{j=1}^{k-1} l_{kj} u_{jk}$$

For $i = k + 1, n$

$$l_{ik} = \left(l_{ik} - \sum_{j=1}^{k-1} l_{ij} u_{jk} \right) \Big/ u_{kk}$$

$$u_{ki} = u_{ki} - \sum_{j=1}^{k-1} l_{kj} u_{ji}$$

Consider now the partition of the matrix as indicated in (5), with **D** of size $n_\mathrm{I} \times n_\mathrm{I}$ (n_I is the number of the internal variables of the subnetwork). After n_I pivot steps, the matrix will be transformed as

$$\begin{bmatrix} \mathbf{D} & \mathbf{C} \\ \mathbf{R} & \mathbf{E} \end{bmatrix} \rightarrow \begin{bmatrix} \mathbf{LU} & \mathbf{C}' \\ \mathbf{R}' & \mathbf{E} \end{bmatrix} \tag{17}$$

Notice that in the remaining pivot steps, only **E** will be modified, with **L**, **U**, **C**′, and **R**′ remaining unchanged. In particular, **R**′ and **C**′ will be a part of the completed LU factors.

Consider now the completed decomposition, with the LU factors partitioned as in (17):

$$\begin{bmatrix} \mathbf{L}^I & 0 \\ \mathbf{R}' & \mathbf{L}^E \end{bmatrix} \begin{bmatrix} \mathbf{U}^I & \mathbf{C}' \\ 0 & \mathbf{U}^E \end{bmatrix} = \begin{bmatrix} \mathbf{L}^I\mathbf{U}^I & \mathbf{L}^I\mathbf{C}' \\ \mathbf{R}'\mathbf{U}^I & \mathbf{R}'\mathbf{C}' + \mathbf{L}^E\mathbf{U}^E \end{bmatrix} = \begin{bmatrix} \mathbf{D} & \mathbf{C} \\ \mathbf{R} & \mathbf{E} \end{bmatrix}$$

From this, we can identify

$$\begin{aligned} \mathbf{L}^I\mathbf{U}^I &= \mathbf{D} \\ \mathbf{L}^E\mathbf{U}^E &= \mathbf{E} - \mathbf{R}'\mathbf{C}' \\ \mathbf{R}'\mathbf{U}^I &= \mathbf{R} \\ \mathbf{L}^I\mathbf{C}' &= \mathbf{C} \end{aligned} \tag{18}$$

The remaining pivot steps after n_I can therefore be performed in two parts:

1. Form $\mathbf{E}' = \mathbf{E} - \mathbf{R}'\mathbf{C}'$.
2. Perform the LU decomposition (Algorithm 1) on $\mathbf{E}'$ to obtain $\mathbf{L}^E$ and $\mathbf{U}^E$.

We have thus found a convenient partition of the LU decomposition algorithm into two parts which follow the partition of the subnetwork into the internal and external variables:

Step 1: (Partial LU decomposition)
Perform the first n_I pivot steps of Algorithm 1.
Form $\mathbf{E}' = \mathbf{E} - \mathbf{R}'\mathbf{C}'$.
Step 2: Perform Algorithm 1 on the submatrix $\mathbf{E}'$.

Let us now turn our attention to the interconnected system whose structure is shown in (15). The LU decomposition has the property that the leading zeros of a row (column) will remain zeros in the decomposition:

$$\begin{aligned} a_{ij} = 0 \quad &\text{implies} \quad l_{ij} = 0 \\ a_{ji} = 0 \quad &\text{implies} \quad u_{ji} = 0 \end{aligned} \qquad (j = 1, 2, \ldots, k < i) \tag{19}$$

From this property, it follows immediately that the structure of the LU decomposition of the connected system (15) will be similar to the original structure, in particular

$$\mathbf{J} = \mathbf{LU} = \begin{bmatrix} \mathbf{L}_1 & & & & \\ & \mathbf{L}_2 & & & \\ & & \cdots & & \\ & & & \mathbf{L}_n & \\ \tilde{\mathbf{R}}'_1 & \tilde{\mathbf{R}}'_2 & \cdots & \tilde{\mathbf{R}}'_n & \mathbf{L}^E \end{bmatrix} \begin{bmatrix} \mathbf{U}_1 & & & & \tilde{\mathbf{C}}'_1 \\ & \mathbf{U}_2 & & & \tilde{\mathbf{C}}'_2 \\ & & \cdots & & \cdots \\ & & & \mathbf{U}_n & \tilde{\mathbf{C}}'_n \\ & & & & \mathbf{U}^E \end{bmatrix}$$

$$= \begin{bmatrix} \mathbf{L}_1\mathbf{U}_1 & & & & \mathbf{L}_1\tilde{\mathbf{C}}'_1 \\ & \mathbf{L}_2\mathbf{U}_2 & & & \mathbf{L}_2\tilde{\mathbf{C}}'_2 \\ & & \cdots & & \cdots \\ & & & \mathbf{L}_n\mathbf{U}_n & \mathbf{L}_n\tilde{\mathbf{C}}'_n \\ \tilde{\mathbf{R}}'_1\mathbf{U}_1 & \tilde{\mathbf{R}}'_2\mathbf{U}_2 & \cdots & \tilde{\mathbf{R}}'_n\mathbf{U}_n & \mathbf{L}^E\mathbf{U}^E + \sum \tilde{\mathbf{R}}'_i\mathbf{C}'_i \end{bmatrix}$$

By comparing (20) with (15), we identify

$$\begin{aligned} \mathbf{L}_i\mathbf{U}_i &= \mathbf{D}_i \\ \tilde{\mathbf{R}}'_i\mathbf{U}_i &= \tilde{\mathbf{R}}_i \\ \mathbf{L}_i\tilde{\mathbf{C}}'_i &= \tilde{\mathbf{C}}_i \\ \mathbf{L}^E\mathbf{U}^E &= \sum \tilde{\mathbf{E}}_i - \sum \tilde{\mathbf{R}}'_i\tilde{\mathbf{C}}'_i \end{aligned} \tag{21}$$

From (16) we see that the rows of the submatrices $\tilde{\mathbf{R}}_i$ in $\mathbf{J}$ in (15) are either zero, or rows of the submatrix $\mathbf{R}_i$ of the component subnetworks, or possibly (if some subnetwork terminals are connected externally) a sum of some of the rows of $\mathbf{R}_i$. [Remember that postmultiplication by $\mathbf{S}^i$ is a gathering (11); the opposite operation of premultiplication by $\mathbf{S}^{iT}$ is a scattering.] From property (19) it follows that the zero rows will remain zero, and in fact

$$\tilde{\mathbf{R}}_i' = \mathbf{S}^{iT}\mathbf{R}_i' \tag{22}$$

or the rows of the submatrices $\tilde{\mathbf{R}}_i'$ in the decomposition of the complete system will be the scattering (same as for the original matrix) of the rows of the submatrices $\mathbf{R}_i'$ in the decomposition of the individual subnetworks.

This fact can be rigorously derived as follows. From (18) we have

$$\mathbf{R}_i'\mathbf{U}_i = \mathbf{R}_i$$

and therefore

$$\mathbf{S}^{iT}\mathbf{R}_i'\mathbf{U}_i = \mathbf{S}^{iT}\mathbf{R}_i \tag{23}$$

From (21)

$$\tilde{\mathbf{R}}_i'\mathbf{U}_i = \tilde{\mathbf{R}}_i \tag{24}$$

But from (11)

$$\tilde{\mathbf{R}}_i = \mathbf{S}^{iT}\mathbf{R}_i$$

and therefore (23) and (24) yield

$$\mathbf{S}^{iT}\mathbf{R}_i'\mathbf{U}_i = \tilde{\mathbf{R}}_i'\mathbf{U}_i$$

and since $\mathbf{U}_i$ is nonsingular, (22) follows immediately.

Similarly we can derive the relation for the columns

$$\tilde{\mathbf{C}}_i' = \mathbf{C}_i'\mathbf{S}^i \tag{25}$$

The columns $\tilde{\mathbf{C}}_i'$ of the LU decomposition of the connected system are obtained from the scattering of the columns $\mathbf{C}_i'$ of the decomposition of the individual subnetworks.

As for the bottom right submatrix of the connected system, we obtain a similar result. From (21)

$$\mathbf{L}^E\mathbf{U}^E = \sum \tilde{\mathbf{E}}_i - \sum \tilde{\mathbf{R}}_i'\tilde{\mathbf{C}}_i' = \sum(\tilde{\mathbf{E}}_i - \tilde{\mathbf{R}}_i'\tilde{\mathbf{C}}_i')$$

Substituting the relations (16), (22), and (25) for $\tilde{\mathbf{E}}_I$, $\tilde{\mathbf{R}}_i'$, and $\tilde{\mathbf{U}}_i'$

$$\begin{aligned}\mathbf{L}^E\mathbf{U}^E &= \sum (\mathbf{S}^{iT}\mathbf{R}_i\mathbf{S}^i - \mathbf{S}^{iT}\mathbf{R}_i'\mathbf{C}_i'\mathbf{S}^i)\\ &= \sum \mathbf{S}^{iT}(\mathbf{E}_i - \mathbf{R}_i'\mathbf{C}_i')\mathbf{S}^i && (26)\\ &= \sum \mathbf{S}^{iT}\mathbf{E}_i'\mathbf{S}^i\\ &= \sum \tilde{\mathbf{E}}_i' && (26)\end{aligned}$$

and $\mathbf{L}^E\mathbf{U}^E$ is found from the decomposition of the matrix in (26) which is the sum of the scattered submatrices $\mathbf{E}'$ contributed by each subnetwork.

The algorithm for LU decomposition of an interconnected system may therefore be stated as follows:

Algorithm 2: Partitioned LU decomposition

1. Perform "partial LU decomposition" for all subnetworks, finding $\mathbf{L}_i$, $\mathbf{U}_i$, $\mathbf{R}'_i$, $\mathbf{C}'_i$, and $\mathbf{E}' = \mathbf{E} - \mathbf{R}'\mathbf{C}'$ for each subnetwork.
2. Form the matrix $\sum \mathbf{S}^{iT}\mathbf{E}'_i\mathbf{S}^i$ by scattering of the entries of $\mathbf{E}'$ of each subnetwork.
3. Decompose this matrix into its factors $\mathbf{L}^E\mathbf{U}^E$.

No ordering is imposed on the decomposition of the subnetworks in step 1, but their partial decomposition must be done before the decomposition of the connection network.

The algorithm just described forms the backbone of the LU decomposition of the recursively BBD matrix of Figure 2.4. To formulate the algorithm, it is convenient to consider the top-down partitioning of a network. Step 1 of Algorithm 2 will consist of recursively applied versions of Algorithm 2 itself. The algorithm can easily be described by a recursive routine:

---

procedure decompose(*circuit*)

1. For all subcircuits (if any) of *circuit*
   —decompose(subcircuit).
2. Form the matrix $\sum \mathbf{S}^{iT}\mathbf{E}'_i\mathbf{S}^i$ by scattering of the entries of $\mathbf{E}'$ of each subnetwork. This matrix will be partitioned according to the internal and external variables of *circuit* as in (5).
3. Perform the pivot steps for the internal variables of *circuit* (find $\mathbf{L}$, $\mathbf{U}$, $\mathbf{R}'$, and $\mathbf{C}'$).
4. Form $\mathbf{E}' = \mathbf{E} - \mathbf{R}'\mathbf{C}'$ (the external part of *circuit*).

end decompose

The procedure is first invoked with the root network as the argument.

The decomposition proceeds bottom-up, since the recursion appears as the first step of the algorithm. If some circuit is a leaf of the tree (i.e., has no subcircuits), step 1 is skipped. Step 2 forms the Jacobian of the subcircuit. For a leaf, the contributions of the elements forming the subnetwork are included at this step. For other tree nodes, any elements of the network at that tree node that are not part of its subnetworks may also be included at this step.

Steps 3 and 4 are the partial LU decomposition. In case of the outermost (root) circuit, there are no terminals, step 3 finishes the decomposition, and step 4 is not performed.

5 FORWARD AND BACK SUBSTITUTION

Let us now consider the problem of solving

$$\mathbf{LUx} = \mathbf{b}$$

by forward and back substitution. We will first point out some relevant properties of the substitution process on a single-level interconnection and then extend the algorithm to the recursive BBD form.

First, let us partition the right-hand-side vector $\mathbf{b}$ according to the subnetwork structure as in (12):

$$\mathbf{b} = \begin{bmatrix} \mathbf{b}^{I_1} \\ \cdots \\ \mathbf{b}^{I_n} \\ \mathbf{b}^{I_C} \end{bmatrix} \tag{27}$$

In most applications, the portion $\mathbf{b}^{I_C}$ corresponding to the connection network can be formed by scattering and superposition of the contributions of the individual subnetworks:

$$\mathbf{b}^{I_C} = \sum \mathbf{S}^{iT}\mathbf{b}^{E_i} \tag{28}$$

Consider now the forward substitution

$$\mathbf{Lz} = \mathbf{b}$$

where $\mathbf{L}$ is partitioned as in (20), $\mathbf{b}$ as in (27), and $\mathbf{z}$ similarly to $\mathbf{b}$:

$$\begin{bmatrix} \mathbf{L}_1 & & & & \\ & \mathbf{L}_2 & & & \\ & & \cdots & & \\ & & & \mathbf{L}_n & \\ \tilde{\mathbf{R}}_1' & \tilde{\mathbf{R}}_2' & \cdots & \tilde{\mathbf{R}}_n' & \mathbf{L}^E \end{bmatrix} \begin{bmatrix} \mathbf{z}^{I_1} \\ \mathbf{z}^{I_2} \\ \cdots \\ \mathbf{z}^{I_n} \\ \mathbf{z}^{I_C} \end{bmatrix} = \begin{bmatrix} \mathbf{b}^{I_1} \\ \mathbf{b}^{I_2} \\ \cdots \\ \mathbf{b}^{I_n} \\ \mathbf{b}^{I_C} \end{bmatrix}$$

By block matrix operations, we obtain

$$\mathbf{L}_i\mathbf{z}^{I_i} = \mathbf{b}^{I_i} \tag{29a}$$

$$\mathbf{L}^E\mathbf{z}^{I_C} = \mathbf{b}^{I_C} - \sum \tilde{\mathbf{R}}_i'\mathbf{z}^{I_i} = \mathbf{b}^{E'} \tag{29b}$$

From (28) and (22), the right-hand side in (29b) can be written as

$$\begin{aligned}\mathbf{b}^{E'} &= \sum \mathbf{S}^{iT}\mathbf{b}^{E_i} - \sum \mathbf{S}^{iT}\mathbf{R}_i'\mathbf{z}^{I_i} \\ &= \sum \mathbf{S}^{iT}(\mathbf{b}^{E_i} - \mathbf{R}_i'\mathbf{z}^{I_i})\end{aligned}$$

or a scattering of "partial forward substitutions." The complete forward substitution can be decomposed into the steps:

Step 1: (Partial forward substitution for all subnetworks)
  a. Do forward substitution on $\mathbf{L}_i\mathbf{z}^{I_i} = \mathbf{B}^{I_i}$ to obtain $\mathbf{z}^{I_i}$.
  b. Form $\mathbf{b}^{E_i'} = \mathbf{b}^{E_i} - \mathbf{R}_i'\mathbf{z}^{I_i}$.
Step 2:
  a. Form the vector $\mathbf{b}^S = \sum \mathbf{S}^{iT}\mathbf{b}^{E_i'}$ by scattering of the entries of $\mathbf{b}^{E'}$ of each subnetwork.
  b. Perform forward substitution on $\mathbf{L}^E\mathbf{z}^{I_C} = \mathbf{b}^S$ to obtain $\mathbf{z}^{I_C}$.

In the case of a recursive BBD form, the same recursion as in the LU decomposition is used to modify the above algorithm:

---

procedure forward(*circuit*)

1. For all subcircuits (if any) of *circuit*
   —forward(subcircuit).
2. Form the vector $\sum \mathbf{S}^{iT}\mathbf{b}^{E_i'}$ (scattering and addition of subcircuits). This vector will be partitioned according to the internal and external variables of *circuit* into $\mathbf{b}^I$ and $\mathbf{b}^E$.
3. Perform forward substitution on the internal variables of *circuit* to obtain $\mathbf{z}^I$ from $\mathbf{L}\mathbf{z}^I = \mathbf{b}^I$.
4. Form $\mathbf{b}^{E'} = \mathbf{b}^E - \mathbf{R}'\mathbf{z}^I$ (the external part of *circuit*).

end forward

Again, if some circuit is a leaf of the tree, step 2 will use the actual contributions for the right-hand side of the subcircuit; for other nodes, any contributions of elements that are not in any subnetwork are also added.

The backward substitution $\mathbf{U}\mathbf{x} = \mathbf{z}$ is analogous. From the partition

$$\begin{bmatrix} \mathbf{U}_1 & & & & \tilde{\mathbf{C}}_1' \\ & \mathbf{U}_2 & & & \tilde{\mathbf{C}}_2' \\ & & \cdots & & \cdots \\ & & & \mathbf{U}_n & \tilde{\mathbf{C}}_n' \\ & & & & \mathbf{U}^E \end{bmatrix} \begin{bmatrix} \mathbf{x}^{I_1} \\ \mathbf{x}^{I_2} \\ \cdots \\ \mathbf{x}^{I_n} \\ \mathbf{x}^{I_C} \end{bmatrix} = \begin{bmatrix} \mathbf{z}^{I_1} \\ \mathbf{z}^{I_2} \\ \cdots \\ \mathbf{z}^{I_n} \\ \mathbf{z}^{I_C} \end{bmatrix}$$

we obtain by block matrix manipulations

$$\mathbf{U}^E\mathbf{x}^{Ic} = \mathbf{z}^{Ic}$$

$$\mathbf{U}_i\mathbf{x}^{I_i} = \mathbf{z}^{I_i} - \tilde{\mathbf{C}}_i'\mathbf{x}^{Ic}$$

From (25), the second expression may be written as

$$\mathbf{U}_i\mathbf{x}^{I_i} = \mathbf{z}^{I_i} - \mathbf{C}_i'\mathbf{S}^i\mathbf{x}^{Ic}$$

and from (11) this becomes

$$\mathbf{U}_i\mathbf{x}^{I_i} = \mathbf{z}^{I_i} - \mathbf{C}_i'\mathbf{x}^{E_i}$$

The steps to be performed are:

Step 1: Perform back substitution on $\mathbf{U}^E\mathbf{x}^{Ic} = \mathbf{z}^{Ic}$.
Step 2:
a. Form $\mathbf{x}^{E_i}$ as a gathering of entries from $\mathbf{x}^{Ic}$.
b. Find $\mathbf{z}^{I_i'} = \mathbf{z}^{I_i} - \mathbf{C}_i'\mathbf{x}^{E_i}$.
c. Perform back substitution on $\mathbf{U}_i\mathbf{x}^{I_i} = \mathbf{z}^{I_i'}$.

For the recursive case, the above algorithm is modified by the addition of recursion in the second step.

---

procedure backward(*circuit*)

1. Perform back substitution on the internal variables of *circuit* to obtain $\mathbf{x}^I$ from $\mathbf{U}\mathbf{x}^I = \mathbf{z}^I$.
2. For all subcircuits (if any) of *circuit*
   a. Form $\mathbf{x}^E = \mathbf{S}^i\mathbf{x}^{Ic}$ as a gathering of entries of $\mathbf{x}^{Ic}$ ($\mathbf{x}^{Ic}$ is the $\mathbf{x}$ of the father of *circuit*).
   b. Set $\mathbf{z}^I \leftarrow \mathbf{z}^I - \mathbf{C}'\mathbf{x}^E$.
   c. Backward(subcircuit).

end backward

---

6 UPDATING OF THE DECOMPOSITION AND SOLUTION

In some applications, only a single subnetwork or a small subset of subnetworks changes before a new solution is required. In this case, a considerable amount of work may be avoided, provided that the LU decomposition and the submatrix $\mathbf{E}'$ for each subnetwork were saved from a previous decomposition. Consider the following points:

1. The LU decomposition proceeds bottom-up in the representation of Figure 2.5, or along the main diagonal in the representation of Figure 2.4.
2. The *order* of processing the subnetworks (diagonal blocks) of a given network is not prescribed.
3. There is no interaction between subnetworks other than through their common ancestors.

It follows that only the decomposition of the network that changed and all its ancestors in the tree representation of the system need be recomputed (Figure 2.7). An addition of the following step to procedure *decompose* will allow the LU decomposition to be updated in such a case:

Procedure decompose(*circuit*)

0. If *circuit* is NOT in the path from the root to some changed subnetwork, return.
1. . . . .

end decompose

If a *single* network changes, a nonrecursive routine to perform the updating may be derived from *decompose*. The procedure is to be called with the changed subnetwork as the argument.

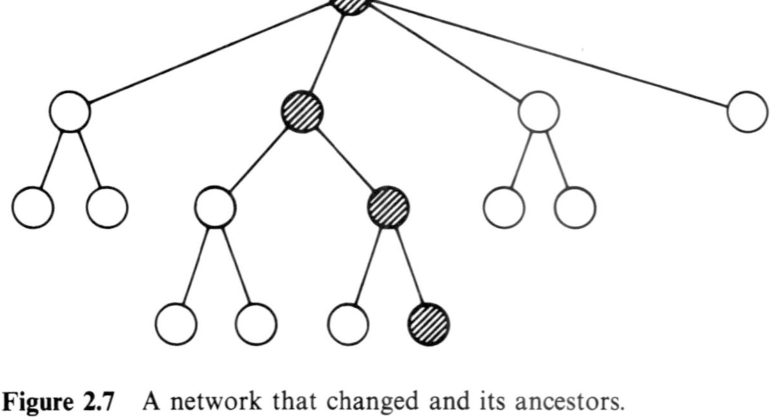

Figure 2.7 A network that changed and its ancestors.

procedure update(*circuit*)

1. Form $\sum \mathbf{S}^{iT}\mathbf{E}_i'\mathbf{S}^i$ (step 2 of *decompose*)
2. Perform the pivot steps for the internal variables of *circuit* (step 3 of *decompose*)
3. Form $\mathbf{E}' = \mathbf{E} - \mathbf{R}'\mathbf{C}'$ (step 4 of *decompose*)
4. If *circuit* is the root, return.
5. Set *circuit* ← parent(*circuit*) and go to step 1.

end update

In terms of the BBD structure of the matrix, this procedure may be interpreted as a reordering of the blocks of the original matrix; only the shaded blocks in Figure 2.8 need be recomputed.

Should it be known *a priori* that a certain network will change several times (e.g., in the case of a blockwise relaxation method or the multilevel Newton iteration), some additional work may be saved in step 1 of procedure *update*. A partial sum is computed and stored, and only the contribution of the changed *circuit* is added to the partial sum at each call to *update*.

In the case of the substitution process, either a network or a right-hand-side vector may change for a subset of the networks. The same changes that were done to procedure *decompose* are then applied to procedure *forward*:

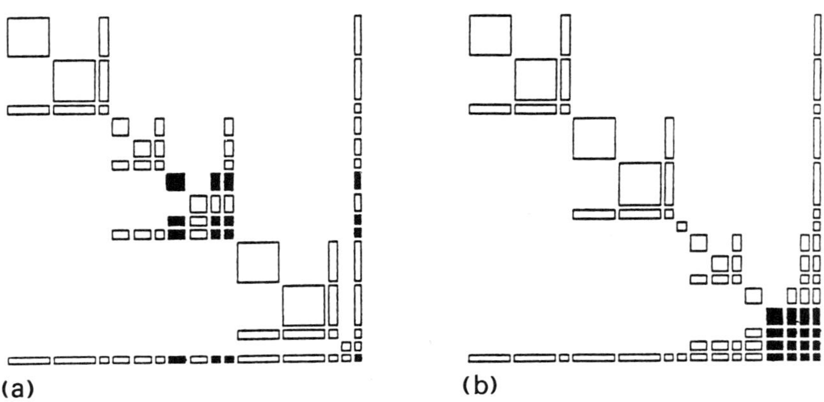

Figure 2.8 Implied reordering of the blocks. (a) The actual structure; (b) the implied reordering.

---

procedure forward(*circuit*)

0. If *circuit* is NOT in the path from the root to some subnetwork that changed, or whose right-hand-side vector changed, return.
1. ....

end forward

In the case of a change in a single network, a nonrecursive routine similar to *update* can be constructed. It will consist of steps 2–4 of *forward* followed by steps 4 and 5 of *update*. The same remark on further savings in case of repeated changes to a single network apply to it as well.

As far as the back substitution is concerned, savings can be realized whenever the solution to only some of the subnetworks is sought. Procedure backward is modified as follows:

---

procedure backward(*circuit*)

0. If a solution is NOT required for *circuit* or for any of its offspring, return.
1. ....

end backward

The nonrecursive version of *backward* to obtain an updated solution to a *single* network is

---

procedure update_*x*(*circuit*)

1. *next* ← root circuit
2. Perform back substitution on the internal variables of *next* (step 1 of *backward*)
3. If *next* is *circuit*, return
4. Set *next* ← the son of *next* which is on the path from the root to *circuit*
5. Find $\mathbf{x}^E$ of *next* (step 2a of *backward*)
6. Set $\mathbf{z}^I \leftarrow \mathbf{Z}^I - \mathbf{C}'\mathbf{x}^E$ (step 2b of *backward*) and go to step 2.

end update–*x*

---

7 STORAGE STRATEGY

In the previous sections, the procedures for the decomposition and forward and back substitution were described solely in terms of the submatrices of the individual networks and their gathering matrices **S**. It is therefore sufficient to represent the block structure of the entire matrix by the tree (Figure 2.5) and the gather/scatter information. Since the rows of the gather matrices **S** consist of elementary unit vectors, a single index per row is sufficient to represent them, and general sparse matrix methods are not required.

The subnetworks themselves should be represented using sparse matrix methods. Each subnetwork will have storage reserved for the matrices **L**, **U**, **R**′, **C**′, and **E**′, and possibly the right-hand-side vectors $\mathbf{b}^I$ and $\mathbf{b}^E$. However, since these submatrices form a partition of the matrix representing the entire subnetwork, existing sparse matrix storage schemes may be used, and a single index (n_I, the number of internal variables) is then sufficient to represent the partition.

In this storage strategy, some duplication exists. The submatrices **E**′ and $\mathbf{b}^E$ will ultimately be scattered into a representation of some higher-level network. (Depending on the application, the **E**′ and $\mathbf{b}^E$ submatrices of each subnetwork may be stored directly in the storage space reserved for some higher-level network. The price is some additional pointer space and the inability to update the decomposition after a subnetwork change.)

8 PREPROCESSING

In any implementation, sparsity must be considered, and the internal variables of each subnetwork must be renumbered according to some strategy. Once the internal variables are ordered, absolute variable (equation) numbers must be assigned.

Renumbering for sparsity should be performed on the "type graph" (Figure 2.6) representation of the system, since the structure of a subnetwork is invariant for different instances of a subnetwork. In order to perform the renumbering, the nonzero entries in the Jacobian must be determined. These will consist of the contributions of the circuit elements (if any) included in the subnetwork, as well as the nonzero contributions of all lower-level networks found from the scattering and superposition in (26). The latter must contain any fill-ins created by an LU decomposition of the lower-level networks. Thus, the renumbering for the complete system description must be done in a specific order of the types (depth-first search); the easiest implementation is by a recursive routine, which is initially called to renumber the type of the "root" circuit:

procedure reorder(type)

—if already renumbered, return
—for all subcircuits referenced
  reorder(subcircuit's type)
—enter nonzero information for all elements
—add nonzero contributions of all subcircuits' external parts $\tilde{\mathbf{E}}$ to the zero/nonzero pattern of the circuit
—renumber the internal variables of the circuit type according to some strategy, marking fill-ins in the external matrix **E** of the circuit

end reorder.

The scheme used for renumbering was minimum local fill-in in the internal part **D** of the subcircuit's Jacobian, with no consideration given to the fill-ins generated in the external parts **C**, **R**, and **E**. In general, **E** will be dense, with little to be gained by special ordering schemes. As implemented, the renumbering required only a simple change in an existing sparse matrix package.

After all the circuit types are renumbered, absolute variable numbers may be assigned. Since this information cannot be shared among circuits, the full representation of the system (as in Figure 2.5) must be used. In order to keep the recursive BBD nature of the overall system matrix, two passes must be used to assign the absolute variable numbers.

procedure assign_internals(*circuit*)

—for all subcircuits,
  assign_internals(subcircuit)
—assign absolute variable numbers to internal variables of circuit as next available in sequence

end assign_internals.

procedure assign_terminals(*circuit*)

—for all subcircuits
  —assign absolute numbers to terminals of the subcircuit from the internal variables of the circuit being processed
  —assign_terminals(subcircuit)

end assign_terminals

As was discussed in the previous sections, the order of the internal variable blocks is of no importance; however, the above numbering keeps the recursive BBD nature of the overall system matrix clearly evident. In a practical implementation, the absolute variable numbers can be assigned in a single preorder traversal of the tree:

---

procedure number(*circuit*)

—assign absolute variable numbers to the internal variables of the circuit as next available in sequence
—for all subcircuits
  —assign absolute variable numbers to the terminals of the subcircuit from the internal variables of its father
  —number(subcircuit)

end number

---

9 NUMERICAL EXPERIMENT

As an example, consider the network and its subnetworks shown in Figure 2.9. The basic building block is a NAND gate (Figure 2.9a) with seven internal and five external nodes. Two of these gates form the SR flip-flop (Figure 2.9b). Notice that it has no internal nodes—it is included only as a convenience in the description of the network and creates some overhead in space and execution time. Three SR flip-flops are connected to form the type-

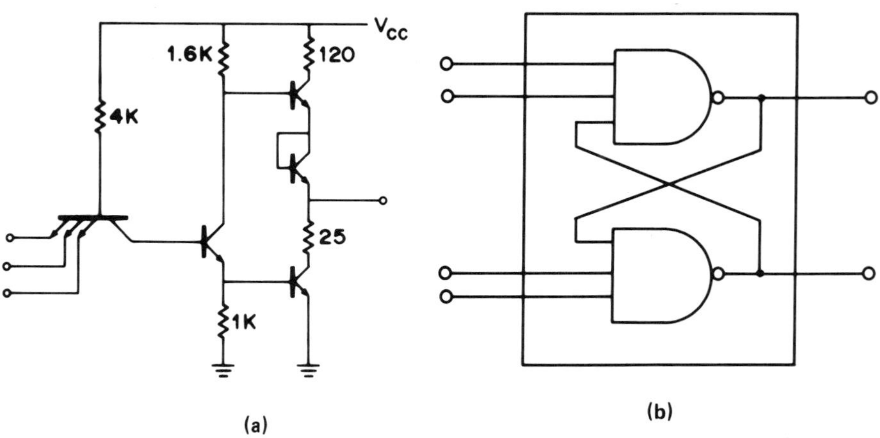

Figure 2.9 Test network and its subnetworks. (a) A TTL NAND gate; (b) an SR flip-flop; (c) a D-type edge-triggered flip-flop; (d) the test network.

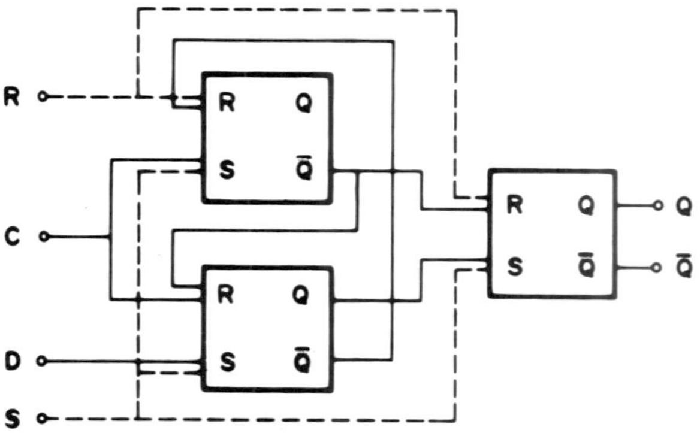

(c)

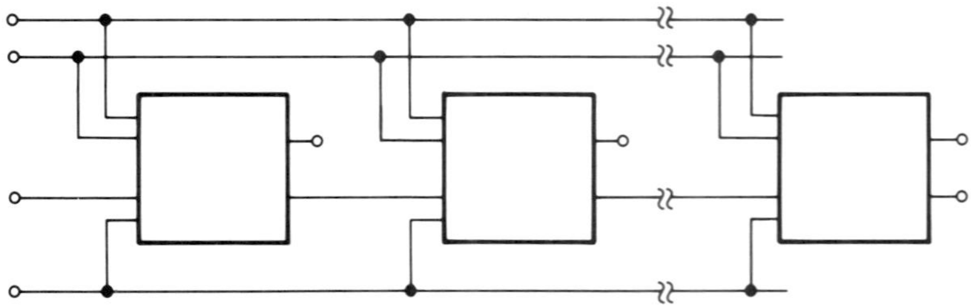

(d)

Figure 2.9 (c), (d)

D edge-triggered flip-flop (Figure 2.9c), with three internal nodes. Finally, these flip-flops are connected in series to form the test network of Figure 2.9d.

The nonzero pattern (including fill-ins) of the matrix for a four-section network of Figure 2.9d, obtained by the structured algorithm, is shown in Figure 2.10a. The recursive BBD nature of the matrix is clearly evident. For comparison, the same matrix, reordered using a minimum local fill-in algorithm [19], is shown in Figure 2.10b.

To give an idea of the behavior of the algorithms, two sets of comparisons summarized in Tables 2.1 and 2.2 were performed. For the first set of results (Table 2.1), the LU decomposition was done for the TTL network of Figure 2.9, with different numbers of sections. The second set of results (Table 2.2) gives comparisons of execution times for different types of networks. The following networks were compared:

TTL 4 bits of the network of Figure 2.9

CMOS a 4-bit shift register latch, Figure 10b in [20], implemented in CMOS

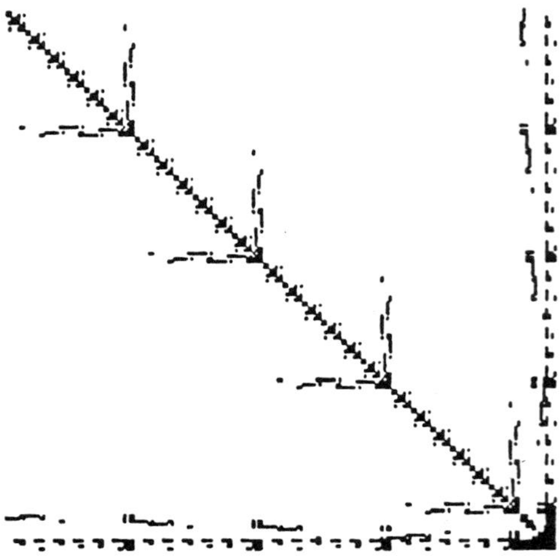

(a)

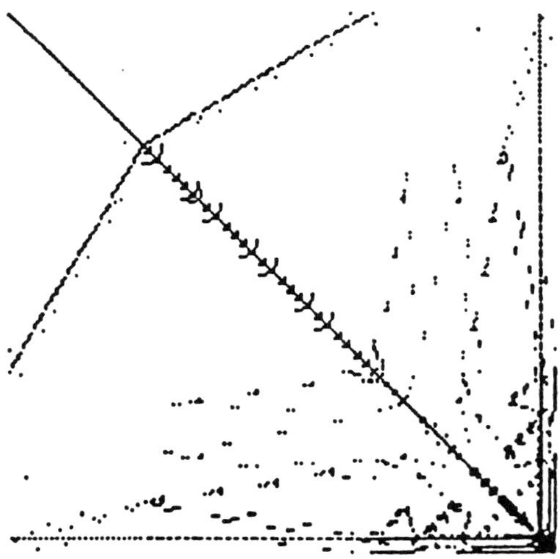

(b)

Figure 2.10 Nonzero pattern for the test network. (a) Structured reordering; (b) minimum local fill-in reordering.

Table 2.1 Execution Times for the LU Decomposition of Networks of Figure 2.9d

			Full LU		Update		Update
No. of sections	Matrix size	Border size	Time (ms)	Overhead (%)	Time (ms)	Overhead (%)	Full (%)
1	53	7	21	16	9.3	26	44
2	101	9	49	17	12.7	22	26
3	149	11	70	12	14.2	21	20.3
4	197	13	88	15	16.5	24	18.7

Table 2.2 Execution Times for the LU Decomposition of Several Different Networks

Network	Matrix size	Full Lu Time (ms)	Full Lu Overhead (%)	Update Time (ms)	Update Overhead (%)	Update/Full (%)
TTL	197	88	15	16.5	24	18.9
CMOS	105	77	16	14.6	38	19.0
ECL	120	172	15	20.4	45	11.9
Analog	104	74	11	13.7	19	18.5

ECL a 4-bit shift register, Figure 8 in [21]
Analog an analog network, including four operational amplifiers, Figure 14 in [10]

In the tables, "overhead" is the proportion of time spent in the scattering process $\sum \mathbf{S}^{iT}\mathbf{E}^{i}\mathbf{S}^{i}$, and "update" time is given for a change in a single lowest-level subnetwork. In Table 2.1, "border size" refers to the number of nodes in the connection (root) network. The times quoted are for an IBM 4341 computer.

Obviously, the structured reordering is not optimal as far as fill-ins are concerned. Table 2.3 summarizes the overhead in fill-ins incurred by the structured reordering. In the case of the logic networks, where the network function forces good partitioning, the overhead is quite small. For the analog network, although substantially more fill-ins are generated, an overall savings in execution time (for updating) can nevertheless be realized.

Table 2.3 Fill-ins Generated by Renumbering for Several Different Networks

Network	Matrix size	Original nonzeros	Minimum local fill-in	Structured renumbering	Increase (%)
TTL	197	1109	512	580	4
CMOS	105	588	369	437	7
ECL	120	671	1037	1155	7
Analog	104	558	224	554	42

Tables 2.1 and 2.2 illustrate the most attractive feature of this partitioning method—the savings realizable when updating is necessary. The trend of decreasing proportion of the updating time is clearly evident from the last column of Table 2.1. The larger the overall system, the bigger the savings from the updating algorithm will be. Even for complete decomposition, the overhead incurred by the extra scattering step (approximately one-sixth of the total execution time) is quite tolerable and the approach is justified by its ability to split a large problem into a series of smaller ones, with possibility of parallel computation.

REFERENCES

1. G. Kron, *Diakoptics*, Macdonald, London, 1963.
2. F. H. Branin, A sparse matrix modification of Kron's method of piecewise analysis, *Proc. 1975 Int. Symp. Circuits and Systems*, Newton, Mass., pp. 383–386, April 1975.
3. F. F. Wu, Solution of large-scale networks by tearing, *IEEE Trans. Circuits Syst.*, vol. CAS-23, no. 12, pp. 706–713, 1976.
4. L. O. Chua and L. K. Chen, Diakoptic and generalized hybrid analysis, *IEEE Trans. Circuits Syst.*, vol. CAS-23, no. 12, pp. 694–705, 1976.
5. I. N. Hajj, Sparsity considerations in network solution by tearing, *IEEE Trans. Circuits Syst.*, vol. CAS-27, no. 5, pp. 357–366, 1980.
6. D. J. Rose and J. R. Bunch, The role of partitioning in the numerical solution of sparse systems, in *Sparse Matrices and Their Applications*, D. J. Rose and R. A. Willoughby, eds., pp. 177–187, Plenum, New York, 1972.
7. B. W. Kernighan, P. J. Plauger, N. B. G. Rabbat, A. L. Sangiovanni-Vincentelli, and H. Y. Hsieh, A multilevel Newton algorithm with macromodeling and latency for the analysis of large scale nonlinear circuits in the time domain, *IEEE Trans. Circuits Syst.* vol. CAS-26, pp. 733–740, Sept. 1979.
8. P. Yang, I. N. Hajj, and T. N. Trick, SLATE: A circuit simulation program with latency exploitation and node tearing, *Proc. 1980 Int. Symp. Circuits and Systems*, Houston, pp. 353–355, April 1980.
9. A. L. Sangiovanni-Vincentelli, Li-Kuan Chen, and L. O. Chua, A new tearing approach—node-tearing nodal analysis, *Proc. 1977 Int. Symp. Circuits and Systems*, Phoenix, Ariz., pp. 143–147, April 1977.
10. A. L. Sangiovanni-Vincentelli, Li-Kuan Chen, and L. O. Chua, An efficient heuristic cluster algorithm for tearing large-scale networks, *IEEE Trans. Circuits Syst.*, vol. CAS-24, no. 12, pp. 709–717, 1977.
11. I. S. Duff, A survey of sparse matrix research, *Proc. IEEE*, vol. 65, no. 4, pp. 500–535, 1977.

12. J. R. Bunch, Block methods for solving sparse linear systems, in *Sparse Matrix Computations*, J. R. Bunch and D. J. Rose, eds., pp. 39–58, Academic Press, New York, 1976.
13. R. Marrett, On The Interconnection of Graphical Systems, Ph.D. Thesis, Univ. of Waterloo, Waterloo, Ontario, 1976.
14. P. Linardis and K. G. Nichols, Partitioning with latency exploitation in the time-domain analysis of large-nonlinear electronic circuits, *Proc. 1979 Int. Symp. Circuits and Systems*, pp. 60–61, Tokyo, July 1979.
15. P. Linardis and K. G. Nichols, Partitioning with latency exploitation in the time-domain analysis of large nonlinear electronic circuits, in *International Conference on Computer Aided Design and Manufacture of Electronic Components, Circuits and Systems*, pp. 105–109, Univ. of Sussex, July 1979.
16. H. Gupta, J. W. Bandler, J. A. Starzyk, and J. Sharma, A hierarchical decomposition approach for network analysis, *Proc. 1982 Int. Symp. Circuits and Systems*, pp. 643–646, Rome, June 1982.
17. M. Zwolinski and K. G. Nichols, The design of an hierarchical circuit-level simulator, in *European Conference on Electronic Design Automation*, pp. 9–12, Univ. of Warwick, March 1984.
18. A. M. Erisman, Decomposition methods using sparse matrix techniques with application to certain electrical network problems, in *Decomposition of Large-Scale Problems*, D. M. Himmelblau, ed., North-Holland, Amsterdam, 1973.
19. J. Vlach and K. Singhal, *Computer Methods for Circuit Analysis and Design*, Van Nostrand-Reinhold, Princeton, N.J., 1983.
20. T. W. Williams and K. P. Parker, Design for testability—a survey, *Proc. IEEE*, vol. 71, pp. 98–112, Jan. 1983.
21. W. L. Engl, R. Laur, and H. K. Dirks, MEDUSA—a simulator for modular circuits, *IEEE Trans. Computer-Aided Design of Integrated Circuits and Systems*, vol. CAD-1, pp. 85–93, April 1982.

3
Piecewise Linear Analysis

Jos T. J. van Eijndhoven

Eindhoven University of Technology
Eindhoven, The Netherlands

1 INTRODUCTION

The use of circuit simulators to check the behavior of electrical circuits before the actual manufacturing is widely accepted in both industry and universities. These programs can give a reasonably accurate prediction of the actual behavior, in only a fraction of the time needed to build a breadboard model. However, the "classical" circuit simulation program still has a great many problems. Here, a classical simulator is a program that solves the set of nonlinear differential equations by an iteration over the time points, using a Newton-Raphson type of iteration to solve the resulting set of nonlinear equations. Typical examples of such programs are (older versions of) SPICE and ASTAP. The problems with programs of this type can be summarized as follows:

1. The Newton-Raphson iteration sometimes does not lead to convergence. Electrical circuits tend to have strongly nonlinear components, with, for instance, exponential behavior, and feedback in order to realize memory circuits, such as flip-flops. For this type of curve, the Newton-Raphson method has severe difficulties. In practice, one tries to find a solution by imposing extremely small time steps for the integration, thus obtaining a good initial estimate for the solution of the Newton-Raphson iteration. However, this is at the cost of strongly increased computational requirements.

2. Because the circuit is solved as a single set of equations, at each time point and at each Newton-Raphson iteration step the whole circuit has to be solved. Thus parts of the circuit in a quiescent state, for which a good solution was already obtained, are repeatedly recomputed. This type of behavior (latency) is found especially in digital circuits, an important class of circuits being analyzed. Expensive computational effort is therefore often wasted.

3. Addition of new component models is quite complicated. The models are required to be at least continuous and preferably continuous differentiable. Furthermore, explicit formulas for all derivatives are often required to speed up simulation. For complex devices such as state-of-the-art metal-oxide-semiconductor (MOS) models, the modeling has become a very difficult problem. Because the models are normally part of the program, individual users are not allowed to add their own (macro) models.

4. Because of the large computational requirements, only relatively small circuits can be analyzed in this way. Depending on the environment, this type of simulation is reasonable for circuits containing up to a few hundred transistors. For larger circuits other simulators are required, such as logic or switch-level simulators, at the cost of a far coarser simulation that yields less information.

Enormous effort has been spent in optimizing these circuit simulators. However, the basic problems as stated above have persisted. Research on different simulation schemes, avoiding some of these problems, does show a few possible solutions. The three main approaches being followed are the waveform relaxation method [12, 3], hierarchical circuit partitioning [18, 17, 5], and piecewise linear analysis [4, 7, 19].

The waveform relaxation method partitions the circuit into modules. Each module is solved over the entire time interval, thus producing updated waveforms of the circuit variables. After all modules have been analyzed, the process is repeated until all waveforms have converged. This relaxation process has only a linear convergence rate, and in practice an initial approximation of the curves is often needed to obtain a reasonable speed. This initial estimation should be given by a fast simulator, such as a logic or a timing simulator. To solve each (small) module independently, a compact and fast circuit simulator is needed. Because each module is solved independently from the others, the time step control is optimized individually, yielding a natural latency evaluation.

Hierarchical circuit partitioning allows a simulator with the normal solution scheme to decide which parts of the circuit need to be solved at which time points. In this way, latency evaluation is fitted in the framework of a conventional simulator. Of course, on the boundaries of the modules, integrity of the data (circuit variables) must be maintained. For this purpose, explicit Jacobians might be used, representing the linearized behavior of the module (subtree). The generation of the Jacobians leads to some overhead, and the more implicit approach of Ref. [18] seems more efficient.

A piecewise linear circuit simulator applies piecewise linear models for all nonlinear components. For the solution of the resulting set of equations, the Newton-Raphson technique is no longer suitable and special algorithms must be applied. It appears that these algorithms normally have remarkably strong global convergence properties, instead of the local convergence of the Newton-Raphson approach. The simulator is thus built on a different mathematical framework, and one of the two partitioning techniques mentioned above can also be applied. It is worth noting that hierarchical circuit partitioning in combination with piecewise linear modeling has less overhead than a conventional nonlinear simulator, because the linear representation of each module changes only at particular discrete time points and not in almost every iteration phase.

For these reasons, piecewise linear analysis has attracted more attention in recent years. The advantages are summarized below:

1. Specialized algorithms to solve sets of piecewise linear equations can have very strong global convergence properties.
2. Piecewise linear modeling is an attractive way to specify macromodels for often used subcircuits. In this way computational effort can be saved by using coarser models if high accuracy is not of primary importance. Experienced users might even add their own models.
3. For complex devices such as short-channel MOS transistors there is no need to express the curves in an analytic way. The measured curves can be used directly in the model.
4. As we will see later, the crossing of one boundary of the piecewise linear system explicitly gives a rank one update on the system matrix. With this update the L/U decomposition of the new system matrix is determined rapidly and efficiently.
5. If desired, piecewise linear simulation can be used in combination with some partitioning method in order to obtain latency evaluation.

In the next sections, we shall see how to efficiently represent piecewise linear models in the computer, how to solve sets of piecewise linear equations, and how a piecewise linear simulator program structure might look.

2 CONTINUITY RESTRICTIONS

For the modeling of electronic components, we are mainly interested in continuous models. The continuity of piecewise linear mappings restricts the amount of freedom we have and hence the amount of data needed to describe the mapping.

2.1 General Description

Assume a general implicit piecewise linear mapping given as N segments σ^i, i = 1, N, and for each segment σ^i:

1. The linear relation for the segment described by the pair $(A^i \quad a^i)$, with A^i a q by m matrix and a^i an m-vector. This defines the linear relation $0 = A^i \cdot x + a^i$ for $x \in R^q$ in this segment.
2. The boundaries of the segment described by the pair $(C^i \quad c^i)$, with C^i a q by p matrix and c^i a p-vector. This defines the domain of this segment as $C^i \cdot x + c^i \geqslant 0$.

In this way we can define all piecewise linear mappings, containing only a finite number of segments. The value of p is taken to be the maximum number of boundary faces found in any segment. The limitation to convex segments in the above description is not a restriction on the mapping, because nonconvex segments can be modeled as a number of adjacent convex segments.

The above definition of a piecewise linear mapping, as a list of linear mappings and domains, wastes a great deal of storage and is difficult to handle when trying to find a solution. Therefore, in practice, the matrices C^i are often chosen identical, except for a sign multiplication of the rows, actually yielding one set of globally (linear) boundary planes partitioning the domain. By additionally restricting these planes to be parallel and equidistant, a mapping with a fast tabular access is created. In contrast to this tabular approach, we will show that the continuity restriction leads to a natural reduction of the data and a compact description.

2.2 Single Boundary Plane

Assume the segment σ^1 and the segment σ^2 have a boundary face in common, denoted by $n \cdot x + c = 0$, with n and x q-vectors and c scalar. Continuity of the mapping is now formulated as

$$\begin{aligned} A^1 \cdot x + a^1 = 0 &\rightarrow A^2 \cdot x + a^2 = 0 \\ n \cdot x + c = 0 &\leftarrow \quad n \cdot x + c = 0 \end{aligned} \tag{1}$$

Therefore equation (2) holds for all x satisfying $n \cdot x + c = 0$:

$$(\Lambda^1 A^1 - \Lambda^2 A^2) \cdot x + (\Lambda^1 a^1 - \Lambda^2 a^2) = 0 \tag{2}$$

for all diagonal matrices Λ^i.

Because (2) holds for all x in the boundary plane, equation (2) must have rank one and

$$\begin{aligned} (\Lambda^1 A^1 - \Lambda^2 A^2) &= w \cdot n^t \\ (\Lambda^1 a^1 - \Lambda^2 a^2) &= w \cdot c \end{aligned} \tag{3}$$

The mapping itself is not affected by the values in Λ^i, so we restrict ourselves here to the identity matrix and obtain:

$$\begin{aligned}(A^1 - A^2) &= w \cdot n^t \\ (a^1 - a^2) &= w \cdot c\end{aligned} \tag{4}$$

Concluding, we can see that with given (A^1, a^1) and a given boundary plane (n, c), we have only the freedom to choose a vector w, to obtain (A^2, a^2).

2.3 Two Boundary Planes

Next we will discuss a piecewise linear mapping for which the segments are bounded by two planes, thus forming four (convex) segments. On their common intersection, the two planes are allowed to cause a breaking of each other's direction. For clarity see Figure 3.1. In this picture, the arrows indicate the direction of the vectors n and the signs of the vector w. Thus an arrow in half-plane k from A^i to A^j indicates that $(A^i - A^j) = w^k \cdot n^{kt}$.

The continuity restriction for this case translates into two different equations. The first equation (5a) ensures that the four half-planes have a common intersection. The second equation (5b) ensures that the net result of the four matrix updates along the path $A^0 \to A^1 \to A^2 \to A^3 \to A^0$ equals zero.

$$\begin{aligned}\begin{bmatrix} n^2 \\ c^2 \end{bmatrix} &= \lambda_{11} \begin{bmatrix} n^0 \\ c^0 \end{bmatrix} + \lambda_{12} \begin{bmatrix} n^1 \\ c^1 \end{bmatrix} \\ \begin{bmatrix} n^3 \\ c^3 \end{bmatrix} &= \lambda_{21} \begin{bmatrix} n^0 \\ c^0 \end{bmatrix} + \lambda_{22} \begin{bmatrix} n^1 \\ c^1 \end{bmatrix}\end{aligned} \tag{5a}$$

$$w^0 \cdot (n^{0t} \quad c^0) - w^1 \cdot (n^{1t} \quad c^1) - w^2 \cdot (n^{2t} \quad c^2) + w^3 \cdot (n^{3t} \quad c^3) = 0 \tag{5b}$$

By substituting (5a) in (5b), and using the independence of $(n^0 \quad c^0)$ and $(n^1 \quad c^1)$, we obtain equation (6):

$$\begin{aligned}w^2 &= \frac{\lambda_{22}}{\Delta} w^0 + \frac{\lambda_{21}}{\Delta} w^1 \\ w^3 &= \frac{\lambda_{12}}{\Delta} w^0 + \frac{\lambda_{11}}{\Delta} w^1\end{aligned} \tag{6}$$

where Δ equals $\lambda_{11} \cdot \lambda_{22} - \lambda_{12} \cdot \lambda_{21}$.

Now still a few more restrictions can be derived. First equation (5a) shows that the independence of $(n^{2t} \quad c^2)$ and $(n^{3t} \quad c^3)$ implies that Δ is nonzero. (We assume that the mapping is really according to Figure 3.1 and does not degenerate with overlapping or empty segments.) We furthermore assumed that each segment was convex, thus restricting the corners of the intersection of the boundary planes. This convexity requirement can be translated into

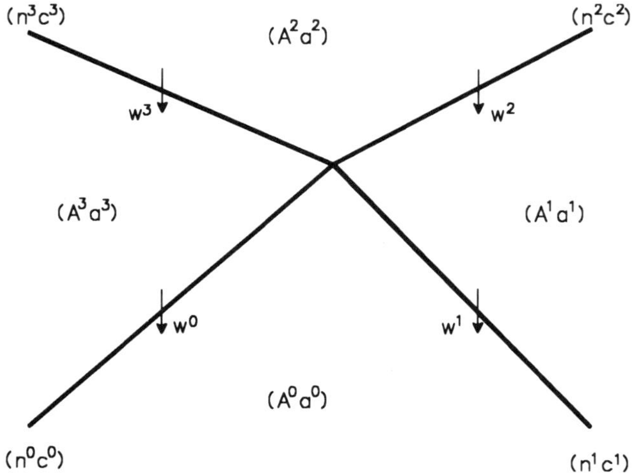

Figure 3.1 Mapping with two boundary planes.

signs of inproducts and leads to the following inequalities:

$$\lambda_{11} > 0, \qquad \lambda_{22} > 0, \qquad \Delta > 0 \tag{7}$$

Whereas we are not interested in the magnitude of the vectors $(n^i \quad c^i)$ and want to control the mapping only, we restrict ourselves to $\lambda_{11} = \lambda_{22} = 1$.

As a conclusion from this section, we can now state that given

$$(A^0 \quad a^0), \quad (n^0 \quad c^0), \quad w^0, \quad (n^1 \quad c^1), \quad w^1, \quad \lambda_{12}, \quad \lambda_{21} \tag{8}$$

the complete (continuous) mapping is defined, and the above equations suffice to derive

$$(A^1 \quad a^1), \quad (A^2 \; a^2), \quad (A^3 \quad a^3), \quad (n^2 \quad c^2), \quad w^2, \quad (n^3 \quad c^3), \quad w^3 \tag{9}$$

Furthermore, it is easily seen from equation (5a) that $\lambda_{12} = \lambda_{21} = 0$ causes the two boundary planes to continue after their intersection, without changing direction. Thus these two numbers actually control the relative influence of the planes on each other.

2.4 Matrix Notation

This section shows a notation method for storing all the necessary data for a continuous mapping in a single matrix. Later we shall see that this matrix not only is suitable for a compact definition of (all the segments of) the mapping but also allows for efficient manipulation. The mapping described in the previous section is defined by

$$\begin{bmatrix} 0 \\ z_1 \\ z_2 \end{bmatrix} = \begin{bmatrix} A^0 & w^0 & w^1 \\ n^{0t} & 1 & -\lambda_{12} \\ n^{1t} & -\lambda_{21} & 1 \end{bmatrix} \cdot \begin{bmatrix} x \\ \bar{z}_1 \\ \bar{z}_2 \end{bmatrix} + \begin{bmatrix} a^0 \\ c^0 \\ c^1 \end{bmatrix}$$

$$z_1 \geqslant 0,\ z^2 \geqslant 0,\ \bar{z}_1 \geqslant 0,\ \bar{z}_2 \geqslant 0,\ z_1 \cdot \bar{z}_1 = 0,\ z_2 \cdot \bar{z}_2 = 0 \qquad (10)$$

Here two new vectors are introduced, z and $\bar{z}$, which are restricted to contain nonnegative elements only, and zero in product. Thus for every index i, $z_i \geqslant 0$ and $\bar{z}_i = 0$, or $z_i = 0$ and $\bar{z}_i \geqslant 0$. These restrictions enable us to solve z and $\bar{z}$ and are actually responsible for the piecewise linear behavior. In the example above the vectors z and $\bar{z}$ have dimension two, thus yielding four possible combinations for the zero/nonzero pairs. By simple matrix operations, it can be shown that each of these four combinations corresponds to one of the segments in Figure 3.1.

When more boundary planes are added, the following data should be provided for the pth plane:

n^p c^p to define the boundary plane in one segment

w^p to define the update on the matrix A for the other side of the boundary plane

$\lambda_{i,p+1}$, $\lambda_{p+1,i}$ for each i, $1 \leqslant i < p$, to define the mutual interaction of this plane with all other boundary planes

These data can be added to equation (10) to extend the matrix with one row and one column. The matrix now defines in general 2^p different segments with their corresponding linear mappings, which are defined by the 2^p different zero/nonzero combinations for z and $\bar{z}$, or, equivalently, 2^p different possibilities for choosing one side of the p (piecewise linear) boundary planes. Of course, some of these segments can be empty in general.

3 DEFINITION OF THE MAPPING

A large class of continuous piecewise linear mappings can be defined in a very compact matrix description. The mappings to be modeled are restricted to a finite number of segments, which are separated by a number of boundary planes. These boundary planes are allowed to change direction when intersecting each other (see Figure 3.1). The mappings are not restricted to functions in the strict sense, and allow the modeling of components with memory such as flip-flops, thyristors, and hysteresis in magnetic materials. The extension to dynamic models will be made later on, as well as the combination of simple models to more elaborate ones.

The matrix notation has an implicit and an explicit form, respectively given by equations (11a) and (11b):

$$\begin{bmatrix} 0 \\ z \end{bmatrix} = \begin{bmatrix} A & B \\ C & D \end{bmatrix} \cdot \begin{bmatrix} x \\ \bar{z} \end{bmatrix} + \begin{bmatrix} a \\ c \end{bmatrix} \qquad z \geqslant 0, \bar{z} \geqslant 0, z^t \cdot \bar{z} = 0 \tag{11a}$$

$$\begin{bmatrix} y \\ z \end{bmatrix} = \begin{bmatrix} A & B \\ C & D \end{bmatrix} \cdot \begin{bmatrix} x \\ \bar{z} \end{bmatrix} + \begin{bmatrix} a \\ c \end{bmatrix} \qquad z \geqslant 0, \bar{z} \geqslant 0, z^t \cdot \bar{z} = 0 \tag{11b}$$

The explicit form (11b) defines a piecewise linear mapping $x \to y$ and is therefore suitable for macromodeling and for checking properties of the mapping. The implicit form is closer to the modeling of electronic components, where we want to define the terminal behavior of the component without explicitly specifying which variables serve as inputs and outputs. However, both forms are easily transformed in each other.

The explicit form is transformed to the implicit form by concatenating x and y into a vector $\tilde{x}$. Furthermore, (A) is extended to $\tilde{A} = (A \quad -I)$ and (C) to $\tilde{C} = (C \quad 0)$. Now these quoted variables can be used in equation (11b) to obtain the desired result.

The implicit form can be transformed into the explicit form, if there exists a segment in which the (linear) mapping $x \to y$ has full rank (rank m). Here x and y result from a partitioning of the original vector x, in inputs and outputs, respectively. By a pivoting process (explained later) the matrix of equation (11a) is transformed so that the intended segment becomes the null segment; that is, all x in this segment yield $\bar{z} = 0$. By linear transformation, the m by m submatrix of A, consisting of the columns of vector y, is transformed to the negative identity matrix and the corresponding columns in C are reduced to (0). Now by moving the vector y to the left-hand side, we obtain (11b).

Because we want to discuss some properties of these piecewise linear mappings and provide a few examples, we will use the explicit form (11b) in the following sections.

With vectors z and $\bar{z}$ of dimension p, the matrix description defines in general 2^p different segments. It is clear that $\bar{z} = 0$ results in the linear mapping $y = A \cdot x + a$ for all x satisfying $0 \leqslant C \cdot x + c$. The linear relation in the other segments is easily obtained by the pivoting process, as explained in the next section. We note that $p = 0$ reduces the system to empty matrices B, C, D and empty vectors z, $\bar{z}$, c, thus resulting in the normal matrix description of linear mappings.

4 THE PIVOTING PROCESS

A piecewise linear mapping is defined as in equation (11b). One segment of the mapping, the so-called null segment σ^0, is explicitly available as

$y = A \cdot x + a$ for all x satisfying $0 \leqslant C \cdot x + c$. Now we assume that x follows a continuous path through the q-dimensional space and crosses one boundary plane of σ^0, thus leaving this segment. The boundary plane that is crossed is determined as one row of the equation $C \cdot x + c$ decreasing and becoming zero. Let us assume that this is the ith row, denoted by $C_{i*\cdot x + c_i}$. Furthermore, assume D_{ii} is positive.

The task of finding the linear relation and the domain of the neighboring segment can be solved by the following steps.

Make $\bar{z}_i$ (from eq. 11b) explicit as

$$\bar{z}_i = -\frac{C_{i*}}{D_{ii}} \cdot x + \frac{1}{D_{ii}} \cdot z_i - \frac{D_{i\bar{i}}}{D_{ii}} \cdot \bar{z}_{\bar{i}} - \frac{1}{D_{ii}} \cdot c_i \tag{12}$$

where the subscript $\bar{i}$ indicates all indices $1, 2, \ldots, p$ except i.

Because we assumed that only one boundary plane is crossed, the components of $\bar{z}_{\bar{i}}$ are positive and the components of $\bar{z}_{\bar{i}}$ are zero. If x is moved to the other side of the boundary plane, the restrictions on z and $\bar{z}$, in combination with equation (12), are solved by $\bar{z}_i > 0$ and $z_i = 0$. Therefore we interchange the positions of the variables z_i and $\bar{z}_i$ in equation (11b), but continue to use the "old" names z for the new left-hand-side vector and $\bar{z}$ for the new right-hand-side vector.

This process actually requires the substitution of equation (12) in all the equations of (11b) except the ith row of C. The ith row of C is replaced by equation (12). As a result of this substitution, an update on the other matrix elements is obtained, yielding among others $\tilde{A}$ and $\tilde{a}$ as

$$\tilde{A} = A - \frac{B_{*i} \cdot C_{i*}}{D_{ii}}, \qquad \tilde{a} = a - \frac{B_{*i} \cdot c_i}{D_{ii}} \tag{13}$$

This update is the rank one vector product update, given earlier as (3) and (4). If D is not the identity matrix (earlier seen as $\lambda_{12}, \lambda_{21} \neq 0$, eq. 8) similar updates affect the matrices B, C, and D, causing a breaking direction of the boundary planes (the other rows of C) without causing a distontinuity (see Section 2.3).

In the above process, the element D_{ii} is called the *pivot*. In general, the pivot can be an off-diagonal element, actually exchanging z_i with $\bar{z}_j$, or a multidimensional pivot (block pivot), exchanging a set of components from z and $\bar{z}$. With diagonal pivoting, we can generate 2^p different representations of the matrix, resulting in a list of all segments with their domain and linear mapping explicitly available. Of course, for some segments the linear inequalities might contradict each other, resulting in an empty domain (segment). An example of a pivot operation is given in Section 9.3.

The pivoting process described above is feasible only if the pivot involved is nonzero, or in the multidimensional case if the determinant of the submatrix of D is nonzero. A zero pivot does not imply the absence of a segment of the mapping, but merely indicates that in the new segment y cannot be written as a (linear) function of x. In these situations, the implicit mapping (11a) has some advantages over (11b).

If the pivot is negative, the new segment is found to be on the same side of the boundary plane, actually overlapping the previous segment and causing a "reflection" of the path x was following. This can occur for mappings that do not model a pure functional relation $x \rightarrow y$. This kind of property of the mappings is the subject of the next section.

5 LINEAR COMPLEMENTARITY

The primary problem to be solved in piecewise linear analysis is stated as:

For a piecewise linear mapping f: $x \rightarrow y$,
given in the form of equation (11b),
find the output y for some given input x.

Once x is given, the product $A \cdot x$ can be added to a, and the product $C \cdot x$ can be added to c. We then have to solve the so-called *linear complementarity problem*, stated as:

For given matrix D and given vector d
find vectors z and $\bar{z}$ satisfying:

$$z = D \cdot \bar{z} + d \qquad z \geqslant 0, \bar{z} \geqslant 0, z^t \cdot \bar{z} = 0 \tag{14}$$

This linear complementarity problem (LCP) is a well-known problem in mathematics, arising for example in game theory, and can be shown to be equivalent to the quadratic minimization problem on a linearly bounded domain [14]. Various algorithms exist to solve this LCP, but they are normally restricted to specific classes of matrices D for which convergence can be ensured. We will present a few of these matrix classes, extracted from a more complete overview in [10].

Positive definite matrices (PD):
D is of class PD if and only if
$\forall z \in R^p$, $z \neq 0$: $z^t D z > 0$

P-matrices (P):
D is of class P if and only if
$\forall z \in R^p$, $z \neq 0 \, \exists k$: $z_k \cdot (Dz)_k > 0$

Strictly copositive matrices (SCP):
D is of class SCP if and only if
$\forall z \in R_+{}^p$, $z \neq 0$: $z^t D z > 0$

Strictly semimonotone matrices (SSM):

D is of class SSM if and only if

$\forall z \in R_+{}^p,\ z \neq 0\ \exists k\colon z_k \cdot (Dz)_k > 0$

L-matrices (L):

D is of class L if and only if

$\forall z \in R_+{}^p,\ z \neq 0\ \exists k\colon z_k > 0 \wedge (Dz)_k \geqslant 0$

and also

$\exists \Lambda, \Omega \geqslant 0\ \forall z \in R_+{}^p,\ z \neq 0,\ Dz \geqslant 0,\ z^t Dz = 0\colon \Omega z \neq 0 \wedge (\Lambda D + D^t \Omega)z = 0$

in which Λ and Ω denote diagonal matrices

From these definitions it can easily be seen that PD is contained in both SCP and P, both SCP and P are contained in SSM, and finally SSM is contained in L. The diagonal elements of class SSM matrices are positive, of class L matrices nonnegative.

Class P is alternatively defined by the property that all principal minors of D are positive. [The principal minors of D are the determinants of submatrices (D_{ij}) with i and j both belonging to one subset of $\{1 \ldots p\}$.] In relation to the LCP it is known that D in class P is a necessary and sufficient condition for the existence of a unique solution for any source vector d. We note that Fig. 3.1 also yielded one solution (segment) for each x, resulting in equations (7) and (10), defining a class P matrix.

For D in class SSM, the LCP has an odd number of solutions for each d. Whereas the class P property is closed under diagonal pivot transformations, the class SSM property is not.

Finally, for D in class L the LCP might not have a solution for some d, there might be a discrete number of solutions, or there might be a whole (bounded) subspace of solutions.

6 SOLUTION ALGORITHM

As stated in the preceding section, the problem of solving a piecewise linear mapping is identical to the linear complementarity problem. For circuit simulation we are interested in finding one solution of a given LCP. For the transient analysis case, we have to solve a sequence of LCPs, leading to a path of z through the p-dimensional space, with parameter t (time).

Many different algorithms exist for the solution of the LCP. The three basic approaches are:

1. Methods based on quadratic minimization. The equivalence of the LCP with (linearly bounded) quadratic minimization is used to solve the LCP. In general, relaxation techniques are used to find the minimum of the function on a bounded domain. The guaranteed convergence of the method is

therefore restricted to mappings that are convex on the specified domain, leading to class PD and P matrices [2, 15].

2. Methods based on integer labeling on a triangular grid. Integer labeling methods are known to be able to solve strongly nonlinear problems and do not depend on convexity requirements [11]. Algorithms of this type can be shown to process the LCP for all class SSM matrices [8]. Where we want to process circuits with memory, such as flip-flops, convergence for class SSM or larger is of primary importance. Both the quadratic minimization and integer labeling methods can solve the LCP by computing matrix vector products only. These algorithms are extremely well suited for fast and compact sparse matrix processing, or for implementation on vector processing machines.

3. Methods relying on pivoting as the basic operation. Sometimes these are referred to as vector labeling algorithms. Many different versions of these algorithms exist, differing in the choice of the pivots and the class of matrices for which convergence can be insured. In practice, these algorithms tend to show fast convergence, solving most problems in only a few steps. However, for large systems complex sparse matrix processing is required, because the algorithm dictates the choice of the pivots, and many fill-ins might occur. Algorithms are devised to solve the LCP for very large classes of matrices, leading to strong global convergence properties for the circuit simulator. A pivoting algorithm that processes the LCP for all class L matrices will be presented below.

A early pivoting-type algorithm was published by C. E. Lemke [13]. In his algorithm the solution is obtained by tracing a continuous path of z, controlled by a monotonic decreasing parameter λ, starting at an artificially generated initial solution and ending at the solution of the problem. This monotonic decrease of λ could be ensured for all class P matrices. In [14] Lemke published a powerful extension of his original algorithm. Now not only the λ-parameter but also components of z and $\bar{z}$ are manipulated in order to trace the path and reach the solution. A description of the algorithm is given below.

1. Assume the problem to be solved is given by $z = D \cdot \bar{z} + d$, $z \geqslant 0$, $\bar{z} \geqslant 0$, $z^t \cdot \bar{z} = 0$. If $d \geqslant 0$, the solution is given by $z = d$, $\bar{z} = 0$. Otherwise some component of d is negative, and we choose a vector e and parameter λ such that $\lambda > 0$ and $z = \lambda \cdot e + d > 0$. Extend the matrix D with the column e, and the vector $\bar{z}$ with the corresponding element λ as $\bar{z}_0$. Set all the other components of $\bar{z}$ equal to zero, and $j = 0$ indicating the only positive component of $\bar{z}$. Now decrease $\lambda = \bar{z}_0$ down to the point where the first component of z, say z_k, reaches zero. Proceed with step 2.

2. Perform a pivot operation on the matrix element D_{kj}, which was found to be nonzero, exchanging the position of the kth element of the left-hand vector with the jth element of the right-hand vector. Proceed with step 3.

3. Set j equal to k. Try to increase the jth element of the right-hand vector until some component of the left-hand vector becomes zero. If no such component becomes zero, the jth element could be increased unlimited, and the algorithm terminates without finding a solution to the LCP. Otherwise some component of the left-hand vector becomes zero, let us say the kth. If this element is the original $\bar{z}_0$, then λ has become zero, and a solution for the LCP is found. Otherwise proceed with step 2.

The algorithm will terminate in a finite number of steps for any matrix D. However, for only a restricted class of matrices, the termination without a solution proves that a solution does not exist. Lemke himself proved this for class CPP (somewhat larger then SCP), but Eaves [6] proved it for all class L matrices.

It is easily seen that the algorithm might use off-diagonal pivots, intermixing the components of z and $\bar{z}$. If a solution is finally found, any original pair $(z_k, \bar{z}_k)$ might be interchanged, but both elements never appear together in the same vector. Especially when a circuit is analyzed as a network of interconnected piecewise linear components with explicit Jacobians, off-diagonal pivots can be cumbersome. As an alternative, Panne [16] describes an algorithm that follows the same path through space as the above algorithm of Lemke, but is restricted to diagonal (block) pivots only. However, the description of the algorithm is considerably more complicated.

7 DYNAMIC SYSTEMS

So far, static piecewise linear mappings have been presented, together with a matrix notation and a solution algorithm. For the simulation of electrical circuits, however, we do need models with time-dependent behavior, to be treated in this section.

Let us start by presenting the matrix notation, extended with vectors u and $\dot{u}$ for a dynamic behavior, to model a piecewise linear dynamic mapping F: $x \to y$.

$$\begin{bmatrix} y \\ \dot{u} \\ z \end{bmatrix} = \begin{bmatrix} A_{11} & A_{12} & A_{13} \\ A_{21} & A_{22} & A_{23} \\ A_{31} & A_{32} & A_{33} \end{bmatrix} \cdot \begin{bmatrix} x \\ u \\ \bar{z} \end{bmatrix} + \begin{bmatrix} a_1 \\ a_2 \\ a_3 \end{bmatrix} \qquad \dot{u} = \frac{\partial u}{\partial t},\ z \geqslant 0,\ \bar{z} \geqslant 0,\ z^t \cdot \bar{z} = 0 \tag{15}$$

The above description (15) can be read as a piecewise linear static mapping f: $(x, u) \to (y, \dot{u})$, in a notation according to (11b), where the inputs u and outputs $\dot{u}$ are connected in a feedback loop with ideal integrators g: $\dot{u} \to u$. If the dimensions of the vectors z and $\bar{z}$ are zero, matrices A_{13}, A_{23}, A_{31}, A_{32}, A_{33} and vector a_3 vanish, and the system (15) degenerates to the conventional description of linear dynamic systems.

By replacing y with the null vector and extending the vector x with these variables, we obtain the implicit description of a piecewise linear dynamic system according to (11a).

An implicit integration rule will now be added to equation (15) in order to show how we can perform the transient integration. The trapezoidal rule (16) is applied as an example.

$$u^k = u^{k-1} + \tfrac{1}{2}h(\dot{u}^{k-1} + \dot{u}^k) \tag{16}$$

Here the superscript k refers to variables at time t, to be solved for, and the superscript $k-1$ to variables at time $t-h$, which are already known.

We assume that equation (15) is valid at time point t and hence assume superscripts k on all the variables involved. Now (16) is substituted in the second row of (15), leading to

$$\dot{u}^k = \Lambda \cdot (A_{22} \cdot \tilde{u}^{k-1} + A_{21} \cdot x^k + A_{23} \cdot \bar{z}^k + a_2) \tag{17}$$

with

$$\tilde{u}^j = u^j + \tfrac{1}{2}h\dot{u}^j \quad \text{and} \quad \Lambda = (I - \tfrac{1}{2}hA_{22})^{-1}$$

We have assumed the inversion for Λ to be feasible, which is always satisfied for small enough h.

Now this value for $\dot{u}^k$ is substituted in (16) and (15), leading to

$$\begin{bmatrix} y^k \\ \tilde{u}^k \\ z^k \end{bmatrix} = \begin{bmatrix} \tilde{A}_{11} & \tilde{A}_{12} & \tilde{A}_{13} \\ \tilde{A}_{21} & \tilde{A}_{22} & \tilde{A}_{23} \\ \tilde{A}_{31} & \tilde{A}_{32} & \tilde{A}_{33} \end{bmatrix} \cdot \begin{bmatrix} x^k \\ u^{k-1} \\ \bar{z}^k \end{bmatrix} + \begin{bmatrix} \tilde{a}_1 \\ \tilde{a}_2 \\ \tilde{a}_3 \end{bmatrix} \qquad z^k \geqslant 0,\ \bar{z}^k \geqslant 0,\ z^{kt} \cdot \bar{z}^k = 0 \tag{18}$$

with

$$\begin{aligned}
\tilde{A}_{ij} &= A_{ij} + \tfrac{1}{2}hA_{i2}\Lambda A_{2j} && \text{for } i, j \in 1, 3 \\
\tilde{A}_{i2} &= A_{i2} \cdot \Lambda && \text{for } i \in 1, 3 \\
\tilde{A}_{2j} &= h\Lambda \cdot A_{2j} && \text{for } j \in 1, 3 \\
\tilde{A}_{22} &= \Lambda \cdot (I + \tfrac{1}{2}hA_{22}) && \\
\tilde{a}_i &= a_i + \tfrac{1}{2}hA_{i2}\Lambda \cdot a_2 && \text{for } i \in 1, 3 \\
\tilde{a}_2 &= h\Lambda a_2 &&
\end{aligned}$$

In this way the transient analysis problem is reduced to the repeated solution of a static piecewise linear problem, to be solved with some LCP algorithm. We assume the inputs x^k are given for all k; the values for $\tilde{u}^{k-1}$ were solved in the previous step.

In order to start this implicit integration scheme, we begin with a DC solution for $k = 0$ of the original equations (15). The initial conditions can be given as values for u or, if preferred, as values for $\dot{u}$ needing a partial inversion of A_{22}. If this LCP is solved, we know the initial solution $(y^0, \dot{u}^0)$ and determine an appropriate value for h. Now $\tilde{u}^0$ is determined as in (17), and the iteration over k can start.

In real-life simulation programs, we often do want a more elaborate integration scheme, however. Therefore the above scheme is to be extended with some step size control mechanism, for the integration of stiff problems; and it is useful to try to synchronize the determination of the time points to solve and the crossing of boundary planes of the mapping, in order to improve the integration accuracy (the local truncation error). This extension will be made in the last section of this chapter on piecewise linear systems. Before going into that theory, we will return for a moment to piecewise linear modeling and show a few examples.

8 MODEL INTERCONNECTION

This section will treat the interconnection of piecewise linear models in order to derive a new model for the interconnected system. The reason for handling this subject is twofold.

First, for analyzing electronic circuits, we want to make use of a library of component models, which are interconnected by the user to form some electrical network (circuit). For the simulation we do need to handle this interconnection in such a way that the resulting piecewise linear system can be solved by the methods discussed earlier.

A second application of the interconnection of piecewise linear models is in the development of new models for (more complex) devices. Whereas the section on continuity treated one way of constructing the matrix (see Fig. 3.1 and eq. 10), the modeling continues to be a tough problem, especially for multidimensional mappings or for mappings that are not functions in the strict sense. In practice, complex models are often developed by combining simpler models.

Assume that f^1: $x^1 \rightarrow 0$ and f^2: $x^2 \rightarrow 0$ are implicit piecewise linear mappings. For notational convenience, we restrict ourselves to static mappings, without losing generality. If these two mappings were given in the explicit form of (11b), they are easily converted to the implicit form (11a) as explained previously. Of course, the combination of more than two mappings proceeds identically. Furthermore, assume that the vector of inputs and outputs of the system after interconnection is given as x^0.

The system can now be given in the form of equation (19):

$$\begin{bmatrix} 0 \\ 0 \\ 0 \\ z^1 \\ z^2 \end{bmatrix} = \begin{bmatrix} S^0 & S^1 & S^2 & 0 & 0 \\ 0 & A^1 & 0 & B^1 & 0 \\ 0 & 0 & A^2 & 0 & B^2 \\ 0 & C^1 & 0 & D^1 & 0 \\ 0 & 0 & C^2 & 0 & D^2 \end{bmatrix} \cdot \begin{bmatrix} x^0 \\ x^1 \\ x^2 \\ \bar{z}^1 \\ \bar{z}^2 \end{bmatrix} + \begin{bmatrix} s \\ a^1 \\ a^2 \\ c^1 \\ c^2 \end{bmatrix}$$

$$z^1 \geqslant 0,\ \bar{z}^1 \geqslant 0,\ z^{1t} \cdot \bar{z}^1 = 0,\ z^2 \geqslant 0,\ \bar{z}^2 \geqslant 0,\ z^{2t} \cdot \bar{z}^2 = 0 \tag{19}$$

Because we assumed that x^0 contains the inputs and outputs of the resulting system, the variables x^1 and x^2 have to be removed from (19). Assume k is the sum of the dimensions of the vectors x^1 and x^2. Now we have to select k rows of the matrix

$$\begin{bmatrix} S^1 & S^2 \\ A^1 & 0 \\ 0 & A^2 \end{bmatrix}$$

covering the space spanned by all the rows of

$$\begin{bmatrix} S^1 & S^2 \\ A^1 & 0 \\ 0 & A^2 \\ C^1 & 0 \\ 0 & C^2 \end{bmatrix}$$

If necessary, this can be done by pivoting on elements in the matrices D^1 and D^2, to change the rank of the matrices mentioned, and actually moving the description to another segment of the mapping.

If these k rows have been determined, linear combinations of them are added to all the other rows to clear the elements in the columns of x^1 and x^2 in all the other rows. Now these k rows and k columns are removed from the matrix description, resulting in a new matrix in the standard form of equation (11a) of the new combined system. An example of the generation of a model by interconnection is presented in Section 9.5.

For circuit simulating the matrices (S^0, S^1, S^2, s) are determined as the Kirchhoff voltage and current equations. However, for model development these matrices are chosen in a special way in order to create the desired effects. The resulting mapping $f^0(x)$ might, for instance, take values $f^1(x^1) + f^2(x^2)$, $f^1(f^2(x^2))$, or even $f^{1^{-1}}(x^1) + f^{2^{-1}}(x^2)$. We want to emphasize that

1. By applying simple linear matrix operations (exchanging the role of inputs and outputs) an explicit description can be obtained for the inverse of a piecewise linear dynamic mapping, without imposing a restriction of being one-to-one. For other nonlinear systems, this is in general not possible.
2. For constructions $f^1(f^2(x^2))$ the resulting number of segments is in general the product of the numbers of segments of f^1 and f^2. However, the dimensions of the vectors z and $\bar{z}$ are just added, which is in accordance with the earlier observation that the modeled number of segments grows exponentially with this dimension. The matrix notation thus remains a very compact definition of the resulting mapping. Had we not adopted this matrix notation, but used a conventional list-oriented approach as in Section 2.1, the resulting mapping after this type of combination would be extremely hard to find and would really grow exponentially in size.

9 MODEL EXAMPLES

This section will present a number of examples of the generation and evaluation of matrix descriptions for the modeling of piecewise linear mappings.

9.1 One-Dimensional Functions

One-dimensional functions $f: x \to y$ are easily and straightforwardly modeled, with the explicit matrix definition (11b). With the construction shown below, the dimension of the vectors z and $\bar{z}$ equals the number of breakpoints in the curve of f. The exponential growth of the number of segments with the size of the matrix is thus not used. It is easy to see that this property cannot be used for a general one-dimensional mapping, because the data for all degrees of freedom cannot be stored in a matrix of logarithmic size.

Let

$$y = a_0 x + b_0 + \sum_{k=1}^{p} a_k[x - b_k]_+ \tag{20}$$

with a_k, b_k $(0 \leqslant k \leqslant p)$ given number numbers and

$$[w]_+ = \begin{cases} 0 & \text{if } w \leqslant 0 \\ w & \text{if } w > 0 \end{cases}$$

Equation (20) clearly defines a one-dimensional continuous piecewise linear function. The corresponding matrix is given as equation (21):

$$\begin{bmatrix} y \\ z_1 \\ z_2 \\ \vdots \\ z_p \end{bmatrix} = \begin{bmatrix} a_0 & a_1 & a_2 & \cdots & a_p \\ -1 & 1 & 0 & \cdots & 0 \\ -1 & 0 & 1 & & 0 \\ \vdots & \vdots & & \ddots & \\ -1 & 0 & 0 & & 1 \end{bmatrix} \cdot \begin{bmatrix} x \\ \bar{z}_1 \\ \bar{z}_2 \\ \vdots \\ \bar{z}_p \end{bmatrix} + \begin{bmatrix} b_0 \\ b_1 \\ b_2 \\ \vdots \\ b_p \end{bmatrix} \tag{21}$$

The matrix D for which the linear complementarity problem must be solved is specified in (21) as the identity matrix, reducing the LCP to a trivial problem ($\bar{z}_k = [x - b_k]_+$). Of course, the identity matrix belongs to class P as defined in Section 5, as was expected for a function in the strict sense.

9.2 Simple MOSFET

An extremely simple model for an MOS transistor is presented as a two-dimensional mapping with two boundary planes. The curves of this piecewise linear model are shown in Figure 3.2.

This mapping is alternatively defined as follows.
The subthreshold region:

$$I\,ds = 0 \qquad \text{if } Vg - Vt - Vs \leqslant 0 \text{ and } Vg - Vt - Vd \leqslant 0$$

The forward saturation region:

$$I\,ds = \beta(Vg - Vt - Vs) \qquad \text{if } Vg - Vt - Vs \geqslant 0 \text{ and } Vg - Vt - Vd \leqslant 0$$

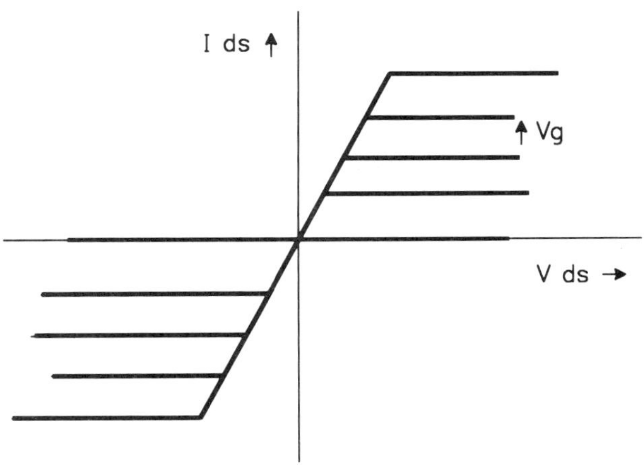

Figure 3.2 Simple MOSFET characteristics.

The backward saturation region:

$$I\,ds = -\beta(Vg - Vt - Vd) \qquad \text{if } Vg - Vt - Vs \leqslant 0 \text{ and } Vg - Vt - Vd \geqslant 0$$

The linear region:

$$I\,ds = \beta(Vd - Vs) \qquad \text{if } Vg - Vt - Vs \geqslant 0 \text{ and } Vg - Vt - Vd \geqslant 0$$

The above description shows how the mapping can be defined with two boundary planes, resulting in four segments as explained in Section 2.3. In the notation of Section 2.3, equation (8), the data for the matrix can be given as

$$x = (I\,ds \quad Vg \quad Vs \quad Vd)^t$$

$$(A^0 \quad a^0) = (-1 \quad 0 \quad 0 \quad 0 \quad 0)$$

$$(n^0 \quad c^0) = (0 \quad -1 \quad 1 \quad 0 \quad Vt)^t, \qquad w^0 = (\beta)$$

$$(n^1 \quad c^1) = (0 \quad -1 \quad 0 \quad 1 \quad Vt)^t, \qquad w^1 = (-\beta)$$

$$\lambda_{12} = \lambda_{21} = 0$$

with Vt and β model parameters.

According to equation (10) the matrix is now given by

$$\begin{bmatrix} 0 \\ z_1 \\ z_2 \end{bmatrix} = \begin{bmatrix} -1 & 0 & 0 & 0 & \beta & -\beta \\ 0 & -1 & 1 & 0 & 1 & 0 \\ 0 & -1 & 0 & 1 & 0 & 1 \end{bmatrix} \cdot \begin{bmatrix} I\,ds \\ Vg \\ Vs \\ Vd \\ \bar{z}_1 \\ \bar{z}_2 \end{bmatrix} + \begin{bmatrix} 0 \\ Vt \\ Vt \end{bmatrix}$$

For a practical relevant model, the above description can be improved, while maintaining compactness, by accounting for resistances in series with the MOSFET terminals and by assuming Vt linearly dependent on Vs and Vd. Furthermore, with the addition of one row and one column for $\partial u/\partial t$ and u, a gate capacitance can be added. Of course, the model remains quite inaccurate and suitable for a fast analysis of digital systems only. A more elaborate model can be found in [7].

9.3 Mapping with Hysteresis

An example of a mapping with hysteresis is given as Figure 3.3. An explicit matrix definition of this mapping can be given as

$$\begin{bmatrix} y \\ z_1 \\ z_2 \end{bmatrix} = \begin{bmatrix} -\frac{1}{3} & \frac{1}{3} & -\frac{1}{3} \\ -\frac{1}{3} & \frac{1}{3} & \frac{2}{3} \\ \frac{1}{3} & \frac{2}{3} & \frac{1}{3} \end{bmatrix} \cdot \begin{bmatrix} x \\ \bar{z}_1 \\ \bar{z}_2 \end{bmatrix} + \begin{bmatrix} \frac{2}{3} \\ -\frac{1}{3} \\ -\frac{2}{3} \end{bmatrix}$$

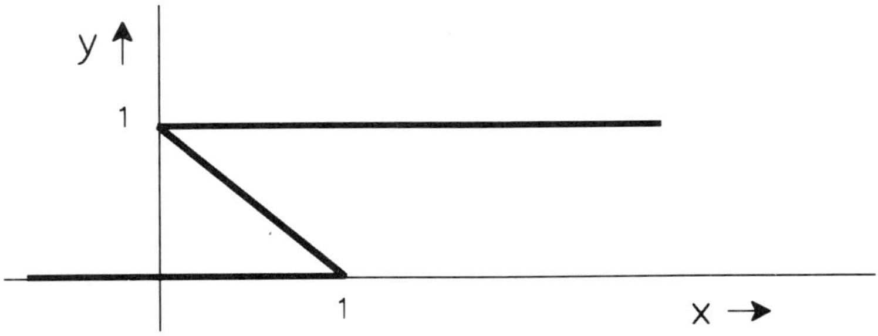

Figure 3.3 Mapping with hysteresis.

The 2 × 2 submatrix D has positive diagonal elements (both $\frac{1}{3}$; however, it has a negative determinant $(-\frac{1}{3})$ and thus does not belong to class P as defined in Section 5. It is easy to check that D does satisfy the class SCP property; hence according to Section 5 the mapping might have an odd number of solutions for some x.

Matching the above matrix description with Figure 3.3 is relatively easy. Whereas D is a 2 by 2 matrix, four possible choices for the zero-nonzero combinations of the vectors z and $\bar{z}$ exist (see Sections 2.4 and 4), yielding four segments with their linear mapping.

The current segment $(\bar{z}_1 = \bar{z}_2 = 0)$ is immediately available as

$$y = -\tfrac{1}{3}\cdot x + \tfrac{2}{3}$$

$$z_1 = -\tfrac{1}{3}\cdot x - \tfrac{1}{3} \geqslant 0$$

$$z_2 = \tfrac{1}{3}\cdot x - \tfrac{2}{3} \geqslant 0$$

The inequalities restricting the domain of this segment contradict each other; thus this segment (this domain) is empty and does not contribute to the mapping.

Performing a pivot operation on element $D_{22} = \frac{1}{3}$ transforms the matrix to another segment, yielding

$$\begin{bmatrix} y \\ z_1 \\ \bar{z}_2 \end{bmatrix} = \begin{bmatrix} 0 & 1 & -1 \\ -1 & -1 & 2 \\ -1 & -2 & 3 \end{bmatrix} \cdot \begin{bmatrix} x \\ \bar{z}_1 \\ z_2 \end{bmatrix} + \begin{bmatrix} 0 \\ 1 \\ 2 \end{bmatrix}$$

Here we have actually denoted the interchange of the elements z_2 and $\bar{z}_2$ as a result of the pivot operation. However, the resulting matrix is functionally equivalent to the previous one, and therefore the left-hand vector normally continues to be called z and the right-hand vector $\bar{z}$.

The solution in this segment is now read as

$$\bar{z}_1 = z_2 = 0$$

$$y = 0$$

$$z_1 = -x + 1 \geqslant 0$$

$$\bar{z}_2 = -x + 2 \geqslant 0$$

The two restrictions on x combine as $x \leqslant 1$, which is the domain for this segment with mapping $y = 0$.

In the same way, ($z_1 = \bar{z}_2 = 0$) yields the segment $y = 1$, $x \geqslant 0$, and ($z_1 = z_2 = 0$) yields $y = -x + 1, 0 \leqslant x \leqslant 1$, corresponding to Figure 3.3. We note that the matrix for the solution $x \leqslant 1$ has a negative diagonal element D_{11}. If x is increased, the boundary $x = 1$ is determined as the first row of D. Trying to cross the boundary by a single pivot on $D_{11} = -1$ causes a reflection, and the new segment is on the same side of the boundary ($y = -x + 1$ for $0 \leqslant x \leqslant 1$; see Figure 3.3).

9.4 Square Wave Generator

As an example of a dynamic system, we extend the (second) matrix of the hysteresis curve with one column u and a corresponding row $\partial u/\partial t = \dot{u}$. The new matrix entries are chosen according to $\dot{u} = 1 - 2 \cdot y$ and $x = u$. Finally, the column of x is deleted from the matrix, yielding

$$\begin{bmatrix} y \\ \dot{u} \\ z_1 \\ \bar{z}_2 \end{bmatrix} = \begin{bmatrix} 0 & 1 & -1 \\ 0 & -2 & 2 \\ -1 & -1 & 2 \\ -1 & -2 & 3 \end{bmatrix} \cdot \begin{bmatrix} u \\ \bar{z}_1 \\ z_2 \end{bmatrix} + \begin{bmatrix} 0 \\ 1 \\ 1 \\ 2 \end{bmatrix}$$

With the start condition $u(t = 0) = 0$, the solution at $t = 0$ is given as $y(0) = 0$ and $\dot{u}(0) = 1$. Thus $u(t) = t$, yielding $z_1 = 1 - t$ and $\bar{z}_2 = 2 - t$. This solution

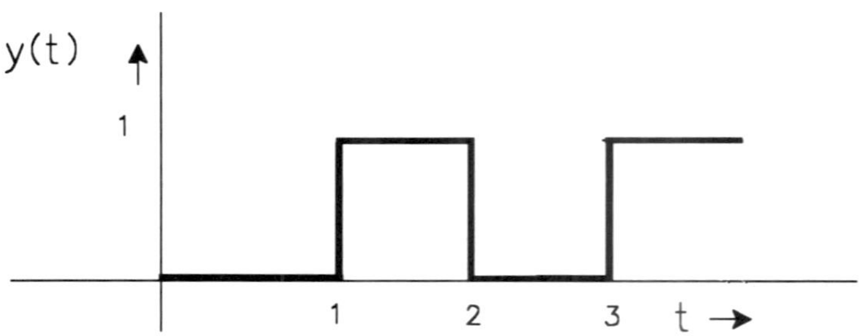

Figure 3.4 Square wave solution.

is valid up to $t = 1$, where z_1 reaches zero. At $t = 1$ a new solution can be found after pivoting on both D_{11} and D_{22}, yielding $y = 1$, $\dot{u} = -1$. The process continues in this way, resulting in a solution for y as depicted in Figure 3.4.

9.5 Logic Gate Model

As an example of an interconnection method to find a new model, a two-input AND gate is used. The model is built from two functions called saturate and min, presented below.

$$\begin{bmatrix} ys \\ zs_1 \\ zs_2 \end{bmatrix} = \begin{bmatrix} 0 & 3 & -3 \\ -1 & 1 & 0 \\ -1 & 0 & 1 \end{bmatrix} \cdot \begin{bmatrix} xs \\ \overline{zs}_1 \\ \overline{zs}_2 \end{bmatrix} + \begin{bmatrix} 0 \\ \frac{1}{3} \\ \frac{2}{3} \end{bmatrix}$$

$$ys = \text{saturate}(xs)$$

The matrix of this mapping is generated with the formulas of Section 9.1, according to the solution

$$ys = \begin{cases} 0 & \text{for } xs \leqslant \frac{1}{3} \\ 3xs - 1 & \text{for } \frac{1}{3} \leqslant xs \leqslant \frac{2}{3} \\ 1 & \text{for } xs \geqslant \frac{2}{3} \end{cases}$$

The function min is given by

$$\begin{bmatrix} ym \\ zm_1 \end{bmatrix} = \begin{bmatrix} 1 & 0 & -1 \\ -1 & 1 & 1 \end{bmatrix} \cdot \begin{bmatrix} xm_1 \\ xm_2 \\ \overline{zm}_1 \end{bmatrix} + \begin{bmatrix} 0 \\ 0 \end{bmatrix}$$

$$ym = \min(xm_1, xm_2)$$

Here ym is the minimum of xm_1 and xm_2; the above matrix is easily derived according to Section 2.2.

The function $y = \text{AND}(x_1, x_2)$ is now defined as $y = \text{saturate}(\min(x_1, x_2))$. This mapping is made as follows:

Rewrite both matrices in the implicit form (11a), and combine them in one new matrix.
Substitute y instead of ys and x_i instead of xm_i.
Add the equation $xs = ym$.
Remove xs and ym by linear matrix operations.
If desired, rewrite the matrix in the explicit form (11b).

After the addition of $xs = ym$ we obtain the following set of equations:

$$\begin{bmatrix} 0 \\ 0 \\ 0 \\ z_1 \\ z_2 \\ z_3 \end{bmatrix} = \begin{bmatrix} 0 & -1 & 0 & 1 & 0 & -1 & 0 & 0 \\ -1 & 0 & 0 & 0 & 0 & 0 & 3 & -3 \\ 0 & -1 & 1 & 0 & 0 & 0 & 0 & 0 \\ 0 & 0 & 0 & -1 & 1 & 1 & 0 & 0 \\ 0 & 0 & -1 & 0 & 0 & 0 & 1 & 0 \\ 0 & 0 & -1 & 0 & 0 & 0 & 0 & 1 \end{bmatrix} \cdot \begin{bmatrix} y \\ ym \\ xs \\ x_1 \\ x_2 \\ \bar{z}_1 \\ \bar{z}_2 \\ \bar{z}_3 \end{bmatrix} + \begin{bmatrix} 0 \\ 0 \\ 0 \\ 0 \\ \frac{1}{3} \\ \frac{2}{3} \end{bmatrix}$$

In this example we can use the first and the third equation to clear the entries in the last two rows and columns of ym and xs. These equations and columns are then removed from the matrix. The second equation is the only equation with a nonzero entry for y, hence y can be moved to the left-hand side without further operations.

This yields the following matrix:

$$\begin{bmatrix} y \\ z_1 \\ z_2 \\ z_3 \end{bmatrix} = \begin{bmatrix} 0 & 0 & 0 & 3 & -3 \\ -1 & 1 & 1 & 0 & 0 \\ -1 & 0 & 1 & 1 & 0 \\ -1 & 0 & 1 & 0 & 1 \end{bmatrix} \cdot \begin{bmatrix} x_1 \\ x_2 \\ \bar{z}_1 \\ \bar{z}_2 \\ \bar{z}_3 \end{bmatrix} + \begin{bmatrix} 0 \\ 0 \\ \frac{1}{3} \\ \frac{2}{3} \end{bmatrix}$$

In the resulting matrix, the 3×3 submatrix D belongs to class P (all the determinants of principal submatrices are equal to 1), hence the matrix

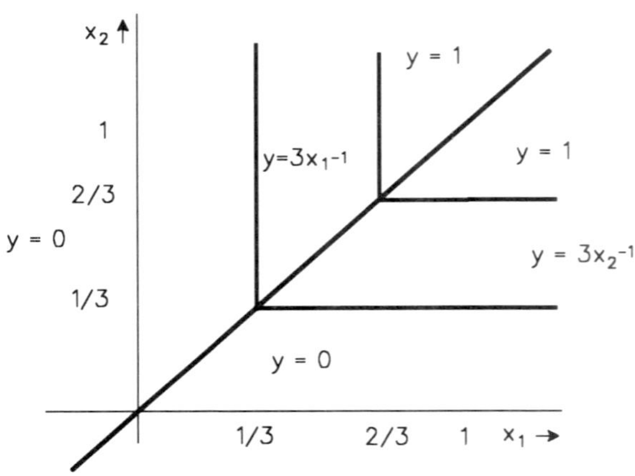

Figure 3.5 The AND function.

defines a function (see Section 5). Whereas the first column of D consists of nonzero numbers, the boundary plane z_1 causes a breaking in the direction of the other two boundary planes (see Section 2.2). A picture of the resulting AND function is given in Figure 3.5.

9.6 Compact Square Function

The final example is a function $f: x \to y$, where y is an approximation of $x \cdot x$. The piecewise linear function is constructed in such a way that a p-dimensional vector z really gives 2^p different segments (intervals) in the function f. The matrix for the mapping $fx: \to y$, in which the domain is partitioned in 16 segments, is given below by applying the four-dimensional vectors z and $\bar{z}$.

$$\begin{bmatrix} y \\ z_1 \\ z_2 \\ z_3 \\ z_4 \end{bmatrix} = \begin{bmatrix} 1 & 2 & 6 & 14 & 30 \\ -1 & 1 & 2 & 2 & 2 \\ -1 & 0 & 1 & 2 & 2 \\ -1 & 0 & 0 & 1 & 2 \\ -1 & 0 & 0 & 0 & 1 \end{bmatrix} \begin{bmatrix} x \\ \bar{z}_1 \\ \bar{z}_2 \\ \bar{z}_3 \\ \bar{z}_4 \end{bmatrix} + \begin{bmatrix} 0 \\ 1 \\ 2 \\ 4 \\ 8 \end{bmatrix}$$

The 4×4 submatrix D belongs to class P, hence the matrix indeed defines a function. Checking whether the function indeed approximates $x \cdot x$ for $0 \leqslant x \leqslant 16$ can be done in the same way as before and is left to the reader.

10 SIMULATION PROGRAM

In the previous sections, piecewise linear mappings were treated. In particular, a matrix notation was presented that is suitable for a compact definition of static and dynamic mappings as well as for a powerful manipulation with these mappings. With these tools a simulation program can be built, having certain advantages over conventional circuit simulation programs. An example program structure that clarifies these advantages is given below.

We assume that a network of components has been processed and circuit equations have been built in some way. All components are specified with a piecewise linear (dynamic) model, for which the linear behavior (the Jacobian) of some segment resides in the network equations, together with connection equations, such as the Kirchhoff voltage and current equations. In this final section the matrix notation for the piecewise linear components is not explicitly required (the list approach of Section 2.1 might suffice); however, we do assume that the vector product update for a crossing of a boundary (see Section 2.2) is explicitly available. For each solumn of the network matrix, we assume a storage location for the value of the associated variable as well as for its time derivative. For given network variables with derivatives, the component models should be able to explicitly determine the allowed time step up to reaching the first boundary plane (see the example in Section 9.4). During transient analysis, the allowed time step is furthermore limited by the step size h of the integration rule. The linear system of interconnected equations and Jacobians is used to solve for the time derivatives, not for the circuit variables.

The simulation program is now given as

```
Compute DC solution
while end of integration-time not reached
{     if new step size needed
      {     Choose and apply new step size and integration rule
            Substitute accordingly modified Jacobians
            Perform full L/U decomposition
      }
      Solve circuit variable derivatives dx/dt
      Determine allowed time step considering integration step size and
            crossing of boundary planes
      Update circuit variables up to the determined time point, and print
            their values
      Update the Jacobian excitation vectors up to this time point
      if time step was limited by the integration accuracy
      {     Determine whether or not to choose a new step size
      }
      else (time step was limited by reaching of boundary)
      {     perform single pivot operation in component model,
            resubstitute the (modified) Jacobian,
            and update L/U decomposition with the external vector product
            if the single pivot did not solve the PWL equation
            {     find multiple pivot solution
            }
      }
}
```

In the above algorithm the Jacobians play a crucial role. Each time one of the Jacobians changes, the L/U decomposition of the (linear) set of equations needs to be recalculated. For dynamic models, the step size h influences the Jacobian (as can be seen in Section 7). For subsequent time steps with equal h, only the Jacobian excitation vector changes, because this vector normally contains among others the dynamic state vector u (also see Section 7). In this case the same L/U decomposition can be used, to solve for the variables in the next time point.

When a boundary of the piecewise linear mapping is crossed for some component model, the Jacobian obtains a vector product update (see Section 2.2). If the model is given by the matrix notation, this corresponds to a single (diagonal) pivot operation (see Section 4), and the vector product update is explicitly available as a row and column of the matrix. The new L/U decomposition is now obtained with an update of the previous one by using the rank one update property on the system matrix. This update can be derived highly efficiently on sparse data structures, which is considerably cheaper than recomputing the full L/U decomposition. For details of the rank one update see Ref. [1] or [9].

Special algorithms for solving sets of piecewise linear equations are required to solve for a DC solution, and during the transient analysis only in case of difficulty, when a single pivot does not provide the solution on the other side of the boundary plane (e.g., see the hysteresis curve, Section 9.3). One such algorithm is the Lemke method, as explained in Section 4. This algorithm has remarkably strong global convergence properties, in contrast to the conventional Newton-Raphson scheme for nonlinear circuits, which has good local convergence only.

Whereas the above algorithm is more or less event-driven, an extension is easily made for individually assigned optimal step sizes h for each (dynamic) component model. Furthermore, when the equations show a hierarchical structuring (for instance, from a hierarchical network specification), this hierarchy can be used to exploit the latency behavior, as explained in Section 1. The full L/U decomposition then reduces to a partial L/U decomposition along a path upward in the hierarchy, and the solution of new circuit variable derivatives proceeds only in the "active" subtree(s) downward. For a more thorough discussion of such a latency evaluation, see, for instance, Refs. [7] and [18].

In a conventional circuit simulator, the while loop over the time points contains an inner loop of the Newton-Raphson iteration, which contains the linearization and the L/U decomposition of the full circuit. For this reason, the L/U decomposition consumes a large amount of the computational effort. In contrast, the above algorithm does not have these nested loops, and the full L/U decomposition will often be skipped in the outer loop. These savings in L/U decomposition can be responsible for a significantly reduced computational effort.

If accurate models are used for nonlinear devices such as transistors, a large number of "events" will be generated within a single time step, and the pivot operation with the rank one update will consume a considerable part of the CPU requirements. In these cases the CPU time will grow linearly with the number of boundaries crossed and hence with the model accuracy. Highly accurate models will therefore slow down the simulation.

The piecewise linear modeling allows good transistor modeling, as well as simple and abstract macromodeling of logic gates, amplifiers, analog-to-digital converters, filters, and so forth. All these models are represented in a uniform way, and therefore mixed level simulation is easily supported. Because of the strong global convergence properties, the simulation program can easily handle the steep transients, as generated by coarse macromodels (see, for instance, Section 9.4).

REFERENCES

1. J. M. Bennett, Triangular factors of modified matrices, *Numer. Math.*, vol. 7, pp. 217–221, 1965.
2. W. M. G. van Bokhoven, Piecewise linear solution techniques, in *Circuit Analysis, Simulation and Design*, Part 2: *VLSI Circuit Analysis and Simulation*, A. E. Ruehli, ed., North-Holland, Amsterdam, 1987.
3. W. K. Chia, T. N. Trick, and I. N. Hajj, Stability and convergence properties of relaxation methods, *Proc. 17th Int. Symp. Circuits and Systems*, Montreal, pp. 530–533, 1984.
4. M. J. Chien, Piecewise linear modelling and simulation of nonlinear networks, *Int. J. Circuit Theory Appl.*, vol. 6, pp. 159–181, 1978.
5. J. A. DeRosie, P. H. Roe, and K. W. Hippel, Hierarchical interconnection of solved subsystems using explicit multiterminal representations, *Proc. 13th Int. Symp. Circuits and Systems*, Houston, pp. 1015–1019, 1980.
6. B. C. Eaves, The linear complementarity problem, *Manage. Sci.*, vol. 17, pp. 612–634, 1971.
7. J. T. J. van Eijndhoven, A piecewise linear simulator for large scale integrated circuits, Ph.D. thesis, Eindhoven Univ. of Technology, Eindhoven, The Netherlands, 1984.
8. J. T. J. van Eijndhoven, Solving the linear complementarity problem in circuit simulation, *SIAM J. Control Optimization*, vol. 24, no. 5, pp. 1050–1062, 1986.
9. T. Fujisawa, E. S. Kuh, and T. Ohtsuki, A sparse matrix method for analysis of piecewise-linear resistive networks, *IEEE Trans. Circuit Theory*, vol. CT-19, pp. 571–584, 1972.
10. S. Karamardian, The complementarity problem, *Math. Program.*, vol. 2, pp. 107–129, 1972.
11. G. van der Laan and A. J. J. Talman, Convergence and properties of recent variable dimension algorithms, in *Numerical Solution of Highly*

Nonlinear Problems: Fixed Point Algorithms and Complementarity Problems, W. Forster, ed., pp. 3–36, North-Holland, Amsterdam, 1980.

12. E. Lelarasmee, A. E. Ruehli, and A. L. Sangiovanni-Vincentelli, The waveform relaxation method for time-domain analysis of large scale integrated circuits, *IEEE Trans. Computer-Aided Design of Integrated Circuits and Systems*, vol. CAD-1, pp. 131–145, 1982.
13. C. E. Lemke, Bimatrix equilibrium points and mathematical programming, *Manage. Sci.*, vol. 11, pp. 681–689, 1965.
14. C. E. Lemke, On complementary pivot theory, in *Nonlinear Programming* (Proceedings of a Symposium) J. B. Rosen, O. L. Mangasarian, and K. Ritter, eds., pp. 349–384, Academic Press, New York, 1968.
15. O. L. Mangasarian, Solution of symmetric linear complementarity problems by iterative methods, *J. Optimization Theory Appl.*, vol. 22, pp. 465–485, 1977.
16. C. van de Panne, A complementary variant of Lemke's method for the linear complementary program, *Math. Program.*, vol. 7, pp. 283–310, 1974.
17. N. B. G. Rabbat, A. L. Sangiovanni-Vincentelli, and H. Y. Hsieh, A multilevel Newton algorithm with macromodeling and latency for the analysis of large-scale nonlinear circuits in the time domain, *IEEE Trans. Circuits Syst.*, vol. CAS-26, pp. 733–741, 1979.
18. M. Vlach, LU decomposition and forward-backward substitution of recursive bordered block diagonal matrices, *Proc. 16th Int. Symp. Circuits and Systems*, Newport Beach, Calif., pp. 427–430, 1984.
19. Q. Yu and O. Wing, PLMAP: A piecewise linear MOS circuit analysis program, *Proc. 17th Int. Symp. Circuits and Systems*, Montreal, pp. 530–533, 1984.

4

Decomposition Techniques in Circuit Simulation

Martin Vlach

Analogy, Inc.
Beaverton, Oregon

Decomposition methods are applied to the problem of solving large networks using piecewise linear approximation. It is shown that the standard Katzenelson algorithm has execution time proportional to the square of the size of the network. Two new methods of structural decomposition and relaxation are described and shown to be superior to the standard algorithm. In particular, the relaxation method exhibits linear growth of execution time with the network size. These results are demonstrated on a metal-oxide-semiconductor (MOS) network.

1 INTRODUCTION

Piecewise linear (PL) approximation has often been used in analyzing nonlinear systems over the last decade and a half. Starting with the original work of Katzenelson [1], many authors have considered the theoretical and practical aspects of the problem [2–11] and several network simulators employing the PL approximation have appeared [12–16]. All of these efforts, however, were concerned with fairly small networks, with several tens of transistors at most.

Here we will take a fresh look at the Katzenelson algorithm from the point of view of large systems, identify its shortcomings, and propose new methods of analyzing large piecewise linear systems.

The first step will be to review and analyze the standard Katzenelson algorithm. We will show that its execution time is proportional to the square of the size of the system. We will then apply decomposition techniques, which were so successfully used in the third-generation simulators [17], to the problem of analyzing large PL systems.

The starting point will be a functional decomposition of the system specified by a hierarchical input language. The two methods of structural decomposition and relaxation (also known as temporal decomposition) will be applied to the problem of next region determination in the Katzenelson algorithm. Structural decomposition of the linear problem (node tearing) is used throughout for the solution of the linear system of equations (see Chapter 2).

We will be able to show that the structural decomposition leads to an algorithm which is faster than n^2. We will also show that the relaxation methods lead to an algorithm those execution time is proportional to the size of the network.

Results of a numerical experiment will be presented to confirm the linear growth of the execution time of the relaxation algorithm with the size of the network, in contrast to the quadratic behavior of the Katzenelson algorithm.

2 THE KATZENELSON ALGORITHM IN REVIEW

In this section we will review the Katzenelson algorithm for solving the nonlinear system of equations

$$\mathbf{f}(\mathbf{x}) = \mathbf{y} \tag{1}$$

where $\mathbf{f}\colon \mathbf{R}^n \to \mathbf{R}^n$ is a continuous PL mapping.

Since $\mathbf{f}$ is piecewise linear, we can represent it as

$$\mathbf{f}(\mathbf{x}) = \mathbf{J}^{(i)}\mathbf{x} + \mathbf{w}^{(i)} \qquad i = 1, 2, \ldots$$

where $\mathbf{J}^{(i)}$ is a constant $n \times n$ matrix and $\mathbf{w}^{(i)}$ is a constant n-vector, each defined in a region R_i of the $\mathbf{R}^n$ space.

In the Katzenelson algorithm a solution to (1) is found by an iterative process starting from an initial guess $\mathbf{x}^{(0)}$ which is in the initial region R_0. Geometrically, the process can be described as follows:

Obtain the image of $\mathbf{x}^{(0)}$ under $\mathbf{f}$:

$$\mathbf{y}^{(0)} = \mathbf{f}(\mathbf{x}^{(0)}) = \mathbf{J}^{(0)}\mathbf{x}^{(0)} + \mathbf{w}^{(0)} \tag{2}$$

Join this point $\mathbf{y}^{(0)}$ to the required right-hand-side vector $\mathbf{y}$ by a straight line in the range space, and trace the inverse image of this line in the $\mathbf{x}$ space. This path in the $\mathbf{x}$ space will join the initial point $\mathbf{x}^{(0)}$ to the solution of (1). The portion of this path in the initial region can be found as follows: From (1) and (2)

$$\mathbf{J}^{(0)}\mathbf{x} + \mathbf{w}^{(0)} = \mathbf{y}$$

$$\mathbf{J}^{(0)}\mathbf{x}^{(0)} + \mathbf{w}^{(0)} = \mathbf{y}^{(0)}$$

Combining,

$$\mathbf{J}^{(0)}(\mathbf{x} - \mathbf{x}^{(0)}) = \mathbf{y} - \mathbf{y}^{(0)}$$

$$\mathbf{x} = \mathbf{x}^{(0)} + \mathbf{J}^{(0)^{-1}}(\mathbf{y} - \mathbf{y}^{(0)})$$

We have thus found the direction of movement

$$\mathbf{d}^{(0)} = \mathbf{J}^{(0)^{-1}}(\mathbf{y} - \mathbf{y}^{(0)}) \tag{3}$$

in the region R_0. If $\mathbf{x} = \mathbf{x}^{(0)} + \mathbf{d}^{(0)}$ lies in the same region as $\mathbf{x}^{(0)}$, R_0, a solution of (1) is found. Otherwise, determine $\lambda^{(0)}$ such that

$$\mathbf{x}^{(1)} = \mathbf{x}^{(0)} + \lambda^{(0)}\mathbf{d}^{(0)} \tag{4}$$

lies on the boundary of R_0. Find the new region R_1 on the other side of this boundary, let $\mathbf{y}^{(1)} = \mathbf{J}^{(1)}\mathbf{x}^{(1)} + \mathbf{w}^{(1)}$, and obtain the new direction of movement

$$\mathbf{d}^{(1)} = \mathbf{J}^{(1)^{-1}}(\mathbf{y} - \mathbf{y}^{(1)})$$

This process of finding a λ which brings the trajectory to a new boundary of the current region and updating to the new region is repeated until a solution is found. As a shortcut to determining $\mathbf{y} - \mathbf{y}^{(1)}$, it can be shown that

$$\mathbf{y} - \mathbf{y}^{(1)} = (1 - \lambda^{(0)})(\mathbf{y} - \mathbf{y}^{(0)}) \tag{5}$$

This follows easily from the continuity of the PL functions, since on the boundary between regions 0 and 1

$$\mathbf{J}^{(0)}\mathbf{x}^{(1)} + \mathbf{w}^{(0)} = \mathbf{J}^{(1)}\mathbf{x}^{(1)} + \mathbf{w}^{(1)}$$

Necessary and sufficient conditions for the algorithm to converge to a unique solution from any initial point $\mathbf{x}^{(0)}$ are as follows:

1. The $\mathbf{J}$ matrices in all the regions are nonsingular.
2. Their determinant signs do not change.
3. The trajectory does not reach a corner (an intersection of two or more boundaries).
4. There is a finite number of regions which cover the entire $\mathbf{x}$ space $\mathbf{R}^n$.

The reasons for these conditions, briefly stated, are that they

1. Guarantee that the direction $\mathbf{d}$ is uniquely defined.

2. Guarantee that the direction is away from a just-crossed boundary and into a new region. It is also a necessary condition for the existence of a unique solution.
3. Guarantee that the new region to be entered is uniquely determined.
4. Guarantee that a solution is found in a finite number of steps, since it can be shown that no region will be reeentered.

In practice, the most restrictive is condition 2, but a simple modification to the algorithm is possible in the case when 2 is violated. In the modified algorithm, the direction of movement in a new region R_i is determined from

$$\mathbf{d}^{(i)} = +\mathbf{J}^{(i)(i)^{-1}}(\mathbf{y} - \mathbf{y}^{(i)}) \qquad \text{if} \quad \text{sign}(\det \mathbf{J}^{(0)}) = \text{sign}(\det \mathbf{J}^{(i)})$$

$$\mathbf{d}^{(i)} = -\mathbf{J}^{(i)^{-1}}(\mathbf{y} - \mathbf{y}^{(i)}) \qquad \text{if} \quad \text{sign}(\det \mathbf{J}^{(0)}) \neq \text{sign}(\det \mathbf{J}^{(i)}) \tag{6}$$

In this modified algorithm, the convergence is no longer guaranteed for all initial points $\mathbf{x}^{(0)}$, but looping occurs rarely in practical problems and can be detected.

Complete discussions of the algorithm and proofs can be found in Refs. [6] and [8]. The "corner problem" (condition 3) and singular Jacobian matrices (condition 1) are also treated and relaxed there.

3 ANALYSIS OF THE KATZENELSON ALGORITHM

Let us summarize the algorithm for easy reference:

The Katzenelson algorithm

1. Choose an initial point $\mathbf{x}^{(0)}$.
2. Find the corresponding R_0 and the PL coefficients $\mathbf{J}^{(0)}$ and $\mathbf{w}^{(0)}$.
3. Perform initial processing:
   Obtain $\mathbf{r}^{(0)} = \mathbf{y} - \mathbf{w}^{(0)}$.
   Perform LU decomposition on $\mathbf{J}^{(0)}$.
   Set $i = 0$.
4. Solve $\mathbf{J}^{(i)}\tilde{\mathbf{x}} + \mathbf{w}^{(i)} = \mathbf{y}$ for $\tilde{\mathbf{x}}$, that is,

$$\tilde{\mathbf{x}} = \mathbf{J}^{(i)^{-1}}(\mathbf{y} - \mathbf{w}^{(i)}) = \mathbf{J}^{(i)^{-1}}\mathbf{r}^{(i)} \tag{7}$$

   Let

$$\mathbf{d}^{(i)} = \pm(\tilde{\mathbf{x}} - \mathbf{x}^{(i)}) \tag{8}$$

   where the plus sign is used if the signs of $\det \mathbf{J}^{(0)}$ and $\det \mathbf{J}^{(i)}$ are the same, the minus sign otherwise.
5. Find positive $\lambda^{(i)} \leqslant 1$ such that

$$\mathbf{x}^{(i+1)} = \mathbf{x}^{(i)} + \lambda^{(i)}\mathbf{d}^{(i)} \tag{9}$$

   is on a boundary of R_i.

If no such $\lambda^{(i)}$ exists, $\tilde{\mathbf{x}}$ is in R_i and a solution is found. Stop. Else

6. Update information for the new region. This includes identifying the new region R_{i+1}, finding the new coefficients $\mathbf{J}^{(i+1)}$ and $\mathbf{w}^{(i+1)}$, and updating the LU decomposition of $\mathbf{J}^{(i+1)}$ and the vector $\mathbf{r}^{(i+1)}$.
7. Set $i = i + 1$ and go to step 4.

This algorithm differs slightly from the classical one in the choice of the right-hand side in the linear system (7), and therefore in the computation of $\mathbf{d}^{(i)}$, although the direction is the same as in (3):

$$\begin{aligned}\mathbf{d}^{(i)} = \pm(\tilde{\mathbf{x}} - \mathbf{x}^{(i)}) &= \pm[\mathbf{J}^{(i)^{-1}}(\mathbf{y} - \mathbf{w}^{(i)}) - \mathbf{x}^{(i)}] \\ &= \pm\mathbf{J}^{(i)^{-1}}[\mathbf{y} - (\mathbf{J}^{(i)}\mathbf{x}^{(i)} + \mathbf{w}^{(i)})] \\ &= \pm\mathbf{J}^{(i)^{-1}}(\mathbf{y} - \mathbf{y}^{(i)})\end{aligned}$$

We will postpone the discussion of the reasons for this modification for the moment.

Let us now look at some details of the algorithm when applied to a solution of piecewise linear networks.

Consider first the choice of the initial point $\mathbf{x}^{(0)}$ (step 1 in the algorithm). The two analyses we are interested in are finding the operating point of a network (DC analysis) and obtaining its transient behavior (transient analysis).

For the operating point analysis, the system to be solved is

$$\mathbf{g}(\mathbf{x}) = \mathbf{j} \tag{10}$$

For purposes of the discussion, we will assume that the modified nodal formulation was used to describe the system consisting of an interconnection of linear and nonlinear elements. Then in (10) $\mathbf{x}$ represents the independent variables, which include the nodal voltages and certain branch currents; $\mathbf{g}(\cdot)$ describes the resistive elements and their interconnections; and $\mathbf{j}$ contains the independent current and voltage source values. The initial point $\mathbf{x}^{(0)}$ may be specified by the user, in which case it is likely to be a previous solution with a somewhat different right-hand side $\mathbf{j}$. In the absence of such guidance, $\mathbf{x}^{(0)} = 0$ is a good practical choice.

For the transient analysis, integration must be performed on the system of differential-algebraic equations

$$\frac{d\mathbf{q}(\mathbf{x})}{dt} + \mathbf{g}(\mathbf{x}) = \mathbf{j}(t)$$

where $\mathbf{J}$ is now a function of time, and $\mathbf{q}$ models the dynamic properties of the network and includes charges and fluxes. A numerical integration algorithm must be used to obtain the transient response. For simplicity, we will use the Euler backward differentiation formula. At each time step, the following nonlinear system of equations must be solved:

$$\frac{1}{h}\mathbf{q}(\mathbf{x}_n) + \mathbf{g}(\mathbf{x}_n) = \mathbf{j}(t_n) + \frac{1}{h}\mathbf{q}(\mathbf{x}_{n-1})$$

or

$$\mathbf{f}(\mathbf{x}) = \mathbf{y} \tag{11}$$

where $\mathbf{f}(\mathbf{x}) = (1/h)\mathbf{q}(\mathbf{x}_n) + \mathbf{g}(\mathbf{x}_n)$ is a piecewise linear function and $\mathbf{y} = \mathbf{j}(t_n) + (1/h)\mathbf{q}(\mathbf{x}_{n-1})$ is a constant right-hand-side vector at each time step. We dropped the subscript n in writing $\mathbf{f}(\mathbf{x})$ since our problem is now the solution of the nonlinear system (11). The initial point $\mathbf{x}^{(0)}$ may be reasonably chosen either as the solution from the previous time step, $\mathbf{x}^{(0)} = \mathbf{x}_{n-1}$, or from a predictor algorithm.

Notice that in all of these cases convergence of the Katzenelson algorithm is *not* guaranteed if the sign(det $\mathbf{J}^{(i)}$) is not the same in all regions [8]. In practice, choosing a "theoretically approved" initial point as discussed in [8] may be expensive, and would in general require a great deal of additional work in solving the system, especially in cases where $\mathbf{x}^{(0)}$ is close to the solution, as in the integration algorithm.

The next step is to find the initial region R_0 corresponding to the initial point $\mathbf{x}^{(0)}$. In our approach, each nonlinear element is described (possibly as an approximation to a smooth function) by a PL function. A region for the global PL function $\mathbf{f}$ consists of a union of the regions for each nonlinear element. Finding R_0 therefore consists of finding the initial region for each element in turn, and is proportional to the number of elements, n_e. (Strictly speaking, it is proportional to the total number of independent variables for all of the nonlinearities, but this is not important for the purposes of the present discussion.) During transient analysis without predictor, the region is already known from a previous time step ($\mathbf{x}_n{}^{(0)} = \mathbf{x}_{n-1}$) and step 2 can be skipped.

Because special updating techniques may be used later, the LU decomposition of $\mathbf{J}^{(0)}$ and the vector subtraction $\mathbf{r}^{(0)} = \mathbf{y} - \mathbf{w}^{(0)}$ needed in step 4 are also performed before the iteration loop is entered. Each of these steps is proportional to n_n, the number of variables in the network.

Inside the iterative loop starting with step 4, $\tilde{\mathbf{x}}$ is found by forward and back substitution, based on the LU decomposition of $\mathbf{J}^{(i)}$ and $\mathbf{r}^{(i)}$, and $\mathbf{d}^{(i)}$ is evaluated. These steps are all proportional to n_n.

The next boundary to be crossed, or equivalently the new region to be entered, must now be determined (step 5) by finding $\lambda^{(i)}$. Just as in the initial region determination, the λ parameter for each element must be found, and the overall λ is obtained from

$$\lambda = \min_{\text{all elements}} \lambda_{\text{single element}} \tag{12}$$

Determining λ at each iteration is thus proportional to the number of elements n_e (same remark as for finding the initial region applies).

Once λ is found, the next region to be entered must be determined, new coefficients **J** and **w** found, and the LU decomposition and the right-hand-side vector updated. Finding the new PL coefficients requires evaluation of the model for a single device and is independent of the size of the problem. Since $\mathbf{J}^{(i+1)}$ and $\mathbf{J}^{(i)}$ differ by (at most) a dyad, special updating of the LU decomposition may be performed [18] to save execution time. However, the process can become unstable, especially with multiple updates, and an occasional full decomposition should be done. In our implementation, the updating technique available with the hierarchical decomposition is used. It is of order less than n_n.

The difference between the two right-hand sides is

$$\mathbf{r}^{(i+1)} - \mathbf{r}^{(i)} = (\mathbf{y} - \mathbf{w}^{(i+1)}) - (\mathbf{y} - \mathbf{w}^{(i)}) = \mathbf{w}^{(i)} - \mathbf{w}^{(i+1)}$$

and so

$$\mathbf{r}^{(i+1)} = \mathbf{r}^{(i)} + (\mathbf{w}^{(i)} - \mathbf{w}^{(i+1)})$$

However, since only a single element changed a region,

$$\mathbf{w}^{(i)} - \mathbf{w}^{(i+1)}$$

is very sparse, having only as many nonzero entries as there are terminals for the element which changed region, and only a few additions are involved in updating **r** irrespective of the size of the problem. The cost of updating **r** is thus insignificant.

Let us recapitulate some of the points. The preliminary steps of finding R_0, the LU decomposition, and $\mathbf{r}^{(0)}$ are proportional to n_e and n_n. In a single iteration loop, obtaining $\tilde{\mathbf{x}}$ and $\mathbf{d}^{(i)}$ is proportional to n_n, finding λ is proportional to n_e, and updating for the next iteration is of order less than n_n.

In networks, n_e is proportional to n_n: at least two elements are connected at each node, and the maximum number of elements connected at a node may depend on the function of the network, but not on its size.

We can therefore say that a single iteration is proportional to the size of the network, measured by the number of nodes or the number of elements.

Unfortunately, the number of iterations necessary to find a solution are also proportional to the number of elements: in general, each element will cross several region boundaries before a solution is found. The exact number of regions crossed depends, of course, on the behavior of the network and in time domain sections of the network may be idle at times, but ultimately each nonlinear element will change region—otherwise it would perform no useful function.

The execution time of the Katzenelson algorithm is proportional to the square of the size of the network. The bottleneck, as observed on many simulation runs, is the determination of λ at each iteration.

4 STRUCTURAL DECOMPOSITION

One possible avenue of approach to speeding up an algorithm is to decompose the problem into smaller subproblems, solve each separately, and combine the results to obtain an overall solution. We will now analyze such an approach to speeding up the λ determination in a Katzenelson algorithm applied to partitioned networks.

By applying partitioning, the overall network is split into subnetworks, each of which may be further subdivided into lower-level subnetworks, and so on to an arbitrary depth. The determination of λ, which is found according to (12) when no partitioning is applied, can be found from

$$\lambda = \min_{\text{all subnetworks}} \lambda_{\text{single subnetwork}} \tag{13}$$

when the network is partitioned. For each subnetwork, λ is determined according to (13) or (12), depending on whether a given subnetwork is further subdivided into lower-level subnetworks or not.

This recursive algorithm may be easily visualized on graphical representation of the network. The hierarchical structure of a network is described by a tree (Figure 4.1). Each tree node has a λ association with it. The λ at each node is the minimum of the λ's associated with all of its sons [expression (13)]. For the leaves, (12) is used to obtain their λ.

The effort needed to determine the overall λ can be reduced substantiallv if it can be determined *a priori* that a λ for some tree node does not change from one iteration to the next, or if the new λ for a subnetwork can be found cheaply. By partitioning the network, we are also forcing a partition of the independent variables $\mathbf{x}$ into sets of independent variables $\mathbf{x}^k$, one for each subnetwork. The overall λ at iteration i is found from

$$\lambda^{(i)} = \min_k \lambda^{k(i)} \tag{14}$$

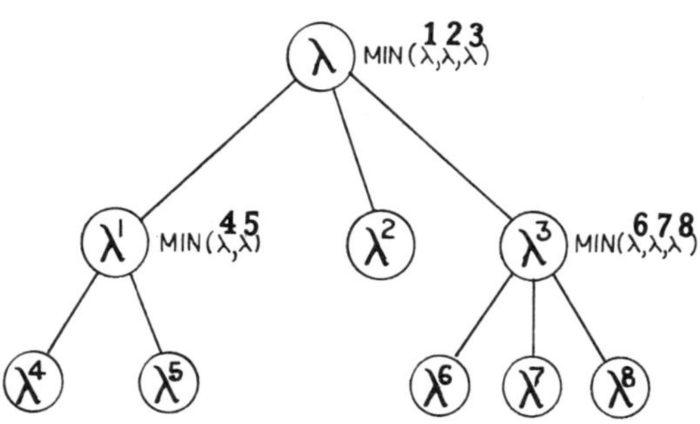

Figure 4.1 Tree representation of a partitioned network.

where each λ^k is such that [see (13) and (9)]

$$\mathbf{x}^{k(i)} + \lambda^{k(i)}(\tilde{\mathbf{x}}^{k(i)} - \mathbf{x}^{k(i)}) \tag{15}$$

is on a boundary in subcircuit k. Since the new point $\mathbf{x}^{k(i+1)}$ is strictly inside the current region except for that subnetwork for which the minimum in (14) is attained, the λ^k in the next iteration is easily obtained, *provided* $\tilde{\mathbf{x}}^k$ *did not change*, and the direction of movement is the same [sign(det $\mathbf{J}^{(i)}$) does not change]. The next iteration's λ^k is obtained from the condition that the point

$$\mathbf{x}^{k(i+1)} + \lambda^{k(i+1)}(\tilde{\mathbf{x}}^{k(i+1)} - \mathbf{x}^{k(i+1)}) \tag{16}$$

is on a boundary of subcircuit **k** [compare (15)]. Recall that from the algorithm

$$\mathbf{x}^{k(i+1)} = \mathbf{x}^{k(i)} + \lambda^{(i)}(\tilde{\mathbf{x}}^{k(i)} - \mathbf{x}^{k(i)}) \tag{17}$$

and so $\mathbf{x}^{k(i+1)}$ lies on the line joining $\mathbf{x}^{k(i)}$ and $\tilde{\mathbf{x}}^{k(i)}$. Now, if $\tilde{\mathbf{x}}^{k(i+1)} = \tilde{\mathbf{x}}^{k(i)}$, the boundary intersection found in (15) is the same point as that to be determined from (16), and so we can equate (15) and (16):

$$\mathbf{x}^{k(i+1)} + \lambda^{k(i+1)}(\tilde{\mathbf{x}}^{k(i+1)} - \mathbf{x}^{k(i+1)}) = \mathbf{x}^{k(i)} + \lambda^{k(i)}(\tilde{\mathbf{x}}^{k(i)} - \mathbf{x}^{k(i)}) \tag{18}$$

Substituting (17) into (18) and noting that $\tilde{\mathbf{x}}^{k(i+1)} = \tilde{\mathbf{x}}^{k(i)}$,

$$\mathbf{x}^{k(i)} + \lambda^{(i)}(\tilde{\mathbf{x}}^{k(i)} - \mathbf{x}^{k(i)}) + \lambda^{k(i+1)}(\tilde{\mathbf{x}}^{k(i)} - \mathbf{x}^{k(i)} - \lambda^{(i)}(\tilde{\mathbf{x}}^{k(i)} - \mathbf{x}^{k(i)}))$$
$$= \mathbf{x}^{k(i)} + \lambda^{k(i)}(\tilde{\mathbf{x}}^{k(i)} - \mathbf{x}^{k(i)})$$

Canceling the leading $\mathbf{x}^{k(i)}$ on both sides and dividing throughout by $(\tilde{\mathbf{x}}^{k(i)} - \mathbf{x}^{k(i)})$,

$$\lambda^{(i)} + \lambda^{k(i+1)}(1 - \lambda^{(i)}) = \lambda^{k(i)}$$

$$\lambda^{k(i+1)} = \frac{\lambda^{k(i)} - \lambda^{(i)}}{1 - \lambda^{(i)}} \tag{19}$$

Expression (19) gives the λ for subnetwork k at iteration $i + 1$ from the λ for subnetwork k at iteration i and the overall λ used at iteration i, *provided the solution* $\tilde{\mathbf{x}}^k$ *for subnetwork k did not change.*

From (19), we can derive an expression for $\lambda^{k(i+n)}$ which will prove useful in a hierarchical algorithm. First, write (19) as

$$1 - \lambda^{k(i+1)} = 1 - \frac{\lambda^{k(i)} - \lambda^{(i)}}{1 - \lambda^{(i)}} = \frac{1 - \lambda^{k(i)}}{1 - \lambda^{(i)}}$$

It is easy now to see that

$$1 - \lambda^{k(i+2)} = \frac{1 - \lambda^{k(i+1)}}{1 - \lambda^{(i+1)}} = \frac{1 - \lambda^{k(i)}}{(1 - \lambda^{(i)})(1 - \lambda^{(i+1)})}$$

and by induction

$$1 - \lambda^{k(i+n)} = \frac{1 - \lambda^{k(i)}}{\Pi_{j=0}^{n-1} (1 - \lambda^{(i+j)})}$$

Finally

$$\lambda^{k(i+n)} = 1 - \frac{1 - \lambda^{k(i)}}{\Pi_{j=0}^{n-1} (1 - \lambda^{(i+j)})} \tag{20}$$

which gives λ for a subcircuit when $\tilde{\mathbf{x}}^k$ did not change for several iterations.

4.1 Hierarchical Determination of λ

In a hierarchical system, whenever $\tilde{\mathbf{x}}^k$ for circuit k remains unchanged, so do *all* $\tilde{\mathbf{x}}^j$ for all lower-level subsystems, and when $\tilde{\mathbf{x}}^k$ does change, *some* of the $\tilde{\mathbf{x}}^j$ may remain unchanged. To fully utilize the potential savings, some way must be found to keep track of the product indicated in (20) for each subnetwork. Overall λ may be obtained by the recursive procedure *lambda* below. In the procedure, the following variables defined for each subnetwork k are needed:

$\bar{\lambda}^k$	is $1 - \lambda^{k(i)}$ determined when $\tilde{\mathbf{x}}^k$ last changed.
p^k	is the product of the $(1 - \lambda)$ terms from the iteration when $\tilde{\mathbf{x}}^k$ last changed to the iteration when $\tilde{\mathbf{x}}^{(\text{parent of } k)}$ last changed. p^k is initialized to 1.
update^k	is a flag which is set when $\bar{\lambda}^k$ is valid. It is reset initially and also when subnetwork k reaches a boundary. This is necessary since it may happen that $\mathbf{J}^{(i)} = \mathbf{J}^{(i+1)}$, in which case $\bar{\mathbf{x}}^k$ would not change but $\bar{\lambda}^k$ is no longer valid. In this case, the update flag is reset for circuit k and all its ancestors.
p	is the product of the $(1 - \lambda)$ terms from the iteration when $\tilde{\mathbf{x}}^{(\text{parent of } k)}$ last changed to the present iteration.

The procedure is first invoked for the root network with $p = 1 - \lambda^{(i)}$ for the current iteration i.

---

procedure lambda(k, p)

  $p^k = p^k \times p$ Note 1

  if ($\tilde{\mathbf{x}}^k$ is unchanged and update^k is set) then

$$\lambda = 1 - \frac{\bar{\lambda}^k}{p^k} \qquad \text{Note 2}$$

  else

    $\lambda = 1$

determine λ for all nonlinear elements of circuit k Note 3
for all subcircuits j of circuit k (if any) Note 4

$\lambda = \min(\lambda, \text{lambda}\ (j, p^k)$

$p^k = 1$
$\bar{\lambda}^k = 1 - \lambda$
update^k = set
end if
end lambda

Note 1: Assures that p^k includes all the $1 - \lambda$ terms in the product.
Note 2: Determines λ if updating according to (20) is possible.
Note 3: All nonlinearities of circuit k are scanned, λ determined for each, and their minimum is taken.
Note 4: Determines λ according to (13); for the leaf circuits, this step is in effect skipped.

4.2 Discussion of the Structural Decomposition

The structural decomposition algorithm depends for its efficiency on the assumption that $\tilde{\mathbf{x}}^k$ will remain unchanged from one iteration to the next for most of the subsystems.

This in turn depends on the kind of the system being analyzed and the type of modeling and approximation used. From the point of view of structural decomposition, a change in a subnetwork ideally should not affect any other subnetworks, but then no useful function would be performed. The best one can hope for is that a change in a subnetwork will influence only some of the other subnetworks in the system. Such behavior is exhibited by systems built from one-way macromodels of logic gates: A change at an output of a gate cannot influence its inputs. With one-way models, however, a change can propagate forward arbitrarily far, and when feedback is present in the system as a whole it may even reach the inputs of the gate under consideration. In order to restrict the influence of a change of a PL region of a gate to only a small set of surrounding gates, we must restrict the gate models to what we shall call isolating gates.

In an isolating gate, a change in input does not influence the output except in some transition region. As an example, consider a simple inverter, whose transfer characteristic is shown in Figure 4.2: In both the ON and OFF regions, the output is constant and within each region is thus independent of the input. We can relax the one-way property somewhat along similar lines, and require that the output influences the input only in a part of the

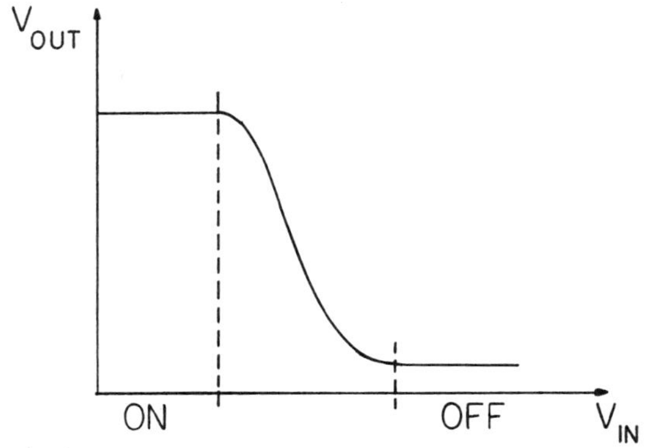

Figure 4.2 An isolating inverter.

operating region of the subnetwork. If a system consists of such "mostly one-way" isolating gates, a change in the behavior of a subnetwork due to a boundary crossing will have a ripple effect through surrounding subnetworks until some gate is reached which blocks this signal propagation.

The hierarchical λ determination may reduce the total execution time substantially if the system being simulated has the properties outlined above. If a change in a region of a gate is confined to some small set of topologically near gates for *all* iterations and *all* gates, the execution time will no longer be proportional to n^2. Although the same number of iterations will be needed, each iteration will now be of order less than n.

With hierarchical representation of the system matrix, the forward substitution is needed only for that subnetwork which changed last and its ancestors. By assumption, there will be a part of the system whose solution $\tilde{\mathbf{x}}^k$ does not change, and the backward substitution will not be needed for any of the offspring of network k. Step 4 of the Katzenelson algorithm is thus of order less than n.

The hierarchical determination of λ in step 5 is again of order less than n, since by assumption there are subnetworks whose λ can be updated rather than evaluated in full. As already discussed, step 6 is of order less than n in hierarchical systems.

In the operating point (DC) analysis of MOS digital circuits it was observed that a change in one gate is indeed confined to its vicinity; that is, there are networks at each iteration whose $\tilde{\mathbf{x}}^k$ does not change. This is due to the one-way behavior of MOS transistors and the fact that in the model used in the analyses $I_{ds} = 0$ for $V_{gs} < V_T$ (the isolation property). The DC analysis of these networks is thus a good candidate for structural decomposition.

In the transient analysis, however, the C_{gs} and C_{gd} capacitances provide a bidirectional path through every transistor in every region of operation. A change in a region in one gate is not confined to the vicinity of the gate, and λ must be recalculated for all gates.

5 RELAXATION DECOMPOSITION

Relaxation or indirect methods [19] are usually called "temporal decomposition" methods in the context of third-generation circuit simulators [17]. In relaxation methods, a given problem is subdivided into subproblems and each subproblem is solved separately, keeping the independent variables of all the other subproblems fixed. Well-known examples include the Jacobi and Gauss-Seidel iterations for linear or nonlinear systems. Classically, systems of equations are solved one equation at a time for a single variable; examples include simulators such as MOTIS [20] and SPLICE [21]. In some simulators, like DIANA [22], block relaxation methods are used, where small blocks of equations are solved simultaneously, applying the relaxation to these blocks.

5.1 Introduction

In this section we will describe a block relaxation algorithm applied to the solution of piecewise linear systems of equations. The relaxation method relies on the fact that when a PL region where the solution lies is known, finding the solution involves only solving a linear system. In the algorithm, the parameters which are kept constant for each block are the PL *coefficients* of the inactive blocks, rather than their independent variables.

We can give the following interpretation of the algorithm in terms of networks and nodal analysis. Figure 4.3 shows the classical case, where a single equation (Kirchhoff's current law at a node) is solved for that nodal voltage, with all other nodal voltages kept constant. Only those elements connected to the node are considered, with the rest of the network in effect replaced by constant independent voltage sources. In classical block relaxation algorithms, a block of equations may be solved simultaneously for several node voltages, but the external network is still modeled by constant sources.

In the proposed algorithm, the basic block consists of several nonlinear elements forming, for example, a gate, and usually includes several internal nodes. All the remaining blocks in the network are then linearized according to their current region, and a solution is obtained for the active nonlinear block embedded in this linear network. The situation is as shown in Figure 4.4. The external network is modeled by constant independent voltage sources *and* a resistive network. The resistive part of the external linearized

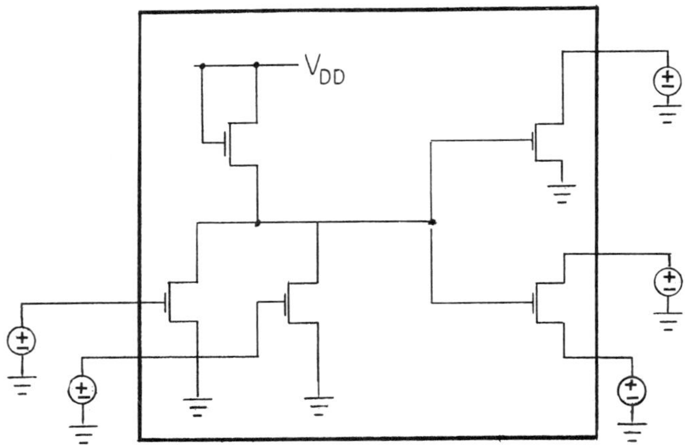

Figure 4.3 Illustration of a classical relaxation algorithm.

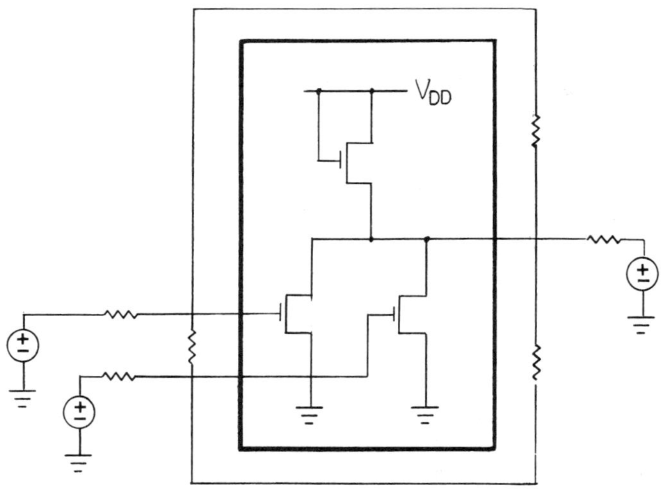

Figure 4.4 Illustration of the PL relaxation algorithm.

network approximates the loading effects on the block under consideration, and any of the external resistors may be zero (short circuit) or infinite (open circuit). In the MOS example, there will be nonzero loading of the output node in transient analysis. It is due to the companion models of the capacitances associated with the various devices.

Before describing the relaxation algorithm in detail, we will establish some ideas about partitioning of a network and some related notation. Consider a system which is built from subsystems. The variables of each subsystem i may be partitioned into internal and external variables $\mathbf{x}^{I_i}$ and $\mathbf{x}^{E_i}$

$$\mathbf{x}^i = \begin{bmatrix} \mathbf{x}^{I_i} \\ \mathbf{x}^{E_i} \end{bmatrix}$$

The description of the subsystem may be similarly partitioned into

$$\mathbf{g}^i(\mathbf{x}^i) = \begin{bmatrix} \mathbf{g}^{I_i}(\mathbf{x}^{I_i}, \mathbf{x}^{E_i}) \\ \mathbf{g}^{E_i}(\mathbf{x}^{I_i}, \mathbf{x}^{E_i}) \end{bmatrix} = 0$$

where the internal part $\mathbf{g}^{I_i}$ includes KCL equations for each internal node and possibly additional equations arising from the modified nodal (MN) formulation, and the external part $\mathbf{g}^{E_i}$ gives the terminal currents. When we interconnect N of these blocks in a network, the description becomes

$$\begin{aligned} &\mathbf{g}^{I_1}(\mathbf{x}^{I_1}, \mathbf{x}^{E_1}) = 0 \\ &\qquad \cdots \\ &\mathbf{g}^{I_N}(\mathbf{x}^{I_N}, \mathbf{x}^{E_N}) = 0 \\ &\sum_{i=1}^{N} \mathbf{S}^{i^T} \mathbf{g}^{E_i}(\mathbf{x}^{I_i}, \mathbf{x}^{E_i}) = 0 \end{aligned} \tag{21}$$

where the $\mathbf{S}^{i^T}$ are scattering matrices which define where the terminals of the blocks are connected. The last system of equations in (21) contains a KCL equation for each node in the interconnection network. In addition, we have a number of conditions relating the terminal voltages $\mathbf{x}^{E_i}$ via a set of nodal voltages in the interconnection network, $\mathbf{x}^C$:

$$\begin{aligned} &\mathbf{x}^{E_1} - \mathbf{S}^1\mathbf{X}^C = 0 \\ &\qquad \cdots \\ &\mathbf{x}^{E_N} - \mathbf{S}^N\mathbf{x}^C = 0 \end{aligned} \tag{22}$$

The system of equations (21) and (22) taken together describe the interconnected system; the independent variables of the entire system of equations are the internal variables $\mathbf{x}^{I_i}$ and the external nodal voltages $\mathbf{x}^{E_i}$ for each subnetwork plus the nodal voltages of the interconnection network $\mathbf{x}^C$:

$$\mathbf{x} = \begin{bmatrix} \mathbf{x}^{I_i} \\ \cdots \\ \mathbf{x}^{E_i} \\ \cdots \\ \mathbf{x}^C \end{bmatrix}$$

Notice that if equations (22) are substituted into (21), the modified nodal formulation results, with the equations and variables partitioned according to the subdivision into subnetworks.

We will also need notation for the linearization of a substystem. At iteration m, the values of the variables of a network are denoted by $\mathbf{x}^{i(m)}$. The *linearization* of subsystem i based on $\mathbf{x}^{i(m)}$ is

$$\mathbf{g}^i(\mathbf{x}^i) \approx \mathbf{J}^{i(m)}\mathbf{x}^i + \mathbf{w}^{i(m)}$$

and when split according to internal and external parts, this in turn becomes

$$\mathbf{g}^i(\mathbf{x}^i) \approx \begin{bmatrix} \mathbf{J}^{II_i(m)} & \mathbf{J}^{IE_i(m)} \\ \mathbf{J}^{EI_i(m)} & \mathbf{J}^{EE_i(m)} \end{bmatrix} \begin{bmatrix} \mathbf{x}^{I_i} \\ \mathbf{x}^{E_i} \end{bmatrix} + \begin{bmatrix} \mathbf{w}^{I_i(m)} \\ \mathbf{w}^{E_i(m)} \end{bmatrix} \tag{23}$$

Note that as long as $\mathbf{x}^i$ is in the same region as $\mathbf{x}^{i(m)}$, the expression in (23) is exact; only when $\mathbf{x}^i$ is in a new region will an approximation be involved.

5.2 The Relaxation Algorithm

With this notation, the block relaxation algorithm may now be stated:

PL block relaxation algorithm

1. Choose an initial vector $\mathbf{x}^{(0)}$. Set $m = 0$.
2. For $k = 1, 2, \ldots, N$ solve the system of equations (24) for $\mathbf{x}^{k(m+1)}$ by the Katzenelson algorithm, starting with the initial guess $\mathbf{x}^{k(m)}$:

$$[\mathbf{J}^{II_i(m+1)} \quad \mathbf{J}^{IE_i(m+1)}] \begin{bmatrix} \mathbf{x}^{I_i} \\ \mathbf{x}^{E_i} \end{bmatrix} + \mathbf{w}^{I_i(m+1)} = 0 \qquad \text{for } i = 1, \ldots, k-1 \tag{24a}$$

$$\mathbf{g}^{I_k}(\mathbf{x}^{I_k}, \mathbf{x}^{E_k}) = 0 \tag{24b}$$

$$[\mathbf{J}^{II_i(m)} \quad \mathbf{J}^{IE_i(m)}] \begin{bmatrix} \mathbf{x}^{I_i} \\ \mathbf{x}^{E_i} \end{bmatrix} + \mathbf{w}^{I_i(m)} = 0 \qquad \text{for } i = k+1, \ldots, N \tag{24c}$$

$$\sum_{i=1}^{k-1} \mathbf{S}^{i^T} \left\{ [\mathbf{J}^{EI_i(m+1)} \quad \mathbf{J}^{EE_i(m+1)}] \begin{bmatrix} \mathbf{x}^{I_i} \\ \mathbf{x}^{E_i} \end{bmatrix} + \mathbf{w}^{E_i(m+1)} \right\}$$
$$+ \sum_{i=k+1}^{N} \mathbf{S}^{i^T} \left\{ [\mathbf{J}^{EI_i(m)} \quad \mathbf{J}^{EE_i(m)}] \begin{bmatrix} \mathbf{x}^{I_i} \\ \mathbf{x}^{E_i} \end{bmatrix} + \mathbf{w}^{E_i(m)} \right\} + \mathbf{g}^{E_k}(\mathbf{x}^{I_k}, \mathbf{x}^{E_k}) = 0 \tag{24d}$$

$$\mathbf{x}^{E_i} - \mathbf{S}^i\mathbf{x}^C = 0 \qquad i = 1, \ldots, N \tag{24e}$$

3. If any region changed in any of the N subproblems of step 2, set $m = m + 1$ and go to 2.
4. Stop.

Let us now discuss the various steps involved. First of all, as (24a)–(24e) show, the algorithm uses "successive displacement" rather than "simultaneous displacement." The results of solving one subsystem are used immediately within the same iteration. This strategy is in fact easier to implement and saves storage, since only one version of $\mathbf{J}^i$ and $\mathbf{w}^i$ need be kept for each subsystem.

When solving the system (24), (24e) is substituted into (24a)–(24d), and the system is solved by hierarchical modified nodal formulation for the interconnected network. Only a sequence of $\mathbf{x}^{I_i(m)}$ and $\mathbf{x}^{E_i(m)}$ is ever calculated.

Notice that at any intermediate point in the execution of the algorithm, (24e) are not necessarily satisfied even if they were satisfied for the initial point $\mathbf{x}^{(0)}$. At termination of the algorithm, however, they will be satisfied automatically.

The algorithm depends for its efficiency on the success of the linearization approximation (23). If during step k of iteration m the solutions $\hat{\mathbf{x}}^i$ of (24), $i \neq k$, do not differ too much from the point where the linearization was taken ($\mathbf{x}^{i(m+1)}$ for $i < k$ and $\mathbf{x}^{i(m)}$ for $i > k$), the approximation (23) will be reasonable, and therefore $\mathbf{x}^{k(m+1)}$ will be a good approximation to the solution of the system (21). In fact, if all $\hat{\mathbf{x}}^i$ are in the same region as their corresponding linearization points, the solution of (21) has been found. This kind of behavior in turn will depend on the analysis being performed, the type of network simulated, and the approximation used.

In the transient analysis, the initial vector $\mathbf{x}^{(0)}$ of step 1 of the Katzenelson algorithm will be close to the solution, and its distance from the solution can be controlled by the selection of the time step.

The type of network and block selection also play an important role. In digital networks, the output of a gate is primarily governed by its inputs (and possibly its internal state), and a change in the loading will not affect the output value significantly. In the context of the relaxation algorithm, the linearization of the load at each iteration is reasonable.

The level of the piecewise linear approximation also will have an important effect: the larger the PL regions, the more likely it is that $\hat{\mathbf{x}}^i$ will remain in the same region as the linearization point.

There are of course cases when the algorithm does not converge. This has been observed on networks where there are feedback paths, and the external resistive network imposes no limit on the distance by which $\mathbf{x}^{k(m+1)}$ can move from $\mathbf{x}^{k(m)}$. A race condition where a gate moves to one extreme on one iteration and is then forced to the other extreme on the next iteration can then occur.

A particular example is the determination of an equilibrium point (DC analysis) of a ring oscillator. *This is of course an unstable equilibrium point.* In this case, since there is no loading on the inverter, it will be either completely

ON or completely OFF, with the opposite state on the next iteration. The undesirable property here is the "isolation property" of the network, described in a previous section, and the feedback path. It should be pointed out that in the transient analysis, when the isolation property is destroyed by the companion models of the various capacitances, the algorithm converges with any time step.

Let us now consider the advantages of the relaxation algorithm. As pointed out earlier, the bottleneck of the Katzenelson algorithm is the determination of λ at each iteration, since with hierarchical decomposition the other steps are of order less than n. The relaxation algorithm in effect decouples the problem into a series of smaller problems, each of size n_k. Although, as stated in (24), the system appears to have size n, the hierarchical decomposition allows us to view it as solving a system of size (24b) plus (24d). The λ determination problem is of course proportional to n_k. Each iteration of the relaxation algorithm is thus proportional to

$$\sum_{k=1}^{N} n_k{}^2 < \max_{1 \leqslant k \leqslant n} n_k \sum_{k=1}^{N} n_k = \alpha n$$

and therefore is proportional to the size of the overall system, since n_k (the size of a single block) depends on the type of the network but not on its size. The number of iterations needed in the relaxation will depend on the local interfaces between the subnetworks and therefore on their properties but *not* on their overall number.

The execution time of the relaxation algorithm is proportional to the size of the system.

6 NUMERICAL EXPERIMENT

To confirm the analyses of the Katzenelson and relaxation algorithms, transient analysis of the shift register latch (SRL) [23] was performed several times for different numbers of register bits.

The network is shown in Figure 4.5, with the details of the gates in Figure 4.6. The simulation was performed with piecewise linear approximation to the MOS transistors in each of the gates. To clearly bring out the properties of the algorithm and not mask them by details of the network operation, the simulated network did not include coupling between adjacent bits, which would normally be present for the shift register operation.

The transient analysis consisted of thirty 1-ns steps, with the clock going up once, and all other inputs remaining at zero. Each bit of the SRL contains 48 devices, 22 internal nodes, and 8 external terminals (including V_{DD}). The four-section network contained 192 MOS transistors and 114 variables. For

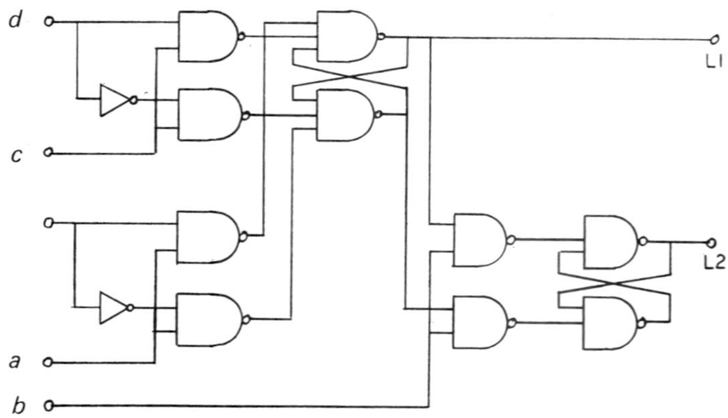

(a)

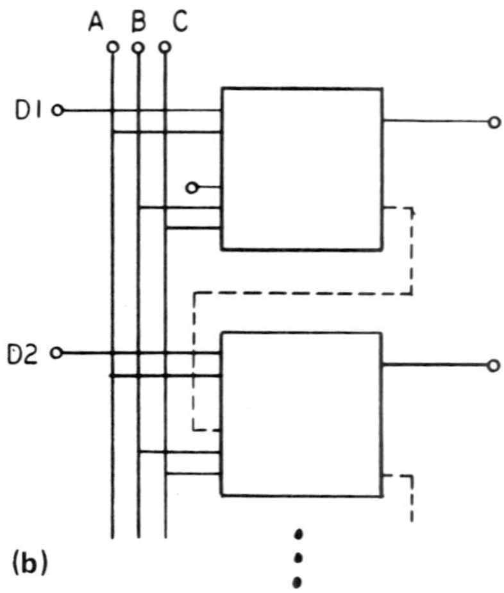

(b)

Figure 4.5 Shift register latch. (a) NAND implementation of an SRL; (b) test network.

the relaxation algorithm, the basic block was a single gate—an inverter and two- and three-input NAND gates.

The results of the execution time measurements are summarized in Table 4.1 for the relaxation algorithm and in Table 4.2 for the Katzenelson algorithm. The meaning of the various columns for the two tables is as follows:

# of bits	gives the number of the SRL register bits included in the network.

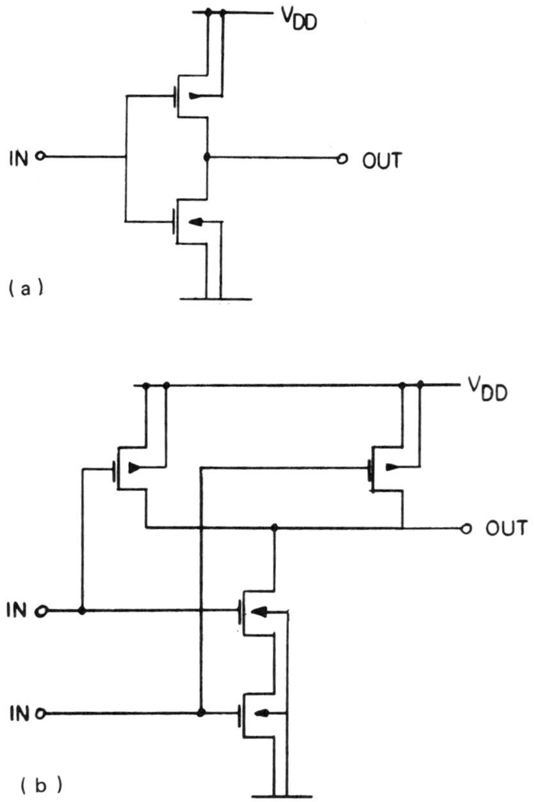

Figure 4.6 Details of the gates in the SRL. (a) Inverter; (b) two-input NAND.

Table 4.1 Execution Times for the Relaxation Algorithm

# of bits	# of iters	Total time (s)	% time for λ	Time for λ (s)	Time/iter (ms)	Time/λ (ms)
1	376	9.45	6.0%	0.57	25.1	1.52
2	752	21.08	4.9%	1.03	28.0	1.37
3	1128	34.02	5.3%	1.80	30.2	1.60
4	1504	49.03	5.0%	2.45	32.6	1.63

Table 4.2 Execution Times for the Katzenelson Algorithm

# of bits	# of iters	Total time (s)	% time for λ	Time for λ (s)	Time/iter (ms)	Time/λ (ms)
1	354	13.26	18.2%	2.41	37.5	6.8
2	708	38.30	27.9%	10.67	54.1	15.1
3	1062	75.85	32.4%	24.56	71.4	23.1
4	1416	125.39	35.5%	44.51	88.6	31.4

\# of iters — gives the total number of Katzenelson iterations used. For the relaxation algorithm, this is the sum of all the iterations needed in all relaxation step and all Katzenelson subproblems.

Total time — gives the total CPU execution time on an IBM 4341 computer.

% time for λ — gives the percentage of the total time spent in the λ determination routine.

Time for λ — is the total CPU execution time for λ determination.

Time/iter — is the CPU time per iteration.

Time/λ — is the CPU time per λ determination.

The last column of the tables illustrates perfectly the dependence of the λ determination on the size of the network for the two algorithm. For the relaxation algorithm, the time is indeed independent of the size of the system. For the Katzenelson algorithm, the time is indeed proportional to the size of the system. The "time for λ" column illustrates the overall behavior of the λ determination: linear with n in the relaxation algorithm, and quadratic with n for the Katzenelson algorithm.

The "total time" column does not reflect the predicted behavior for the following reasons: For the relaxation algorithm, the dominant portion of the algorithm is in fact the LU updating and forward and back substitution, which is somewhat worse than linear. The total execution time depends on the properties of the hierarchical decomposition rather than on the properties of the λ determination, which accounts for only a twentieth of the total CPU time. For the Katzenelson algorithm, the reason is somewhat similar. The λ determination is not yet completely dominant, and the better than n^2 behavior of the hierarchical decomposition improves the total CPU time dependence on the size of the system.

Comparison of the number of iterations of the two methods illustrates the success of the relaxation algorithm. The overhead of only $376 - 354 = 22$

iterations, or 6%, is due to the different paths in the **x** space taken by the two algorithms and indicates in a sense an "overshoot" in the relaxation process. This is, of course, a small price to pay considering the overall savings in the execution time of the relaxation algorithm.

REFERENCES

1. J. Katzenelson, An algorithm for solving nonlinear resistor networks, *Bell Syst. Tech. J.*, vol. 44, pp. 1605–1620, 1965.
2. E. S. Kuh and I. N. Hajj, Nonlinear circuit theory: Resistive networks, *Proc. IEEE*, vol. 59, no. 3, pp. 340–355, 1971.
3. L. O. Chua, Efficient computer algorithms for piecewise-linear analysis of resistive nonlinear networks, *IEEE Trans. Circuit Theory*, vol. CT-18, no. 1, pp. 73–84, 1971.
4. T. Ohtsuki and N. Yoshida, DC analysis of nonlinear networks based on generalized piecewise-linear characterization, *IEEE Trans. Circuit Theory*, vol. CT-18, no. 1, pp. 146–151, 1971.
5. T. Fujisawa, E. S. Kuh, and T. Ohtsuki, A sparse matrix method for analysis of piecewise-linear resistive networks, *IEEE Trans. Circuit Theory*, vol. CT-19, no. 6, pp. 571–584, 1972.
6. T. Fujisawa and E. S. Kuh, Piecewise-linear theory of nonlinear networks, *SIAM J. Appl. Math.*, vol. 22, no. 2, pp. 307–328, 1972.
7. I. N. Hajj, D. J. Roulston, and P. R. Bryant, Three-terminal piecewise-linear modelling approach to DC analysis of transistor circuits, *Circuit Theory Appl.*, vol. 2, pp. 133–147, 1974.
8. M. J. Chien and E. S. Kuh, Solving piecewise-linear equations for resistive networks, *Circuit Theory Appl.*, vol. 4, no. 3, pp. 3–24, 1976.
9. M. J. Chien and E. S. Kuh, Solving nonlinear resistive networks using piecewise-linear analysis and simplicial subdivision, *IEEE Trans. Circuits Syst.*, vol. CAS-24, no. 6, pp. 305–317, 1977.
10. S. N. Stevens and Pen-Min Lin, Analysis of piecewise-linear resistive networks using complementary pivot theory, *IEEE Trans. Circuits Syst.*, vol. CAS-28, no. 5, pp. 429–441, 1981.
11. L. O. Chua and R. L. P. Ying, Canonical piecewise-linear analysis, *IEEE Trans. Circuits Syst.*, vol. CAS-30, no. 3, pp. 125–140, 1983.
12. J. Katzenelson, AEDNET: A simulator for nonlinear networks, *Proc. IEEE*, vol. 54, pp. 1536–1552, 1966.
13. L. O. Chua and P. A. Medlock, MECA—A User Oriented Computer Program for Analyzing Resistive Nonlinear Networks, Vol. 1: User's Manual, Tech. Rep. TR-EE-69-7, Purdue Univ. Lafayette, Ind., April 1969.

14. K. Kawakita and T. Ohtsuki, NECTAR2—a circuit analysis program based on piecewise linear approach, *Proc. 1975 Int. Symp. Circuits and Systems*, Newton, Mass., pp. 92–95, April 1975.
15. I. N. Hajj, K. Singhal, J. Vlach, and P. R. Bryant, WATAND—a program for the analysis and design of linear and piecewise linear networks, *16th Midwest Symp. Circuit Theory*, pp. VI.4.1–VI.4.9, April 1973.
16. M. Vlach, WATAND User's Manual, Version VI.09, 2nd ed., Tech. Rep. UW-EE-82-01, Univ. of Waterloo, Jan. 1983.
17. G. D. Hachtel and A. L. Sangiovanni-Vincentelli, A survey of third-generation simulation techniques, *Proc. IEEE*, vol. 69, no. 10, pp. 1264–1280, 1981.
18. I. N. Hajj, Updating method for LU factorisation, *Electron. Lett.*, vol. 8, no. 7, pp. 186–188, 1972.
19. J. M. Ortega and W. C. Rheinboldt, *Iterative Solution of Nonlinear Equations in Several Variables*, Academic Press, New York, 1970.
20. B. R. Chawla, H. K. Gummel, and P. Kozak, MOTIS—an MOS timing simulator, *IEEE Trans. Computer-Aided Design of Integrated Circuits and Systems*, vol. CAS-22, no. 12, pp. 901–909, 1975.
21. A. R. Newton, Techniques for the simulation of large-scale integrated circuits, *IEEE Trans. Computer-Aided Design of Integrated Circuits and Systems*, vol. CAS-26, no. 9, pp. 741–749, 1979.
22. H. DeMan et al., DIANA: Mixed mode simulator with a hardware description language for hierarchical design of VLSI, *Proc. IEEE, ICCC'80*, Rye, N.Y., October 1980.
23. T. W. Williams and K. P. Parker, Design for testability—a survey, *Proc. IEEE*, vol. 71, pp. 98–112, Jan. 1983.

5
Waveform Relaxation Algorithms

Sadatoshi Kumagai

Department of Electronic Engineering, Osaka University, Suita, Osaka, Japan

1 INTRODUCTION

In the design of very large scale integrated (VLSI) circuits, each component of the logic networks obtained through the logic design phase should be converted into electronic circuits which meet all design specifications, such as logic operations, speed, power consumption, and signal levels. Unfortunately, there exist no such design tools that automatically accomplish the conversion and specify parameters which will be used in the next layout design. Designers have to assess the electrical performance of the electronic circuits using appropriate simulation programs and modify the design parameters so that the circuits satisfy all requirements at least within the accuracy guaranteed by the simulation program. The dynamic behavior of electronic circuits is simulated by solving the differential equations with specified initial states and inputs, which is called transient analysis. Transient analysis is necessary for assessing the delay, or overshoot in digital circuits, and various types of performance in analog circuits.

A numerical transient simulation is composed of two iteration loops as shown in Figure 5.1. The outer loop corresponds to the time-discretized integration for the specified simulation interval. Implicit integration formulas such as the backward Euler or trapezoidal integration formula should be used to deal with the stiff differential equations encountered in circuit analysis. The inner loop corresponds to solving the resulting nonlinear

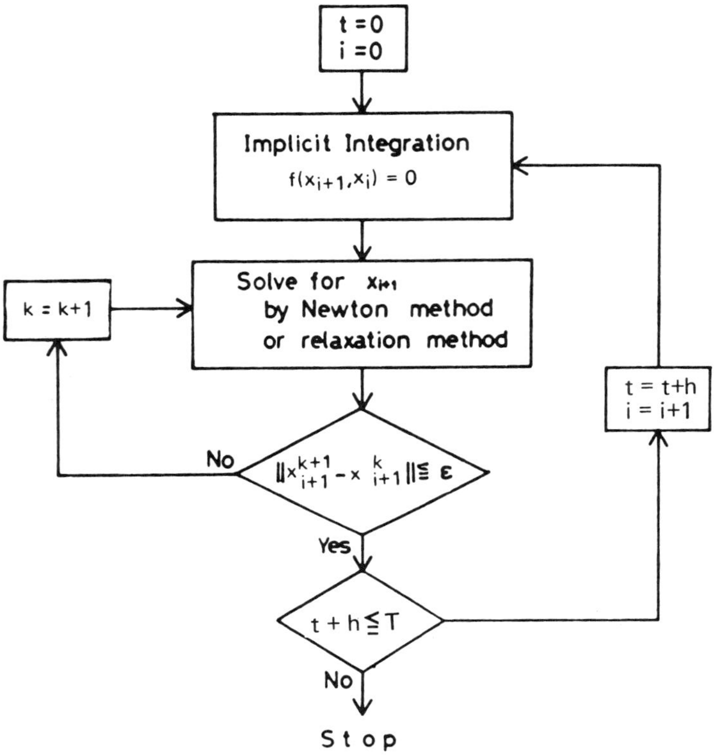

Figure 5.1 Numerical transient analysis.

algebraic equations at each time point by the Newton-Raphson method or by relaxation methods. Transient analysis is one of the most time-consuming design phases. For example, 50 to 80% of the overall design period for a standard dynamic memory cell is consumed in the transient analysis.

In the 1970s, circuit simulation was established as a significant design aid and also a major cost item. Many simulation programs such as SPICE [1] and ASTAP [2] have been developed and embellished where sparse Gaussian elimination and stiff implicit integration approaches are the common tools. A number of speed improvement techniques have been implemented in these circuit simulators. The use of latency [3] can avoid the expense of simulating modules which are not active at a simulated time point. The time cost for evaluating nonlinear device models has been reduced by using table lookup models [4]. In order to perform repetitive calculations of sparse linear equations, microcode generators are used for efficient pivoting and LU decomposition. Circuit simulators with these facilities are called "standard" or "second-generation" simulators [5]. The second-generation simulators have been used successfully for circuits containing a few hundred transistors. However, the spectacular growth in the scale of integrated circuits (ICs) based on metal-oxide-semiconductor (MOS) technology made the second-generation simulators economically infeasible because of their large simulation time cost and memory storage requirement. For example, it is reported that a 700-MOSFET circuit, analyzed by SPICE2 for 4 μs of simulated time with a 2-ns time step, takes approximately 4 CPU hours on a VAX 11/780 VMS computer with floating-point accelerator hardware [6]. Considering the usual environment of a multiuser workstation, it would take the equivalent of 2 or 3 days running on a computer to obtain just one simulated waveform.

In late 1970s, searches for third-generation simulators started and efforts to resolve the time and storage problems in the design of VLSI circuits were intensified. Third-generation simulators are characterized by their common use of tearing and temporal decomposition techniques. Tearing implies the decomposition of circuits so that the coefficient matrix of the linearized circuit equations can be permuted into a special form, for example, into a bordered block triangular form. The analysis of the whole circuit is reduced to the iterated analysis of each subcircuit corresponding to a diagonal block. IC simulators such as SLATE [7] and MACRO [8] employ this technique.

In tearing methods, the decomposition is performed inside the Newton iteration at a simulation time point. In temporal decomposition, circuit partitioning is performed before the linearization so that the relaxation is needed at the nonlinear equation level. An equivalent nonlinear resistive subcircuit is independently analyzed with the decoupling vectors between adjacent subcircuits made equal to the updated values. The speed of convergence depends on the strength of the electrical coupling between subcircuits and the order of the analysis. A family of simulators, called timing simulators or mixed-mode simulators, such as MOTIS [9], SPLICE [4], and DIANA [10], are examples of those which use this technique. Exploiting the quasi-unidirectional property of MOS circuits and scheduling algorithms such as the selective-trace method, these simulators can achieve speed improvement of two orders of magnitude compared to the standard ones, at the cost of accuracy.

More recently, a different relaxation algorithm, called the waveform relaxation algorithm, was proposed [11], where the relaxation is applied at the differential equation level; in each iteration, each decoupled subcircuit is independently analyzed through the overall simulation interval. The main feature of the waveform relaxation method is its easy exploitation of the quasi-unidirectional and multirate nature of large-scale integrated circuits. RELAX [12] is the first simulator based on waveform relaxation techniques.

Waveform relaxation algorithms are particularly advantageous for parallel computation because the calculation of each subcircuit is continued through the overall simulation interval and thus the communication overhead for data acquisition is negligible compared to the total time cost. The aim of this chapter is to introduce the properties of waveform relaxation, abbreviated WR hereafter. For practical use of WR algorithms, it is most important to investigate the numerical convergence, which depends on the circuit partitioning. In Section 2, the difference between analytical convergence and numerically meaningful convergence is clarified. In Section 3, a circuit partitioning that guarantees rapid numerical convergence is discussed. In Section 4, we introduce parallel implementation of circuit simulation based on WR algorithms. Although WR algorithms can also be used for bipolar transistor circuits, emphasis is placed on their practical use in the efficient simulation of MOS circuits. Pros and cons of WR methods are summarized in the last section.

2 CONVERGENCE PROPERTIES OF WR ALGORITHMS

Consider the following differential equations.

$$\mathbf{f}(\mathbf{x}, \dot{\mathbf{x}}, \mathbf{u}(t)) = 0 \tag{1}$$

where $\mathbf{x}(t) \in R^n$ is a state vector, $\mathbf{u}(t) \in R^m$ is an input vector, and $\mathbf{f}$ is a mapping from $R^n \times R^n \times R^m$ to R^n. Let $\mathbf{x}$ and $\dot{\mathbf{x}}$ be decomposed into p, $1 < p < n$, subvectors such that

$$\mathbf{x}^t = [\mathbf{x}_1{}^t, \mathbf{x}_2{}^t, \ldots, \mathbf{x}_p{}^t]^t \tag{2}$$

and

$$\dot{\mathbf{x}}^t = [\dot{\mathbf{x}}_1{}^t, \dot{\mathbf{x}}_2{}^t, \ldots, \dot{\mathbf{x}}_p{}^t]^t \tag{3}$$

Correspondingly, $\mathbf{f}$ is decomposed as

$$\mathbf{f}^t = [\mathbf{f}_1{}^t, \mathbf{f}_2{}^t, \ldots, \mathbf{f}_p{}^t]^t \tag{4}$$

Two types of WR algorithms for solving the initial-value problem of the differential equations (1) are written as follows.

Block Gauss-Jacobi WR algorithm

Let $i := 0$; $\mathbf{x}^0(t) := \mathbf{x}^0$ for $t \in [0, T]$
Repeat $i := i + 1$
  For all k, $k = 1, 2, \ldots, p$
  Solve for $\mathbf{x}_k{}^i(t)$, $t \in [0, T]$

$$\mathbf{f}_k(\mathbf{x}_1{}^{i-1}, \ldots, \mathbf{x}_{k-1}{}^{i-1}, \mathbf{x}_k{}^i, \mathbf{x}_{k+1}{}^{i-1}, \ldots, \mathbf{x}_p{}^{i-1}, \dot{\mathbf{x}}_1{}^{i-1}, \ldots, \dot{\mathbf{x}}_{k-1}{}^{i-1}, \dot{\mathbf{x}}_k^i, \dot{\mathbf{x}}_{k+1}{}^{i-1}, \ldots, \dot{\mathbf{x}}_p{}^{i-1}, \mathbf{u}) = 0$$

with

$$\mathbf{x}^i(0) = \mathbf{x}^0(0) \tag{5}$$

until

$$\max_k \max_{t \in [0,T]} \|\mathbf{x}_k{}^i(t) - \mathbf{x}_k{}^{i-1}(t)\| \leqq \varepsilon \tag{6}$$

Here $\|\ \|$ is a norm in real Euclidean space R^n.

Block Gauss-Seidel WR algorithm:

Let $i := 0$; $\mathbf{x}^0(t) = \mathbf{x}^0$ for $t \in [0, T]$
Repeat $i := i + 1$
For $k = 1, 2, \ldots, p$
Solve for $\mathbf{x}_k{}^i(t)$, $t \in [0, T]$

$$\mathbf{f}_k(\mathbf{x}_1{}^i, \ldots, \mathbf{x}_k{}^i, \mathbf{x}_{k+1}{}^{i-1}, \ldots, \mathbf{x}_p{}^{i-1}, \dot{\mathbf{x}}_1{}^i, \ldots, \dot{\mathbf{x}}_k{}^i, \dot{\mathbf{x}}_{k+1}{}^{i-1}, \ldots, \dot{\mathbf{x}}_p{}^{i-1}, \mathbf{u}) = 0$$

with

$$\mathbf{x}^i(0) = \mathbf{x}^0(0) \tag{7}$$

until

$$\max_k \max_{t \in [0,T]} \|\mathbf{x}^i(t) - \mathbf{x}^{i-1}(t)\| \leqq \varepsilon \tag{8}$$

The original initial-value problem is reduced to iteratively solving much smaller differential equations for each subvector while other subvector waveforms updated in the preceding analysis are considered as known inputs. These virtual input vectors are called the decoupling vectors. We consider the convergence of the WR algorithms. The derivation follows the approach presented in Ref. [11].

For simplicity, we assume that equations (1) are put into the normal form, that is,

$$\dot{\mathbf{x}} = \mathbf{f}(\mathbf{x}, \mathbf{u}) \tag{9}$$

and assume that the block Gauss-Jacobi WR algorithm is applied to equation (9). The ith iteration is expressed as solving, for $\mathbf{y}_k(t)$, $t \in [0, T]$,

$$\dot{\mathbf{y}}_k = \hat{\mathbf{f}}_k(\mathbf{y}_k, \mathbf{x}, \mathbf{u}) \qquad k = 1, 2, \ldots, p \tag{10}$$

where $\mathbf{x}$ is set equal to the $(i-1)$st iterated waveforms, $\mathbf{x}^{i-1}(t)$, and $\hat{\mathbf{f}}_k$ is defined as

$$\hat{\mathbf{f}}_k(\mathbf{y}_k, \mathbf{x}, \mathbf{u}) = \mathbf{f}_k(\mathbf{x}_1, \mathbf{x}_2, \ldots, \mathbf{x}_{k-1}, \mathbf{y}_k, \mathbf{x}_{k+1}, \ldots, \mathbf{x}_p, \mathbf{u}) \tag{11}$$

Define a mapping $\mathbf{F}$ in the space of differentiable waveforms such that, for $\mathbf{x}(t)$, $t \in [0, T]$,

$$\mathbf{F}(\mathbf{x}(t)) = \mathbf{y}(t) \tag{12}$$

where $\mathbf{y}(t)$ is the solution of equation (10) for $\mathbf{x}(t)$. Let $\mathbf{y}^1$ and $\mathbf{y}^2$ be the images of $\mathbf{F}$ for waveforms $\mathbf{x}^1$ and $\mathbf{x}^2$, respectively, that is,

$$\mathbf{y}^1 = \mathbf{F}(\mathbf{x}^1) \tag{13}$$

and

$$\mathbf{y}^2 = \mathbf{F}(\mathbf{x}^2) \tag{14}$$

Now we assume that the mapping $\mathbf{f}$ of equation (9) is Lipschitz-continuous with respect to $\mathbf{x}$; for any $\mathbf{x}^1(t)$ and $\mathbf{x}^2(t)$, there exists a positive number r such that

$$\|\mathbf{f}(\mathbf{x}^1(t), \mathbf{u}) - \mathbf{f}(\mathbf{x}^2(t), \mathbf{u})\| \leqq r\|\mathbf{x}^1(t) - \mathbf{x}^2(t)\| \tag{15}$$

Then, for $\mathbf{y}^1(t)$ and $\mathbf{y}^2(t)$ defined in (13) and (14),

$$\begin{aligned} \frac{d}{dt}\|\mathbf{y}^1(t) - \mathbf{y}^2(t)\| &\leqq q\|\dot{\mathbf{y}}^1(t) - \dot{\mathbf{y}}^2(t)\| \\ &= q\|\mathbf{f}(\mathbf{y}^1, \mathbf{x}^1, \mathbf{u}) - \mathbf{f}(\mathbf{y}^2, \mathbf{x}^2, \mathbf{u})\| \\ &\leqq r_1\|\mathbf{y}^1(t) - \mathbf{y}^2(t)\| + r_2\|\mathbf{x}^1(t) - \mathbf{x}^2(t)\| \end{aligned} \tag{16}$$

where q, r_1, and r_2 are some positive integers. From the well-known Bellman-Gronwall formula,

$$\|\mathbf{y}^1(t) - \mathbf{y}^2(t)\| \leqq r_2 \int_0^t e^{r_1(t-\tau)}\|\mathbf{x}^1(\tau) - \mathbf{x}^2(\tau)\|\, d\tau \tag{17}$$

We define a norm $\| \; \|_f$ in the space of waveforms such that

$$\|\mathbf{x}\|_f = \max_{t\in[0,T]} e^{-\alpha t}\|\mathbf{x}(t)\| \tag{18}$$

for a positive number α. Rewrite inequality (17) as

$$\|\mathbf{y}^1(t) - \mathbf{y}^2(t)\| \leqq r_2 e^{\alpha t}\int_0^t e^{(r_1-\alpha)(t-\tau)}e^{-\alpha\tau}\|\mathbf{x}^1(t) - \mathbf{x}^2(\tau)\|\, d\tau \tag{19}$$

Then we obtain

$$\max_{t\in[0,T]} e^{-\alpha t}\|\mathbf{y}^1(t) - \mathbf{y}^2(t)\| \leqq k \max_{t\in[0,T]} e^{-\alpha t}\|\mathbf{x}^1(t) - \mathbf{x}^2(t)\|$$

or

$$\|\mathbf{y}^1 - \mathbf{y}^2\|_f \leqq k\|\mathbf{x}^1 - \mathbf{x}^2\|_f \tag{20}$$

where

$$k = \frac{r_2}{\alpha - r_1} \tag{21}$$

With sufficiently large α, inequality (20) implies that $\mathbf{F}$ is a contraction mapping in the norm defined in (18). This guarantees the convergence of the waveforms to the fixed point of $\mathbf{F}$ which is the solution of equation (9). As shown above, the convergence of the WR algorithm is analytically ensured under a mild condition; it is sufficient for $\mathbf{f}$ to be Lipschitz-continuous. However, the convergence in the norm as defined in (18) may take a very large amount of time to meet the stop criterion (6) or (8) for a long simulation interval $[0, T]$, that is, for large T. The convergence of waveforms in the norm as defined in (6) or (8) is called monotone convergence [13].

For practical use of WR algorithms, we should find more stringent conditions which guarantee monotone convergence. Let us consider the following linear differential equations:

$$\begin{aligned} \dot{\mathbf{x}} &= A\mathbf{x} + B\mathbf{u} \\ \mathbf{x}(0) &= \mathbf{x}^0 \end{aligned} \tag{22}$$

Assume that $\mathbf{x}$ is decomposed into p numbers of subvectors and A and B are accordingly decomposed into

$$A = \begin{bmatrix} A_{11} & A_{12} & \cdots & A_{1p} \\ A_{21} & A_{22} & & \\ \vdots & & \ddots & \vdots \\ A_{p1} & & \cdots & A_{pp} \end{bmatrix} \tag{23}$$

and

$$B = \begin{bmatrix} B_1 \\ B_2 \\ \vdots \\ B_p \end{bmatrix} \tag{24}$$

respectively. Suppose that the block Gauss-Jacobi WR algorithm is applied to (22) and each of the decoupled differential equations is numerically integrated by the backward-Euler integration formula with a fixed time step h. The instantaneous values at a time point $t \in [0, T]$ of the $(i + 1)$st and ith iterated waveforms are related by

$$\mathbf{x}^{i+1}(t) = \mathbf{x}^{i+1}(t - h) + h(D\mathbf{x}^{i+1}(t) + C\mathbf{x}^i(t)) + hB\mathbf{u}(t) \tag{25}$$

where

$$D = \begin{bmatrix} A_{11} & & & \\ & A_{22} & & \\ & & \ddots & \\ & & & A_{pp} \end{bmatrix} \tag{26}$$

and

$$C = A - D \tag{27}$$

Let H be defined as

$$H = I - hD \tag{28}$$

where I is an identity matrix. For sufficiently small h, H can be considered nonsingular and, from equation (25),

$$\mathbf{x}^{i+1}(t) = H^{-1}\mathbf{x}^{i+1}(t-h) + hH^{-1}C\mathbf{x}^{i}(t) + hH^{-1}B\mathbf{u}(t) \tag{29}$$

Then

$$\begin{aligned} \|\mathbf{x}^{i+1}(t) - \mathbf{x}^{i}(t)\| &\leqq h\|H^{-1}C\|\,\|\mathbf{x}^{i}(t) - \mathbf{x}^{i-1}(t)\| \\ &\quad + \|H^{-1}\|\,\|\mathbf{x}^{i+1}(t-h) - \mathbf{x}^{i}(t-h)\| \\ \|\mathbf{x}^{i+1}(t-h) - \mathbf{x}^{i}(t-h)\| &\leqq h\|H^{-1}C\|\,\|\mathbf{x}^{i}(t-h) - \mathbf{x}^{i-1}(t-h)\| \\ &\quad + \|H^{-1}\|\,\|\mathbf{x}^{i+1}(t-2h) - \mathbf{x}^{i}(t-2h)\| \\ &\vdots \\ \|\mathbf{x}^{i+1}(h) - \mathbf{x}^{i}(h)\| &\leqq h\|H^{-1}C\|\,\|\mathbf{x}^{i}(h) - \mathbf{x}^{i-1}(h)\| \\ &\quad + \|H^{-1}\|\,\|\mathbf{x}^{i+1}(0) - \mathbf{x}^{i}(0)\| \end{aligned} \tag{30}$$

Multiply the both sides of inequalities (30) by 1, $\|H^{-1}\|$, $\|H^{-1}\|^2, \ldots, \|H^{-1}\|^q$. Note that $t = (q+1)h$ and $\mathbf{x}^{i+1}(0) = \mathbf{x}^{i}(0) = \mathbf{x}^{0}(0)$. By adding all the resulting inequalities, we obtain

$$\begin{aligned} \|\mathbf{x}^{i+1}(t) - \mathbf{x}^{i}(t)\| \leqq h\|H^{-1}C\|\{&\|\mathbf{x}^{i}(t) - \mathbf{x}^{i-1}(t)\| \\ &+ \|H^{-1}\|\,\|\mathbf{x}^{i}(t-h) - \mathbf{x}^{i-1}(t-h)\| \\ &\vdots \\ &+ \|H^{-1}\|^{q}\|\mathbf{x}^{i}(h) - \mathbf{x}^{i-1}(h)\|\} \end{aligned} \tag{31}$$

Now let $\|D\| = d_1$ and assume that there exists a positive number d_2 such that

$$\|H^{-1}\| = \|(I - hD)^{-1}\| = \frac{1}{1 + d_2} \tag{32}$$

If D is negative diagonal, we can easily find such a d_2. Define a norm $\| \ \|_f$ for $\mathbf{x}(t)$, $t \in [0, T]$, as

$$\|\mathbf{x}\|_f = \max_{t \in [0,T]} \|\mathbf{x}(t)\| \tag{33}$$

Then, from (31) and (32),

$$\|\mathbf{x}^{i+1} - \mathbf{x}^i\|_f < \left(\frac{d_1}{d_2}\right) \|D^{-1}A - I\| \, \|\mathbf{x}^i - \mathbf{x}^{i-1}\|_f \tag{34}$$

If the inequality

$$\|D^{-1}A - I\| < \frac{d_2}{d_1} \tag{35}$$

is satisfied, then for some r, $0 < r < 1$,

$$\|\mathbf{x}^{i+1} - \mathbf{x}^i\|_f < r\|\mathbf{x}^i - \mathbf{x}^{i-1}\|_f \tag{36}$$

This implies that the waveforms generated by the WR iterations converge monotonically to the solution irrespective of the time step h and the initial waveform $\mathbf{x}^0(t)$. We call r in (36) the iteration factor of the WR algorithm. For the case where D is a negative diagonal matrix and $\| \ \|$ is L_∞-norm, the condition (35) reduces to

$$\min_i |a_{ii}| > \max_i \sum_{j \neq i} |a_{ij}| \tag{37}$$

which is stronger than the diagonal dominance of matrix A.

For the Gauss-Seidel WR algorithm, we can derive similar conditions on the iteration matrix $L^{-1}U$, where L and U are the lower block triangular part and the strict upper block triangular part of A, respectively. It should be noted that the iteration factor r, or the speed of the convergence, depends heavily on the norm of the iteration matrix. For a given matrix A, this in turn implies that it depends on the decomposition of A according to which the decoupled differential equations are solved independently. In the next section, we apply the above discussion to the partitioning of MOS circuits through which WR algorithms are used effectively to obtain correct waveforms.

3 CIRCUIT PARTITIONING

MOS circuits are formulated by a nodal approach into

$$\frac{d}{dt}\mathbf{c}(\mathbf{v}, \mathbf{u}) + \mathbf{g}(\mathbf{v}, \mathbf{u}) = 0 \tag{38}$$

where $\mathbf{c}(\mathbf{v}, \mathbf{u})$ is the node charge vector for node voltage vector $\mathbf{v}$ and input voltage vector **u**. In circuit simulation, a numerical integration formula is applied directly to equation (38). For analytical purposes, we assume that (38) is put into a normal form such that

$$\dot{\mathbf{v}} = -C^{-1}(\mathbf{v}, \mathbf{u})\mathbf{g}(\mathbf{v}) + \mathbf{b}(\mathbf{u}) \tag{39}$$

where C is a capacitance matrix with positive nonzero entries. For the simple case where C is positive diagonal with almost equal nonzero entries, the iteration factor of the WR algorithms can be evaluated by the conductance matrix $G(\mathbf{v}) = \partial g/\partial \mathbf{v}$. For instance, consider a circuit as shown in Figure 5.2. The nodal equations are written as

$$\dot{v}_1 = -C^{-1}(g_1 + g)v_1 + C^{-1}g_1 v_2$$

$$\dot{v}_2 = -C^{-1}(g_1 + g)v_2 + C^{-1}g_1 v_1$$

If the Gauss-Jacobi WR algorithm is applied according to the partitioning of node 1 and node 2, then the iteration factor r is easily evaluated by

$$r = \|D^{-1}A - I\|_\infty = \frac{g_1}{g_1 + g}$$

Thus, the speed of convergence becomes lower as the conductance g_1 becomes larger.

Let us examine a more realistic example. Figure 5.3 shows a two-stage CMOS inverter chain. If we partition the circuit at terminal nodes of r_1 and r_2 in the second inverter, the equivalent subcircuits analyzed by the WR algorithm are as shown in Figure 5.4. The simulation results obtained by the Gauss-Seidel WR algorithm are shown in Figure 5.5, where (a) and (b) correspond to the cases $r_1 = r_2 = 50\,\Omega$ and $r_1 = r_2 = 500\,\Omega$, respectively, and k denotes the iteration counts. It is noted that the speed of convergence is affected significantly by the conductances between the partitioned node pairs. The iteration factor depends on the block diagonal dominance of the

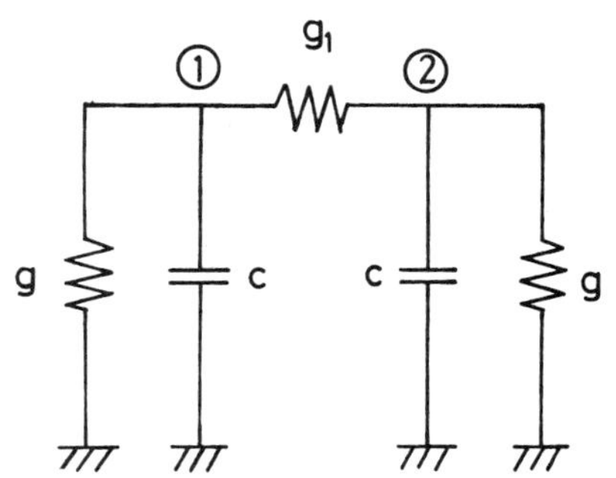

Figure 5.2 A partitioning and the iteration factor.

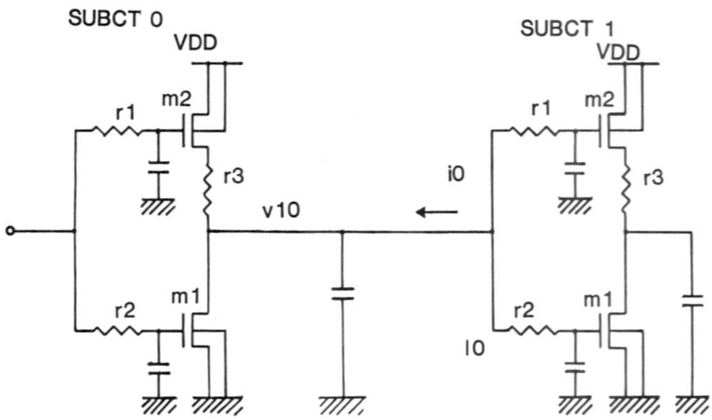

Figure 5.3 Inverter chain.

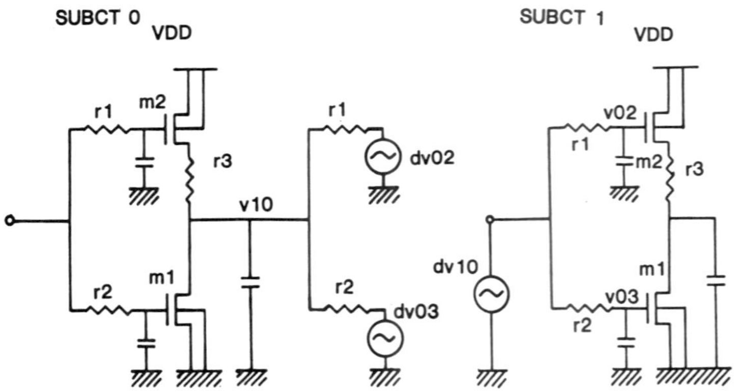

Figure 5.4 Partitioning at resistor terminals.

conductance matrix, as shown in the preceding section. Thus, qualitatively, the circuit should be partitioned at weak coupling branches with small conductances compared to the other branches, which contain a set of nodes with larger conductances.

Unfortunately, it is difficult to derive quantitative criteria for general circuits which specify the relation between the circuit partitioning and the iteration factor. So far there exists no efficient method for obtaining the optimal partitioning which satisfies both the requirement for fast convergence and the size restriction on subcircuits for taking advantage of WR algorithms. A heuristic partitioning algorithm based on the node merging criterion has been proposed [14]. In MOS circuits, the equivalent resistance between gate and drain or source terminal is orders of magnitude larger than

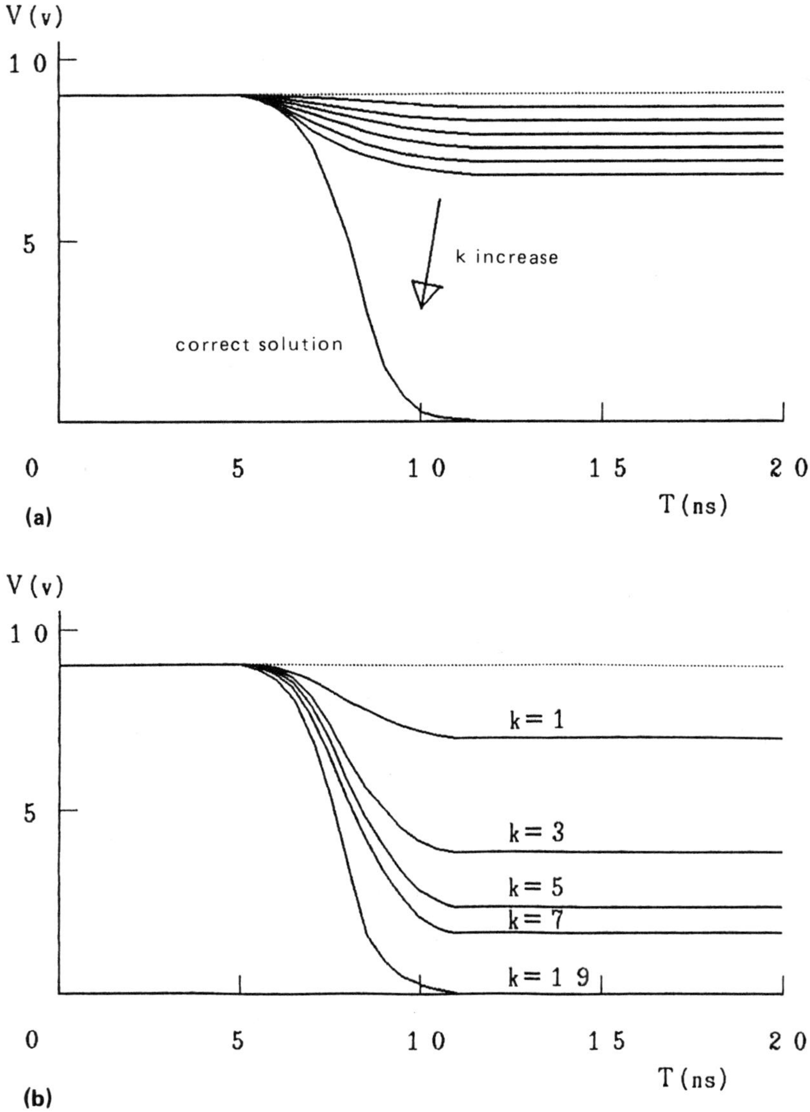

Figure 5.5 Iterated waveforms of voltage V10. (a) $r_1 = r_2 = 50\,\Omega$; (b) $r_1 = r_2 = 500\,\Omega$.

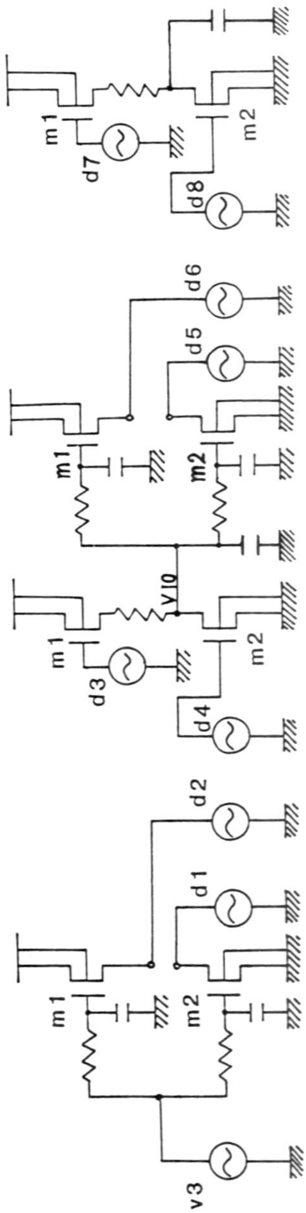

Figure 5.6 Overlapped partitioning at input MOSFETs.

other resistances. Figure 5.6 shows the decoupled subcircuits obtained from the partitioning of the circuit shown in Figure 5.3 at the MOS transistor gates. Note that each input MOS transistor is overlapped in two succeeding subcircuits. The overlapped partitioning is robust in the sense that the speed of convergence is affected less by the variation of the circuit parameters [15]. When we apply the Gauss-Seidel WR algorithm using this partitioning, the solution waveform has been determined in one iteration.

In the above discussion, we neglected the effect of the capacitances between gate and drain or source terminals. In fact, even in the case where these capacitances are made three orders of magnitude as large as the nominal values, the solution can be obtained in four iterations. The circuit partitioning scheme is summarized as follows.

1. Decompose the whole circuit into functional blocks by cutting each lead line incident on the gate of the input MOSFET. (See Figure 5.7.)
2. Attach to each block the input MOSFETs of the fan-out blocks and define the resulting circuit as the corresponding subcircuit. (See Figure 5.6.)
3. Define the decoupling vector of the subcircuit as the gate voltages of the input MOSFETs of the subcircuit and the floating source and drain voltages of the attached MOSFETs. (See Figure 5.6.)

Note again that the inner nodes of input MOSFETs are analyzed twice in two subcircuits.

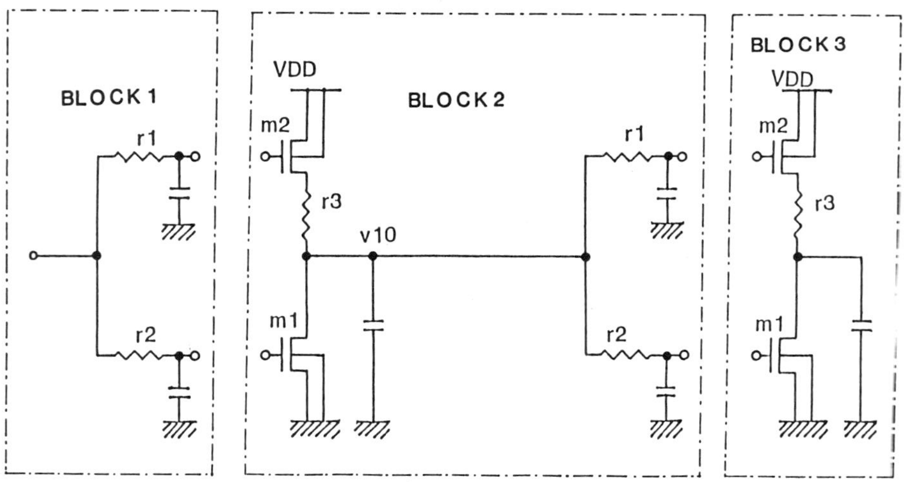

Figure 5.7 Functional block decomposition.

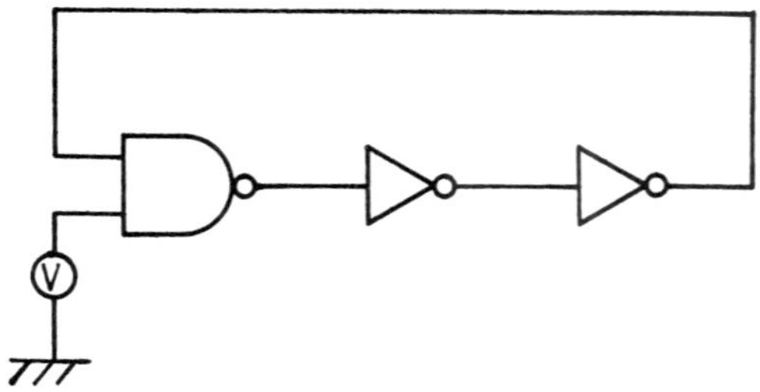

Figure 5.8 Ring oscillator.

The serious drawback of WR algorithms is the weak convergence when they are applied to circuits with large feedback loops. For example, when applied to a ring oscilator as shown in Figure 5.8, the Gauss-Seidel WR algorithm requires more than 20 iterations to converge. Such a tightly coupled portion of a large-scale circuit should be contained in one subcircuit; that is, subcircuits on a feedback loop are merged into one big subcircuit. If the resulting subcircuit becomes too large, it may fail to take advantage of WR algorithms. At the present stage, there exists no good strategy for overcoming this difficulty. It should also be mentioned that the prediction of a good initial waveform by, say, a timing simulation cannot alleviate the slow convergence problem. This unexpected phenomenon is due to the multirate effect, that is, the effect of the accumulated error caused by the difference between the time step width for the initial waveform and that determined independently in the numerical integration for each subcircuit. Recall that multirate integration is a typical feature of WR methods. On the other hand, a windowing technique [14] decomposes the simulation time interval into subintervals so that in each subinterval we can obtain rapid convergence. But it is still not known how to determine the optimal length of subintervals.

Finally, it should be emphasized that WR methods can be used as vehicles for parallel simulation of VLSI circuits. An example of the parallel implementation based on WR algorithms is introduced in the next section.

4 WR-BASED PARALLEL SIMULATION

Suppose that the whole circuit is partitioned into p subcircuits of equal size and each subcircuit is analyzed by one of m node computers in a multicomputer system. The computation time of sparse Gaussian elimination is roughly proportional to $N^{1.5}$, where N is the size of the circuit. Thus, the partitioning can reduce the time cost for each subcircuit to $1/p^{1.5}$. Let k be the iteration counts necessary for convergence, and let q be the percentage of busy node computers in parallel execution. If we can ignore the communication overhead, the speed-up factor F of the parallel simulation is estimated from

$$F = \frac{\sqrt{pmq}}{100k} \tag{40}$$

For example, if $p = 100$, $m = 10$, $q = 80$, and $k = 4$, then there is a factor of 20 speed-up compared to the standard circuit simulation. For quasi-unidirectional circuits, the Gauss-Seidel algorithm with the partitioning scheme described in the preceding section can determine the solution waveform usually in one iteration. For such a case, the speed-up factor is 80. In this section, a parallel circuit simulator called PNAP (Parallel Network Analysis Program) is introduced [16].

PNAP adopts the block Gauss-Seidel WR algorithm as the vehicle of the parallel simulation. The program is implemented on the multicomputer system LINKS-1 [17]. The hardware configuration of LINKS-1 is shown in Figure 5.9. The host computer (HC), operating on UNIX, mainly manages the file system. The root computer (RC) and node computer (NC) are of the same structure, having a CPU, an arithmetic processing unit, and a 1- to 4-MB memory unit. In PNAP, the RC supervises all waveforms calculated in NCs and checks the convergence. The scheduler on the RC selects a set of subcircuits for the next iteration and transfers the updated decoupling vectors

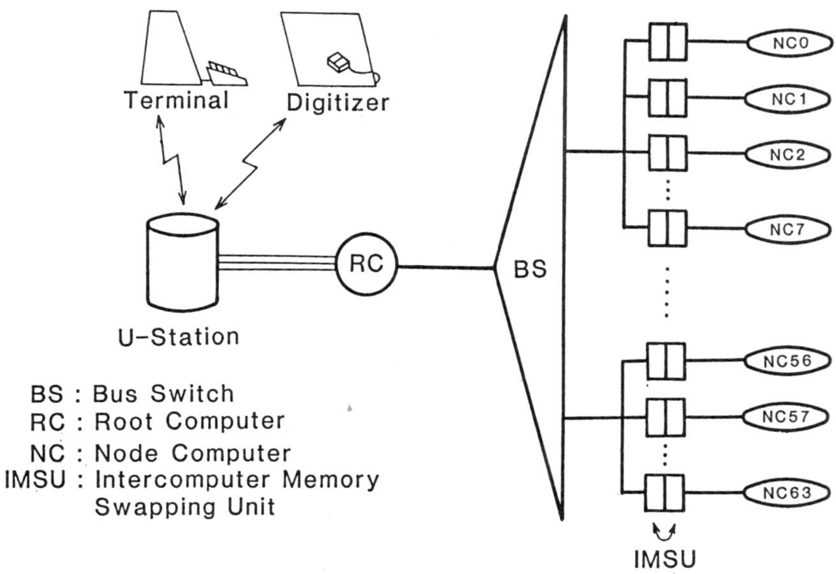

Figure 5.9 Hardware configuration of LINKS-1.

to available NCs, which analyze the allotted subcircuit. Each NC possesses circuit data for all subcircuits and can analyze any assigned subcircuit with the updated decoupling vector transferred from the RC. After the calculation, the waveforms are transferred to the RC to check the convergence and update decoupling vectors. An intercomputer memory swapping unit (IMSU) transfers these data by exchange of a memory block through the use of a bus exchange switch. The communication overhead is negligible compared to the computation time for each subcircuit.

When a functional-level circuit description is input to the HC, the program DECOMPOSITION automatically partitions the circuit and creates circuit data CTDATA of subcircuits, which are copied to the RC and each NC. CTDATA contains the name of the function block and the specifications of input voltage sources and the decoupling vector for each subcircuit. A level is defined for each subcircuit according to the associated flow graph of the circuit, and the HC creates SJDATA, which is used for the scheduling in the RC. GTELIB and MOSLIB on the HC are the libraries of gate models and MOSFET models, respectively, which are linked together with CTDATA to set up subcircuit equations in each NC. Parameters for numerical analysis, such as the simulation interval, the error criterion for checking convergence and time step control, and the types of integration formulas used, are specified in ACOM on the HC. The flow of these data is depicted in Figure 5.10.

Since we adopt the Gauss-Seidel WR algorithm, subcircuits should be analyzed in the proper order to attain fast convergence. For example, a unidirectional inverter chain as depicted in Figure 5.11 should be analyzed from the leftmost subcircuit to the rightmost subcircuit. Good scheduling is required to establish efficient parallelism in the ordered computation. For a circuit such as that shown in Figure 5.11, the acyclic flow graph is constructed as shown in Figure 5.12. The level of a subcircuit is defined as the longest path length to its corresponding node from the input node in the flow graph. If there is a feedback loop in the circuit, subcircuits on the loop are merged into one node to make the flow graph acyclic. SCHEDULE in the RC selects subcircuits for the kth iteration according to the following rules.

1. Select subcircuits, in ascending order of levels, such that all subcircuits in lower levels and all subcircuits in higher levels have gone through their kth and $(k - 1)$st iterations, respectively. Assign each selected subcircuit to a free NC for the kth iteration.
2. If there are still more free NCs, then let $k := k + 1$ and return to step 1.

A test circuit is shown in Figure 5.13. The whole circuit is partitioned into 32 subcircuits. The WR process with six node computers is shown in Figure 5.14. The solution was obtained in one iteration. It takes 5 hours to simulate

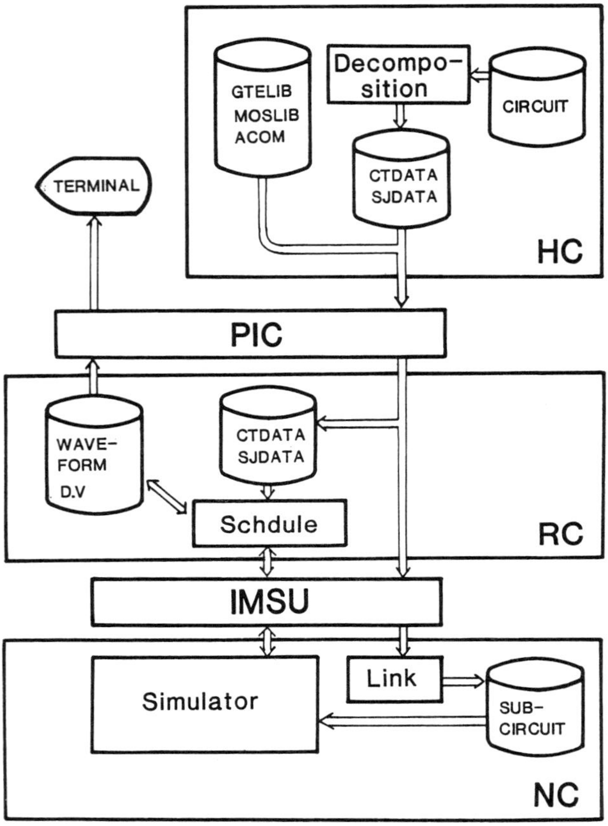

Figure 5.10 Data flow in PNAP.

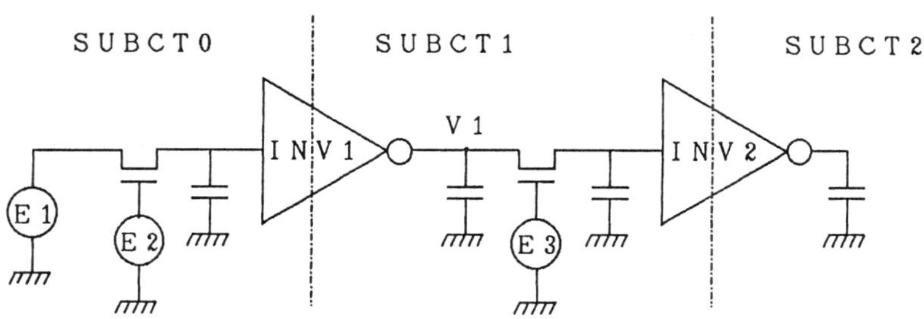

Figure 5.11 Unidirectional circuit.

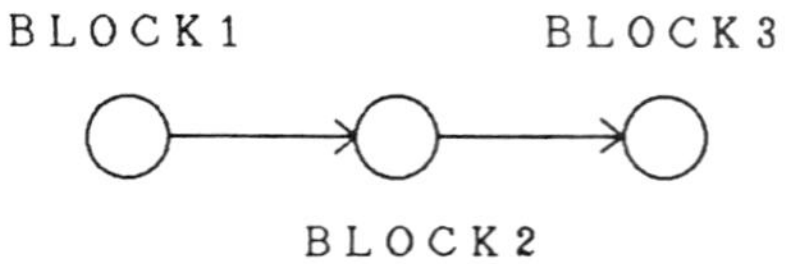

Figure 5.12 Associated flow graph for the circuit in Figure 5.11.

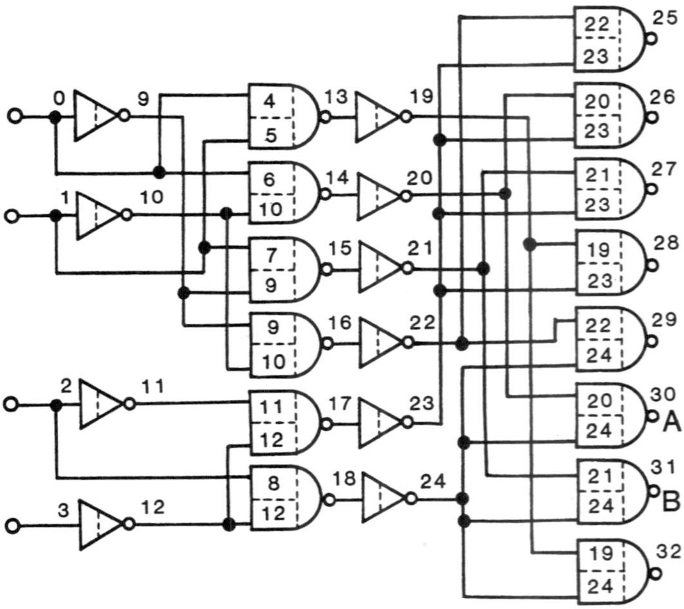

Figure 5.13 Test circuit.

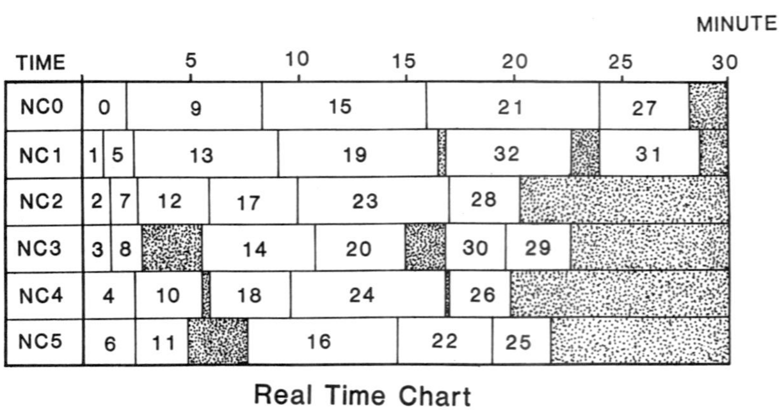

Figure 5.14 Parallel WR process.

the whole circuit by one node computer in which a SPICE-like standard simulation program is implemented. So we obtain about a factor of 20 speed-up in this case compared to the standard circuit simulation. The speed-up factor F calculated with $p = 32$, $m = 6$, $q = 80$, and $k = 1$ is about 27. The difference is due mainly to the overlapped partitioning used in PNAP, which seems to result in reduction of the number of subcircuits, p.

5 SUMMARY

To overcome the speed and memory storage barriers in VLSI circuit simulation, various types of relaxation methods have been proposed. The waveform relaxation methods introduced in this chapter have several advantages over other relaxation-based methods. Convergence is analytically guaranteed for ordinary circuits with Lipschitz-continuous branch characteristics. Since subcircuit waveforms are calculated independently, the latency or partial convergence can easily be employed within each subcircuit. The time-step controller in the numerical integration chooses the best time step for each subcircuit irrespective of the remaining subcircuits. This is a typical feature of multirate integration in waveform relaxation. Above all, waveform relaxation methods are well suited to parallel simulations because of their negligible communication overhead.

The major problem for practical use of WR algorithms is associated with the scheme for partitioning circuits to obtain fast convergence. For MOS circuits, the overlapped partitioning described in Section 3 has been used successfully to achieve efficient simulations. For bipolar circuits, there have been few attempts to use WR algorithms because the couplings between subcircuits vary by orders of magnitude, and thus repartitioning at several operating points is needed [18]. Overlapped partitioning such as that introduced here can take into account the effects of variation of couplings between fan-outs. For circuits with large feedback loops, no good method has been found yet to overcome slow convergence. Experimentally, a windowing technique cannot significantly improve the simulation time cost. Prediction of initial waveforms or, in other words, estimation of the feedback effect does not work well because of the multirate effect inherent in the WR process. At this stage, one is reluctant to use WR algorithms for such circuits.

The parallel simulation scheme based on WR algorithms has been shown to be quite successful for quasi-unidirectional large-scale integrated circuits. The parallel techniques introduced here will be common tools for next-generation simulators.

REFERENCES

1. L. W. Nagel, SPICE2: A computer program to simulate semiconductor circuits, ERL Memo ERL-M520, Univ. of California, Berkeley, May 1975.
2. W. T. Weeks, A. J. Jiminetz, G. W. Mahoney, D. Mehta, H. Qassemzadeh, and T. R. Scott, Algorithms for ASTAP—a network analysis program, *IEEE Trans. Circuit Theory*, vol. CT-20, pp. 628–634, Nov. 1973.
3. N. B. Rabbat and H. Y. Hsieh, A latent macromodular approach to large-scale sparse networks, *IEEE Trans. Circuits Syst.*, vol. CAS-23, pp. 745–752, Dec. 1976.
4. A. R. Newton, Techniques for the simulation of large-scale integrated circuits, *IEEE Trans. Circuits Syst.*, vol. CAS-26, pp. 741–749, Sept. 1979.
5. G. D. Hachtel and A. L. Sangivanni-Vincentelli, A survey of third-generation simulation techniques, *Proc. IEEE*, vol. 69, pp. 1264–1280, Oct. 1981.
6. A. R. Newton and A. L. Sangiovanni-Vincentelli, Relaxation-based electrical simulation, *IEEE Trans. Computer-Aided Design of Integrated Circuits and Systems*, vol. CAD-3, pp. 308–331, Oct. 1984.
7. P. Yang, I. N. Hajj, and T. N. Trick, SLATE: A circuit simulation program with latency exploitation and node tearing, *Proc. IEEE Int. Conf. Circuits and Computers*, Port Chester, N.Y., pp. 976–979, Oct. 1980.
8. N. B. Rabbat, A. L. Sangiovanni-Vincentelli, and H. Y. Hsieh, A multilevel Newton algorithm with macromodeling and latency for analysis of large-scale nonlinear networks in time domain, *IEEE Trans. Circuits Syst.*, vol. CAS-26, pp. 733–741, Sept. 1979.
9. B. R. Chawla, H. K. Gummel, and P. Kozak, MOTIS—an MOS timing simulator, *IEEE Trans. Circuits Syst.*, vol. CAS-22, pp. 901–909, Dec. 1975.
10. P. Reyneart, H. De Man, G. Arnout, and J. Cornelissen, DIANA: A mixed-mode simulator with a hardware description language for hierarchical design of VLSI, *Proc. IEEE Int. Conf. Circuits and Computers*, Rye, N.Y., pp. 356–360, Oct. 1980.
11. E. Lelarasmee, A. E. Ruehli, and A. L. Sangiovanni-Vincentelli, The waveform relaxation method for time domain analysis of large scale integrated circuits, ERL Memo. ERL-M81/75, Univ. of California, Berkeley, June 1981.
12. E. Lelarasmee and A. L. Sangiovanni-Vincentelli, RELAX: A new circuit simulator for large scale MOS integrated circuits, *Proc. 1982 Design Automation Conf.*, pp. 682–690, June 1982.

13. H. Uno, S. Kumagai, I. Shirakawa, and S. Kodama, a parallel analysis of MOS digital circuits, *Trans. IECE*, vol. J70-A, pp. 331–339, March 1987.
14. J. White and A. L. Sangiovanni-Vincentelli, Partitioning algorithm and parallel implementations of waveform relaxation algorithms for circuit simulation, *Proc. IEEE Int. Symp. Circuits Syst.*, Kyoto, Japan, pp. 221–224, June 1985.
15. M. E. Mokari-Bolhassan, D. Smart, and T. N. Trick, A new robust relaxation technique for VLSI circuit simulation, *Proc. IEEE Int. Conf. Computer-Aided Design*, Santa Clara, Calif., pp. 26–28, Nov. 1985.
16. H. Uno, H. Kinoshita, S. Kumagai, I. Shirakawa, and S. Kodama, A parallel implementation of MOS digital circuit simulation, *Proc. IEEE Int. Conf. Computer-Aided Design*, Santa Clara, Calif., pp. 2–4, Nov. 1985.
17. H. Nishimura, H. Ohno, T. Kawata, I. Shirakawa, and K. Omura, LINKS-1: A parallel pipelined multimicrocomputer system for image creation, *Proc. 10th Ann. Int. Symp. Computer Architecture*, pp. 387–394, 1983.
18. G. Marong and A. L. Sangiovanni-Vincentelli, Waveform relaxation and dynamic partitioning for the transient simulation of large scale bipolar circuits, *Proc. IEEE Int. Conf. Computer-Aided Design*, Santa Clara, Calif., pp. 32–34, Nov. 1985.

6

Computer Methods for Analysis of Switched-Capacitor Networks

Jiri Vlach

University of Waterloo
Waterloo, Ontario, Canada

1 INTRODUCTION

In the late 1970s, technological progress made it possible to put large digital networks on one chip but there were considerable difficulties in integrating analog networks: It was not possible to manufacture sufficiently reliable, stable, and compact resistors on the chip. Research conducted to relieve the problem discovered that a very rapidly switched capacitor (SC) behaves approximately as a resistor for signals considerably slower than the switching frequency. It was proposed to use networks composed of transistors and capacitors, the switches being realized by the transistors. Early studies have shown that correct ratio of capacitor values is more important than exact capacitor values, and the fact that the technology can realize exactly such ratios came as an additional bonus.

As long as the switching is done very rapidly compared to the speed of the signals, the SC approximation of a resistor works reasonably well. If the speed of the signals grows, then the approximation becomes less and less satisfactory. It was necessary to develop a new theory which would adequately explain all the inaccuracies. In the time domain, existing analysis programs were able to resolve the problem reasonably well. In the frequency domain, with all elements linear, it was necessary to accept certain simplifications because otherwise the problem became intractable. This chapter follows the standard simplified theory, which assumes that

The switch can be represented by a short circuit when it is conducting and by an open circuit otherwise.
The capacitors are linear and without losses.
The sources are either ideal voltage sources or voltage-controlled voltage sources. Frequency-dependent roll-off is not allowed.
Resistors, inductors, and current sources are not considered.

By accepting the above restrictions we can secure instant transfers of charges between the switched or nonswitched capacitors. Details of the theory were summarized in many publications and we refer here to Refs. [1] and [2]. The reader can also find the derivations in Ref. [3].

We will clarify the principles using the network shown in Figure 6.1a. The switch transfers periodically from position 1 to position 2 and back to position 1. The network is said to have two switching phases. Redrawing the network for both phases we get the networks shown in Figures 6.1b and 6.1c. The input signal is denoted by $w(t)$; numbering of the nodes is in circles. The node voltages have two subscripts: The first one denotes the switching phase, the second one is the number of the node. If the node voltage is varying with time, it is denoted by $v(t)$ with the appropriate subscripts. A fixed value is denoted by v, again with the subscripts. These fixed voltages are equal to the node voltages *just before switching to the next phase* and determine the amount of charge on the capacitor which is transferred into the next phase as initial charge. Writing the charge balance for phase 1 and node 2 we have

$$\begin{aligned} C_1[v_{1,2}(t) - v_{1,1}(t)] &= C_1(v_{2,2} - v_{2,1}) \\ v_{1,1}(t) &= w(t) \qquad t \text{ in phase 1} \end{aligned} \tag{1.1}$$

It was sufficient to write the charge balance equation for node 2 only. The charge transferred from the previous (second) phase depends on the voltages in phase 2 just prior to switching. The transition to phase 2 from phase 1 leads to

$$\begin{aligned} C_1[v_{2,2}(t) - v_{2,1}(t)] + C_2 v_{2,2}(t) &= C_1(v_{1,2} - v_{1,1}) \\ v_{2,1}(t) &= w(t) \qquad t \text{ in phase 2} \end{aligned} \tag{1.2}$$

For computer applications, we must rewrite the equations in matrix form.

Phase 1:

$$\begin{bmatrix} -C_1 & C_1 \\ 1 & 0 \end{bmatrix} \begin{bmatrix} v_{1,1}(t) \\ v_{1,2}(t) \end{bmatrix} = \begin{bmatrix} -C_1 & C_1 \\ 0 & 0 \end{bmatrix} \begin{bmatrix} v_{2,1} \\ v_{2,2} \end{bmatrix} + \begin{bmatrix} 0 \\ 1 \end{bmatrix} w(t) \tag{1.3}$$

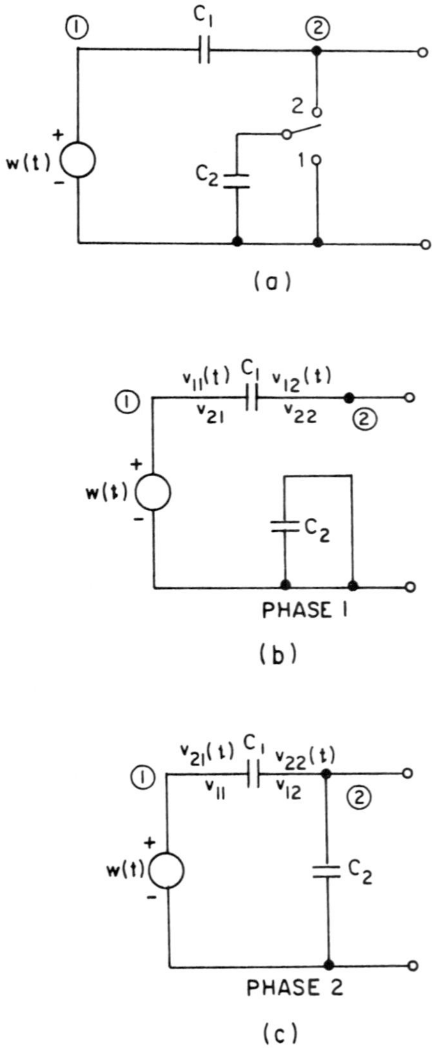

Figure 6.1 A simple switched network.

Phase 2:

$$\begin{bmatrix} -C_1 & (C_1+C_2) \\ 1 & 0 \end{bmatrix} \begin{bmatrix} v_{2,1}(t) \\ v_{2,2}(t) \end{bmatrix} = \begin{bmatrix} -C_1 & C_1 \\ 0 & 0 \end{bmatrix} \begin{bmatrix} v_{1,1} \\ v_{1,2} \end{bmatrix} + \begin{bmatrix} 0 \\ 1 \end{bmatrix} w(t) \tag{1.4}$$

We will denote the matrices on the left by $\mathbf{A}_1$ and $\mathbf{A}_2$, the matrices on the right by $\mathbf{B}_1$ and $\mathbf{B}_2$, and the vectors which take into account the presence of the source by $\mathbf{g}_1$ and $\mathbf{g}_2$, the subscript denoting the switching phase. The system of equations is now written as

$$\begin{aligned} \mathbf{A}_1\mathbf{v}_1(t) &= \mathbf{B}_1\mathbf{v}_2 + \mathbf{g}_1 w(t) \qquad t \text{ in phase } 1 \\ \mathbf{A}_2\mathbf{v}_2(t) &= \mathbf{B}_2\mathbf{v}_1 + \mathbf{g}_2 w(t) \qquad t \text{ in phase } 2 \end{aligned} \tag{1.5}$$

It will be our task to find an automatic and efficient method for writing these matrices and vectors, but first we must introduce a few definitions.

2 DEFINITIONS

General SC networks may have more than two switching phases and the phases may not have equal durations. We thus introduce the following notations: Let T be the duration of the switching period, after which the network returns to the same sequence of switching. Let N be the number of phases. A general phase will always be referred to by the subscript k and the duration of the kth phase will be denoted by τ_k. Their sum is related to the switching period by

$$T = \sum_{i=1}^{N} \tau_i \tag{2.1}$$

It is convenient to introduce another incremental time constant defined as follows:

$$\sigma_k = \sum_{i=1}^{k} \tau_i \tag{2.2}$$

with

$$\sigma_N = T \qquad \text{and} \qquad \sigma_0 = 0 \tag{2.3}$$

Should all the phases have equal durations, then

$$\tau = \frac{T}{N} \tag{2.4}$$

and we omit the subscript. For the kth phase, the matrix equations become

$$\mathbf{A}_k\mathbf{v}_k(t) = \mathbf{B}_k\mathbf{v}_{k-1} + \mathbf{g}_k w(t) \qquad t \text{ in phase } k \tag{2.5}$$

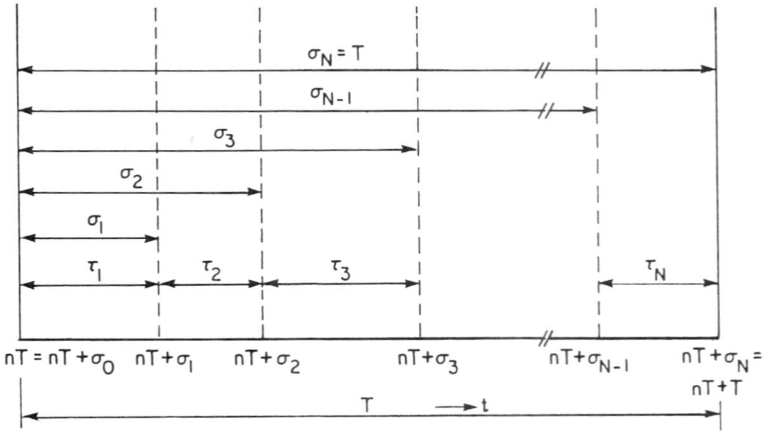

Figure 6.2 Definitions for N-phase network.

with the understanding that if $k - 1 = 0$ then

$$\mathbf{v}_0 = \mathbf{v}_N$$

The definitions are sketched in Figure 6.2.

3 FORMULATION OF MATRICES

The main problem in computerized analysis of SC networks is to find an efficient method to formulate the matrices $\mathbf{A}_k$, $\mathbf{B}_k$ and the vectors $\mathbf{g}_k$. Many methods have been proposed, some leading to large matrices which require sparse matrix solutions,others trying to reduce the sizes of the matrices. We believe that it is best to have the matrices as small as possible. The method we describe here is based on the modified nodal formulation. It uses two types of preprocessing. The first one removes all the switches by replacing them with either short circuits (for closed switches) or open circuits (for open switches). Removal of the switches may lead to different numbers of nodes in the various phases, but this small complication is by far outweighed by the many advantages. In addition to the reduction of the number of nodes, a special two-graph preprocessing reduces the matrices by one row and one column for *each* operational amplifier (OPAMP) or unity gain buffer.

We will indicate the formal background of the two-graph method but emphasis will be given to easy understanding of how to formulate the matrices. The simplifications will be extended to the point that the writing of the matrices becomes automatic.

In the usual graph description of network elements, every one-port is represented by one oriented edge and every two-port by two oriented edges. This makes writing the matrices easy but increases their sizes because many variables, which are in fact known, are to be taken into account as unknowns. This applies, for instance, to the ideal OPAMP, for which we know in advance that the input terminals must be at the same potential. Similarly, in the case of a unity gain buffer, we know that the output voltage must be equal to the input voltage, but they are both kept separately as unknowns in a one-graph formulation.

Such variables can be eliminated topologically by using separate graphs for voltages and currents. If no current flows into the port, the edge can be removed on the *I*-graph but is retained on the *V*-graph. For a short circuit, the nodes are contracted on the *V*-graph but the edge is retained on the *I*-graph. In addition, many variables may be of no interest to us. Usually, we are not interested in the current flowing through the voltage source. The rules for the two types of graphs can be summarized as follows:

If the current in the branch (voltage across the branch) is zero, its edge is deleted (collapsed) on the *I*-graph (*V*-graph).
If the current (voltage) of the branch does not enter the constitutive equations, its edge is collapsed (deleted) on the *I*-graph (*V*-graph).

These rules were applied to all active elements used in analog simulation [4]. At this point we also note that in all practical SC networks all voltage sources, dependent or independent, always have one terminal grounded. This fact, and the rules stated above, are summarized in Figure 6.3. To simplify understanding, we will not talk about current and voltage graphs, but we will discuss the collapsing by writing node numbers in **squares** for the current graphs and in **triangles** for the voltage graphs.

We are, for instance, not interested in the current flowing through any voltage source, dependent or independent. Thus we can collapse the node on the current graph and since the other terminal of the voltage source is grounded, the node number on the current graph (in the square) will be zero, the usual numbering for ground. Since the voltage difference between the input nodes of an ideal differential OPAMP is zero, the edge is collapsed on the *V*-graph. In Figure 6.3, this is indicated by writing the same node number n in the triangle (which denotes the *V*-graph). A similar rule applies to the input and output nodes of a unity gain buffer, since both are at the same potential. In the case of an amplifier with finite gain, the letter m appearing at the output terminal of the amplifier means only that the number of this node, whichever it eventually will be, appears in the constitutive equations of the amplifier, as given in Figure 6.3. Finally, although this is not necessary, we start numbering the nodes from the independent voltage source and thus the

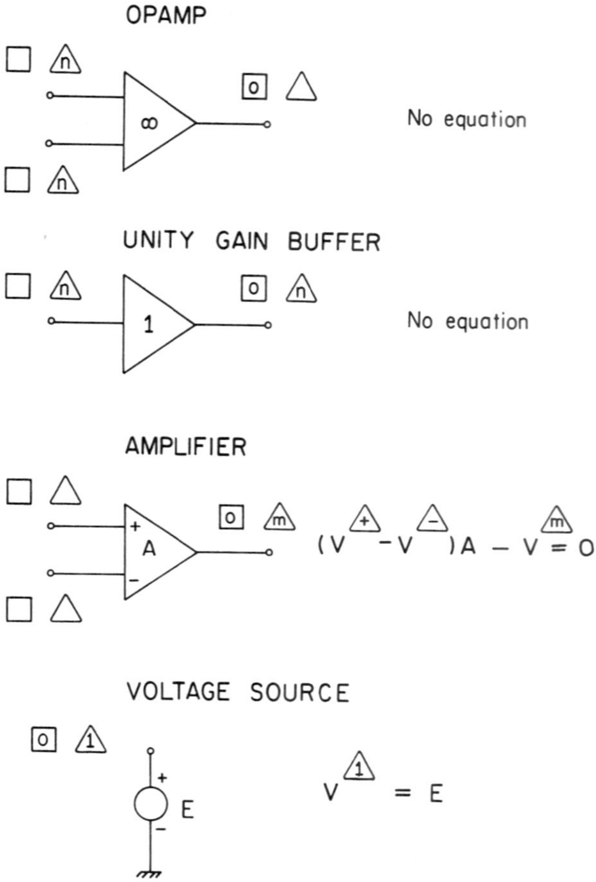

Figure 6.3 Rules for two-graph formulation.

number in the triangle is chosen to be 1. Because we are dealing with two graphs, every node must be given two numbers, one in the square and one in the triangle. Any empty square or triangle in Figure 6.3 simply means that a node number must be given to it. Although this can be done entirely arbitrarily, it is best to do so from left to right and both numberings must be consecutive numbers.

When considering charges of the capacitors, it is very easy to make a mistake, because the charges are coming from the previous phase and switching may change the connections of the capacitor in the network. For this reason we suggest that the reader follow strictly the recommendations summarized below:

1. Draw the network so that the capacitors go either horizontally or vertically.
2. Redraw separately each phase and remove the switches. A short circuit replaces a closed switch, an open circuit replaces an open switch.
3. Indicate the connection of the capacitor in the network by first giving the left or the top node.
4. If in some phase a node, a voltage source, or an amplifier is completely disconnected from the rest of the network, remove it from the drawing of that phase.
5. NEVER remove any capacitor, even if it is floating without any connection or if it is short-circuited.
6. In each phase, every nongrounded node must have two sets of numbers. Numbering in squares refers to the current graph, numbering in triangles refers to the voltage graph. Ground is assigned zero in both sets.

It is convenient to replace the graph by a table of connections and we will show the application of the above steps on an example. Figure 6.4a shows a simple integrator; the network is redrawn for both phases in Figures 6.4b and 6.4c. Each node is assigned a number in a square and a number in a triangle. Using Figure 6.3, we first contract current graph edges of the voltage sources.

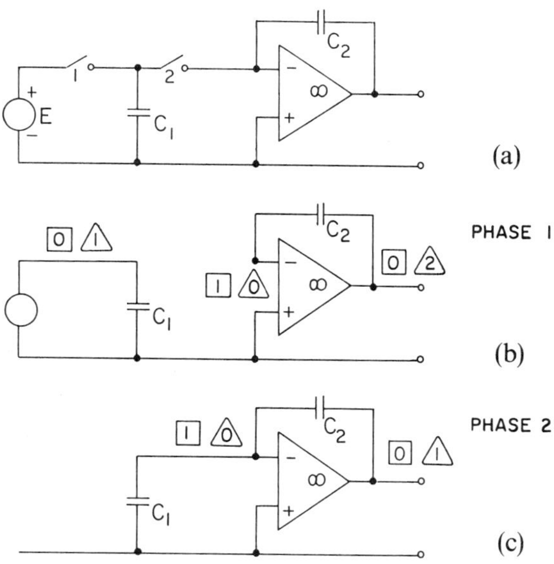

Figure 6.4 Switched-capacitor integrator.

This is equivalent to writing zeros in the squares at the independent voltage source and at the output of the OPAMP. The voltage at the input of the OPAMP is zero, because the other input terminal is grounded. This is recognized by writing zero into the triangle at the input of the OPAMP. All the remaining nodes are numbered independently for both sets. In phase 2, the voltage source is disconnected from the network and is removed from the figure.

The connections of the capacitors are now filled into a table which is equivalent to the two graphs. Follow strictly the rule that the left or top node of each capacitor is given first. For phase 1, the connectivity table is

	$\mathbf{A}_1$	C_1	C_2
I-1	from node	0	1
	to node	0	0
V-1	from node	1	0
	to node	0	2

If we now think for a moment about the usual nodal formulation in analog networks, then we recall that the row indicates the node number where the Kirchhoff current law (KCL) is applied and the column indicates the voltage which multiplies that particular column of the matrix. *The same applies here*, except that the row is given by the current graph number and the column by the voltage graph number. If zero (ground) is in the connectivity table, such an entry does not exist (because in nodal formulation the KCLs are not written for the ground node). Always consider one position from the I-graph and one from the V-graph (altogether four possibilities):

If on both graphs the direction is "from node" or "to node," enter $+C$ into the row indicated by the I-graph and into the column indicated by the V-graph.

If the directions differ, enter $-C$.

If zero appears in the table, the entry does not exist in the matrix.

We now apply the rule to write the matrix $\mathbf{A}_1$. The capacitor C_1 does not appear in the matrix because the table for the I-graph has both entries zero. Capacitor C_2 will appear in row 1 and column 2, and since the directions differ, the entry will be $-C_2$. The remaining three entries do not exist. This completes writing the nodal portion of the matrix but we must still add one row which takes into account the presence of the voltage source $v_{1,1}(t) = w(t)$.

The complete matrix is

$$\mathbf{A}_1 = \begin{bmatrix} 0 & -C_2 \\ 1 & 0 \end{bmatrix} \tag{3.1}$$

The vector $\mathbf{g}_1$ expresses the presence of the source in the appropriate row of the matrix. Since in (3.1) the source is taken care of by the second row, $\mathbf{g}_1$ will have unity in the second row as well:

$$\mathbf{g}_1 = \begin{bmatrix} 0 \\ 1 \end{bmatrix} \tag{3.2}$$

The second phase is redrawn in Figure 6.4c. The connections are given by the table:

	$\mathbf{A}_2$	C_1	C_2
I-2	from node	1	1
	to node	0	0
V-2	from node	0	0
	to node	0	1

Capacitor C_1 does not appear in $\mathbf{A}_2$ since both entries for the V-graph are zero. Capacitor C_2 will be in the position (1, 1) with negative sign, since directions differ. There is no voltage source in phase 2; the matrix has dimension 1×1:

$$\mathbf{A}_2 = [-C_2] \tag{3.3}$$

and

$$\mathbf{g}_2 = [0] \tag{3.4}$$

We still need the **B** matrices, which take into account the charges across the capacitors from the previous phase. All we have to do is copy the connectivity table of the I-graph of the phase we consider and the V-graph connectivity table *of the phase immediately preceding it in time*. In a two-phase network it is always the other phase, but in a network with many phases the above statement is important: Phase 1 is always preceded by phase N, phase 2 by phase 1, phase 3 by phase 2, and so on. The method of getting the matrices is the same as explained above. For $\mathbf{B}_1$ copy the information $I-1$ and $V-2$. The table is

	$\mathbf{B}_1$	C_1	C_2
I-1	from node	0	1
	to node	0	0
V-2	from node	0	0
	to node	0	1

and the matrix is

$$\mathbf{B}_1 = \begin{bmatrix} -C_2 \\ 0 \end{bmatrix} \tag{3.5}$$

Matrices $\mathbf{B}_k$ express the presence of charges on the capacitors. Since they must have the same number of rows as the matrix $\mathbf{A}_k$, zeros are placed in the row corresponding to the presence of the source in the $\mathbf{A}_k$ matrix. The same applies for each finite-gain amplifier.

For the matrix $\mathbf{B}_2$ use the connectivity table with $I-2$ and $V-1$,

	$\mathbf{B}_2$	C_1	C_2
I-2	from node	1	1
	to node	0	0
V-1	from node	1	0
	to node	0	2

The matrix is

$$\mathbf{B}_2 = [C_1 \quad -C_2] \tag{3.6}$$

We will apply the method of setting up the matrices to one more network, shown in Figure 6.5a. It was taken from Ref. [5], p. 175, and is redrawn for

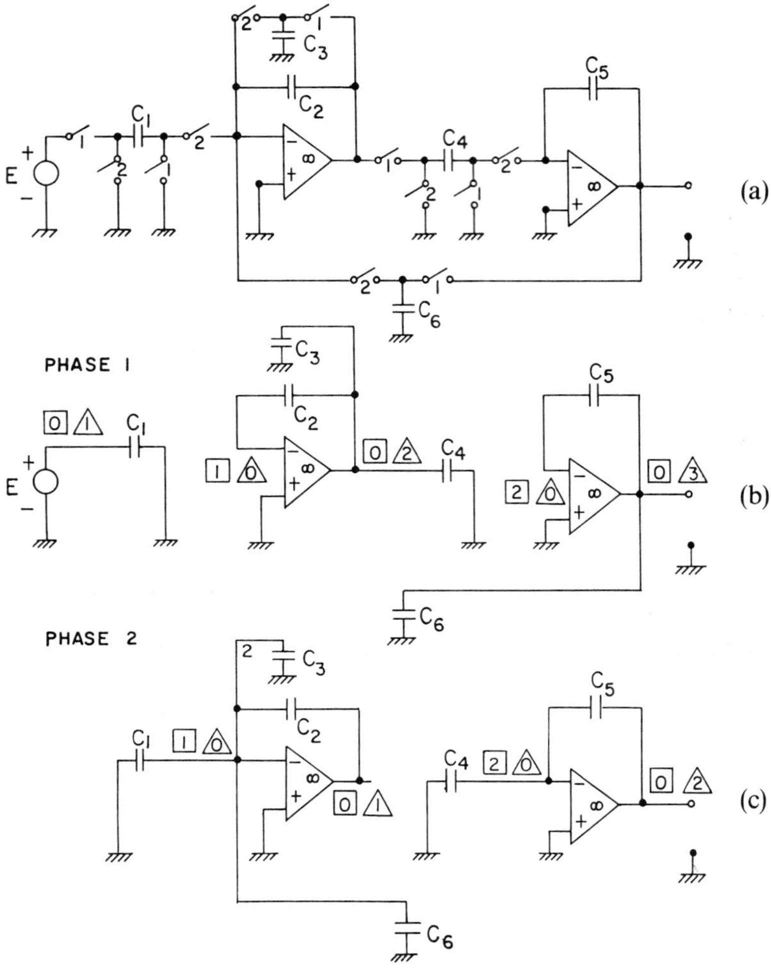

Figure 6.5 Second-order switched-capacitor network.

both phases in Figures 6.5b and 6.5c. For phase 1, the connectivity table is

	$\mathbf{A}_1$	C_1	C_2	C_3	C_4	C_5	C_6
I-1	from node	0	1	0	0	2	0
	to node	0	0	0	0	0	0
V-1	from node	1	0	2	2	0	3
	to node	0	2	0	0	3	0

and matrix $\mathbf{A}_1$ is

$$\mathbf{A}_1 = \begin{bmatrix} 0 & -C_2 & 0 \\ 0 & 0 & -C_5 \\ 1 & 0 & 0 \end{bmatrix} \tag{3.7}$$

Since the influence of the source is taken into account by the third row of $\mathbf{A}_1$, the source vector is

$$\mathbf{g}_1 = \begin{bmatrix} 0 \\ 0 \\ 1 \end{bmatrix} \tag{3.8}$$

for the second phase, the connectivity table is

	$\mathbf{A}_2$	C_1	C_2	C_3	C_4	C_5	C_6
I-2	from node	0	1	1	0	2	1
	to node	1	0	0	2	0	0
V-2	from node	0	0	0	0	0	0
	to node	0	1	0	0	2	0

and the matrix $\mathbf{A}_2$ is

$$\mathbf{A}_2 = \begin{bmatrix} -C_2 & 0 \\ 0 & -C_5 \end{bmatrix} \tag{3.9}$$

No source is connected in phase 2 to the network and the vector $\mathbf{g}_2$ is

$$\mathbf{g}_2 = \begin{bmatrix} 0 \\ 0 \end{bmatrix} \tag{3.10}$$

The table for the $\mathbf{B}_1$ matrix takes the information from $I - 1$ and $V - 2$:

	$\mathbf{B}_1$	C_1	C_2	C_3	C_4	C_5	C_6
$I - 1$	from node	0	1	0	0	2	0
	to node	0	0	0	0	0	0
$V - 2$	from node	0	0	0	0	0	0
	to node	0	1	0	0	2	0

The matrix is

$$\mathbf{B}_1 = \begin{bmatrix} -C_2 & 0 \\ 0 & -C_5 \\ 0 & 0 \end{bmatrix} \tag{3.11}$$

Finally, matrix $\mathbf{B}_2$ takes information from $I-2$ and $V-1$,

$\mathbf{B}_2$		C_1	C_2	C_3	C_4	C_5	C_6
$I-2$	from node	0	1	1	0	2	1
	to node	1	0	0	2	0	0
$V-1$	from node	1	0	2	2	0	3
	to node	0	2	0	0	3	0

and the matrix is

$$\mathbf{B}_2 = \begin{bmatrix} -C_1 & (-C_2 + C_3) & C_6 \\ 0 & -C_4 & -C_5 \end{bmatrix} \tag{3.12}$$

In the above explanation we tried to give sufficient information about the necessary steps without going into complicated theoretical details. The method is quite general and it was actually used to write a general program for the analysis of SC networks, WATSCAD [6, 7].

In the last step we show how to formulate the matrices if the amplifier has finite gain. We will use the network in Figure 6.4. The input terminal of the amplifier is no longer at ground potential and the node numbers in triangles must be changed. In phase 1, the number in a triangle at the input terminal of the amplifier will be 2 and at the output terminal 3. In phase 2, the same nodes will be renumbered to 1 and 2, respectively. Readers should modify their figures accordingly and trace the steps. They should get $\mathbf{g}_1{}^T = [0 \quad 0 \quad 1]$, $\mathbf{g}_2{}^T = [0 \quad 0]$, and

$$\mathbf{A}_1 = \begin{bmatrix} 0 & C_2 & -C_2 \\ 0 & -A & -1 \\ 1 & 0 & 0 \end{bmatrix}$$

$$\mathbf{A}_2 = \begin{bmatrix} (C_1 + C_2) & -C_2 \\ -A & -1 \end{bmatrix}$$

$$\mathbf{B}_1 = \begin{bmatrix} C_2 & -C_2 \\ 0 & 0 \\ 0 & 0 \end{bmatrix}$$

$$\mathbf{B}_2 = \begin{bmatrix} C_1 & C_2 & -C_2 \\ 0 & 0 & 0 \end{bmatrix}$$

4 TIME DOMAIN SOLUTION

Time domain solutions of SC networks are relatively easy once the $\mathbf{A}_k$, $\mathbf{B}_k$ matrices and the $\mathbf{g}_k$ vectors have been prepared. In Section 2, we derived (2.5), repeated here for convenience:

$$\mathbf{A}_k\mathbf{v}_k(t) = \mathbf{B}_k\mathbf{v}_{k-1} + \mathbf{g}_k w(t) \qquad t \text{ in phase } k \tag{4.1}$$

To save on calculations, it is reasonable to premultiply (4.1) by $\mathbf{A}_k{}^{-1}$ and define

$$\mathbf{B}_k^* = \mathbf{A}_k{}^{-1}\mathbf{B}_k \tag{4.2}$$

$$\mathbf{g}_k^* = \mathbf{A}_k{}^{-1}\mathbf{g}_k \tag{4.3}$$

This reduces (4.1) to

$$\mathbf{v}_k(t) = \mathbf{B}_k^*\mathbf{v}_{k-1} + \mathbf{g}_k^* w(t) \qquad t \text{ in phase } k \tag{4.4}$$

The reader should note that the first term on the right side changes only at the switching instant and then stays constant during the whole phase. As the time increases, the system is cyclically reset by changing k from 1 to N and then back to 1 again.

It is convenient here to prepare some steps for the frequency domain solutions. At the moment of switching, $t = nT + \sigma_k$, we denote

$$w_k = w(nT + \sigma_k)$$

$$\mathbf{v}_k = \mathbf{v}(nT + \sigma_k) \tag{4.5}$$

and simultaneously subtract and add $\mathbf{A}_k\mathbf{v}_k$ on the left side and $\mathbf{g}_k w_k$ on the right side of (4.1). We group the terms as follows:

$$\mathbf{A}_k[\mathbf{v}_k(t) - \mathbf{v}_k] + \mathbf{A}_k\mathbf{v}_k = \mathbf{B}_k\mathbf{v}_{k-1} + \mathbf{g}_k[w(t) - w_k] + \mathbf{g}_k w_k \tag{4.6}$$

At the moment of switching, the terms in square brackets on both sides are zero and we can split (4.6) into two equations: a discrete one, valid only at the instants of switching,

$$\mathbf{A}_k\mathbf{v}_k = \mathbf{B}_k\mathbf{v}_{k-1} + \mathbf{g}_k w_k \tag{4.7}$$

and an algebraic one, valid elsewhere,

$$\mathbf{A}_k[\mathbf{v}_k(t) - \mathbf{v}_k] = \mathbf{g}_k[w(t) - w_k] \tag{4.8}$$

This last equation can be simplified by inverting $\mathbf{A}_k$ and inserting (4.3):

$$\mathbf{v}_k(t) = \mathbf{v}_k + \mathbf{g}_k^* r_k(t) \tag{4.9}$$

where we defined for later use

$$r_k(t) = w(t) - w_k \tag{4.10}$$

Independent solutions of (4.7) and (4.9) form the basis for the frequency domain solution of SC networks.

5 FREQUENCY DOMAIN

In the frequency domain we first consider the discrete system for which it is possible to apply the z-transform. Let the switching frequency be defined by

$$\omega_s = \frac{2\pi}{T} \tag{5.1}$$

and the z-variable by

$$z = e^{j\omega T} \tag{5.2}$$

Then the z-domain transformations of the discrete voltages of the respective phases are

$$\mathbf{V}_k = \sum_{n=-\infty}^{\infty} \mathbf{v}(nT + \sigma_k)z^{-n} \qquad k = 1, 2, \ldots, N-1$$

$$\mathbf{V}_N = \sum_{n=-\infty}^{\infty} \mathbf{v}(nT)z^{-n} \tag{5.3}$$

and the signal transformation at the discrete instants is

$$W_k = \sum_{n=-\infty}^{\infty} w(nT + \sigma_k)z^{-n} \qquad k = 1, 2, \ldots, N-1$$

$$W_N = \sum_{n=-\infty}^{\infty} w(nT)z^{-n} \tag{5.4}$$

We also note that

$$\sum_{n=-\infty}^{\infty} \mathbf{v}(nT + \sigma_N)z^{-n} = \sum_{n=-\infty}^{\infty} \mathbf{v}(nT + T)z^{-n} = z\mathbf{V}_N$$

$$\sum_{n=-\infty}^{\infty} w(nT + \sigma_N)z^{-n} = \sum_{n=-\infty}^{\infty} w(nT + T)z^{-n} = zW_N \tag{5.5}$$

Using these definitions, we can transform the N discrete equations into the z-domain and write a matrix equation

$$\begin{bmatrix} \mathbf{A}_1 & 0 & 0 & \cdots & 0 & -\mathbf{B}_1 \\ -\mathbf{B}_2 & \mathbf{A}_2 & 0 & \cdots & 0 & 0 \\ 0 & -\mathbf{B}_3 & \mathbf{A}_3 & \cdots & 0 & 0 \\ \cdots & \cdots & \cdots & \cdots & \cdots & \cdots \\ 0 & 0 & 0 & \cdots & -\mathbf{B}_N & z\mathbf{A}_N \end{bmatrix} \begin{bmatrix} \mathbf{V}_1 \\ \mathbf{V}_2 \\ \mathbf{V}_3 \\ \cdots \\ \mathbf{V}_N \end{bmatrix} = \begin{bmatrix} \mathbf{g}_1 W_1 \\ \mathbf{g}_2 W_2 \\ \mathbf{g}_3 W_3 \\ \cdots \\ \mathbf{g}_N z W_N \end{bmatrix} \tag{5.6}$$

In simplified notation,

$$\mathbf{MV} = \mathbf{H} \tag{5.7}$$

For the right-hand side we can apply the Poisson formula [3]

$$W_k = \sum_{n=-\infty}^{\infty} w(nT + \sigma_k)e^{-jn\omega T} = \frac{1}{T}\sum_{n=-\infty}^{\infty} W(\omega - n\omega_s)e^{j(\omega - n\omega_s)\sigma_k}$$

$$W_N = \sum_{n=-\infty}^{\infty} w(nT)e^{-jn\omega T} = \frac{1}{T}\sum_{n=-\infty}^{\infty} W(\omega - n\omega_s) \tag{5.8}$$

Here $W(\omega)$ is the Fourier transform of the signal $w(t)$. Now define the signal to be

$$w(t) = e^{j\omega_0 t} \tag{5.9}$$

and let the frequency under consideration always be related to the signal and switching frequency by the formula

$$\omega = \omega_0 + n\omega_s \tag{5.10}$$

where n is an integer. Then

$$W(\omega) = 2\pi\delta(\omega - \omega_0)$$

$$W(\omega - n\omega_s) = 2\pi\delta(\omega - \omega_0 - n\omega_s) \tag{5.11}$$

Substituting into (5.8), we obtain the right-hand-side value for any frequency defined by (5.10) as

$$W_k = \frac{2\pi}{T}e^{j\omega_0\sigma_k}, \qquad W_N = \frac{2\pi}{T} \tag{5.12}$$

In the following, we drop the coefficient 2π. In addition, it is convenient *not* to divide by T now. For these reasons we define the right-hand side of (5.6) as

$$\mathbf{H}_{FS} = \begin{bmatrix} \mathbf{g}_1 e^{j\omega_0\sigma_1} \\ \mathbf{g}_2 e^{j\omega_0\sigma_2} \\ \mathbf{g}_3 e^{j\omega_0\sigma_3} \\ \cdots \\ \mathbf{g}_N e^{j\omega_0\sigma_N} \end{bmatrix} \tag{5.13}$$

Here the subscript FS refers to *full signal.*

Consider also the z in the matrix (5.6), in view of the fact that the frequencies are defined by (5.10):

$$e^{j\omega T} = e^{j(\omega_0 + n\omega_s)T} = e^{j\omega_0 T} e^{jn\omega_s T} = e^{j\omega_0 T}$$

This means that both the matrix and the right-hand-side vector remain the same for any frequency defined by (5.10) and the system must be solved only once for all such frequencies; differences will be introduced by special factors, to be derived in the next section.

The situation changes if the signal is sampled and held *in each phase* before it is applied to the network. In such a case, charges flow only during the switching instances and $r_k(t)$, equation (4.10), is identically zero. Moreover, (4.7) simplifies to

$$\mathbf{A}_k \mathbf{v}_k = \mathbf{B}_k \mathbf{v}_{k-1} + \mathbf{g}_k w_{k-1}$$

Tracing the same steps as above, we end up with the vector

$$\mathbf{H}_{SH} = \begin{bmatrix} \mathbf{g}_1 \\ \mathbf{g}_2 e^{j\omega_0\sigma_1} \\ \mathbf{g}_3 e^{j\omega_0\sigma_2} \\ \cdots \\ \mathbf{g}_N e^{j\omega_0\sigma_{N-1}} \end{bmatrix} \tag{5.14}$$

The subscript SH stands for *sampled and held* signal.

In subsequent sections, we will refer to $\mathbf{H}$ only, with the understanding that the proper right-hand-side vector has been chosen for the required type of analysis.

Let us now return to the two examples we prepared earlier and consider the sampled and held signal. In both examples, the networks are operated with a two-phase clock and thus the general expression (5.6) simplifies to

$$\begin{bmatrix} \mathbf{A}_1 & -\mathbf{B}_1 \\ -\mathbf{B}_2 & z\mathbf{A}_2 \end{bmatrix} \begin{bmatrix} \mathbf{V}_1 \\ \mathbf{V}_2 \end{bmatrix} = \begin{bmatrix} \mathbf{g}_1 \\ \mathbf{g}_2 z^{1/2} \end{bmatrix} \tag{5.15}$$

For the network in Figure 6.4 we must solve

$$\begin{bmatrix} 0 & -C_2 & C_2 \\ 1 & 0 & 0 \\ -C_1 & C_2 & -zC_2 \end{bmatrix} \begin{bmatrix} V_{1,1} \\ V_{1,2} \\ V_{2,1} \end{bmatrix} = \begin{bmatrix} 0 \\ 1 \\ 0 \end{bmatrix} \tag{5.16}$$

The first subscript denotes the phase, the second denotes the node number in a triangle. Similarly, for the network in Figure 6.5 we have

$$\begin{bmatrix} 0 & -C_2 & 0 & C_2 & 0 \\ 0 & 0 & -C_5 & 0 & C_5 \\ 1 & 0 & 0 & 0 & 0 \\ C_1 & (C_2 - C_3) & -C_6 & -zC_2 & 0 \\ 0 & C_4 & C_5 & 0 & -zC_5 \end{bmatrix} \begin{bmatrix} V_{1,1} \\ V_{1,2} \\ V_{1,3} \\ V_{2,1} \\ V_{2,2} \end{bmatrix} = \begin{bmatrix} 0 \\ 0 \\ 1 \\ 0 \\ 0 \end{bmatrix} \tag{5.17}$$

6 DETAILED FREQUENCY DOMAIN FORMULAS

Solution of the digital system provides values of the voltages at the switching instances but the output of the network exists between these instances. To take this fact into consideration we define a window function

$$\xi_k(t) = \begin{matrix} 1 & \text{for } nT + \sigma_{k-1} < t < nT + \sigma_k \\ 0 & \text{elsewhere} \end{matrix} \tag{6.1}$$

and multiply by it both sides of (4.9) and (4.10). Without loss of generality we will continue the derivations by using scalar functions. As seen from (4.9), we must find Fourier transforms of three functions:

$$\begin{aligned} \alpha(t) &= \sum_{n=-\infty}^{\infty} v(nT + \sigma_k)\xi_k(t) \\ \beta(t) &= \sum_{n=-\infty}^{\infty} w(nT + \sigma_k)\xi_k(t) \\ \gamma(t) &= \sum_{n=-\infty}^{\infty} w(t)\xi_k(t) \end{aligned} \tag{6.2}$$

The Fourier transform of the first function is

$$\begin{aligned} F[\alpha(t)] &= \sum_{n=-\infty}^{\infty} v(nT + \sigma_k) \int_{nT+\sigma_{k-1}}^{nT+\sigma_k} e^{-j\omega t}\, dt \\ &= \frac{e^{-j\omega\sigma_{k-1}} - e^{-j\omega\sigma_k}}{j\omega} \sum_{n=-\infty}^{\infty} v(nT + \sigma_k)e^{-jn\omega T} \end{aligned} \tag{6.3}$$

The sum on the right is nothing but the solution of the discrete system, $\mathbf{V}_k$. When we consider the last phase, the expression will refer to $nT + \sigma_N$. Because of the original definition in (5.3) we must apply (5.5); this leads to the following frequency-dependent multiplicative factors:

$$D_k = \frac{e^{-j\omega\sigma_{k-1}} - e^{-j\omega\sigma_k}}{j\omega T} \qquad k = 1, 2, \ldots, N-1$$

$$D_N = e^{j\omega T}\frac{e^{-j\omega\sigma_{N-1}} - e^{-j\omega\sigma_N}}{j\omega T} \tag{6.4}$$

Note the division by T; we have now used the division which we omitted in the definition of the right-hand-side vectors (5.13) and (5.14).

The Fourier transform of the second term follows the same steps and the result is the same except for the change of the letter v into w. However, we can continue by applying the Poisson formula (5.8) and by substituting for the signal:

$$F[\beta(t)] = D_k e^{j\omega_0\sigma_k} 2\pi \sum_{n=-\infty}^{\infty} \delta(\omega - \omega_0 - n\omega_s) \tag{6.5}$$

Proceeding similarly for the last phase and taking the steps involving (5.3) and (5.5), we obtain

$$\mu_k = D_k e^{j\omega_0\sigma_k} \qquad k = 1, 2, \ldots, N-1$$

$$\mu_N = D_N \tag{6.6}$$

The third function for which we are seeking the Fourier transform is

$$F[\gamma(t)] = \sum_{n=-\infty}^{\infty} \int_{nT+\sigma_{k-1}}^{nT+\sigma_k} e^{j\omega_0 t} \cdot e^{-j\omega t}\, dt$$

$$= \frac{e^{-j(\omega-\omega_0)\sigma_{k-1}} - e^{-j(\omega-\omega_0)\sigma_k}}{j(\omega-\omega_0)} \sum_{n=-\infty}^{\infty} e^{-j(\omega-\omega_0)nT} \tag{6.7}$$

We now note that the expression after the sum can be replaced by $(2\pi/T)\delta(\omega - \omega_0 - n\omega_s)$. Dropping the term 2π, we get for each frequency expressed by (5.10)

$$\Theta_{k,n} = \frac{e^{-jn\omega_s\sigma_{k-1}} - e^{-jn\omega_s\sigma_k}}{jn\omega_s T} \qquad k = 1, 2, \ldots, N,\ n \neq 0$$

$$\Theta_{k,0} = \frac{\sigma_k - \sigma_{k-1}}{T} = \frac{\tau_k}{T} \qquad k = 1, 2, \ldots, N,\ n = 0 \tag{6.8}$$

Let us now summarize our results. First we collect (6.6) and (6.8) into one formula:

$$R_{k,n} = \Theta_{k,n} - D_k e^{j\omega_0 \sigma_k} \qquad k = 1, 2, \ldots, N-1$$
$$R_{N,n} = \Theta_{N,n} - D_N \tag{6.9}$$

The frequency domain equivalent of (4.9) for a full signal is

$$V_{k,FS} = D_k \mathbf{V}_k + \mathbf{g}_k^* R_{k,n} \tag{6.10}$$

and for a sampled and held signal

$$V_{k,SH} = D_k \mathbf{V}_k \tag{6.11}$$

In both cases we assume that the correct right-hand-side vector (5.13) or (5.14) has been used to solve (5.6).

We still need a formal way to get the output of the network from the vector (6.10) or (6.11); for better understanding we use the example in Figure 6.5. In phase 1, the output voltage is $V_{1,3}$ (the second subscript is the node number in a triangle). In order to select this voltage from the vector $\mathbf{V}_1$ we can define a transpose vector $\mathbf{d}_1{}^t = [0 \quad 0 \quad 1]$, and the output voltage is then obtained as the product $V_{3,\text{out}} = \mathbf{d}_1{}^t\mathbf{V}_1$. In the second phase, the output voltage is $V_{2,2}$. In order to select this voltage from the vector, we define $\mathbf{d}_2{}^t = [0 \quad 1]$ and form the product $V_{2,\text{out}} = \mathbf{d}_2{}^t\mathbf{V}_2$. We are now in the position to define the overall output algebraically:

$$\Phi_{FS} = \sum_{k=1}^{N} \mathbf{d}_k{}^t[D_k \mathbf{V}_k + \mathbf{g}_k^* R_{k,n}] \tag{6.12}$$

$$\Phi_{SH} = \sum_{k=1}^{N} \mathbf{d}_k{}^t D_k \mathbf{V}_k \tag{6.13}$$

The above formulas are general, but most practical networks have equal phase durations. In such a case significant simplifications result: The vector (5.14) reduces to

$$\mathbf{H}_{SH,\text{equal}} = \begin{bmatrix} \mathbf{g}_1 z^{0/N} \\ \mathbf{g}_2 z^{1/N} \\ \mathbf{g}_3 z^{2/N} \\ \cdots \\ \mathbf{g}_N z^{N-1} \end{bmatrix} \tag{6.14}$$

and

$$\mathbf{H}_{FS,\text{equal}} = z^{1/N}\mathbf{H}_{SH,\text{equal}} \tag{6.15}$$

The coefficients D_k also simplify to

$$D_{k,\mathrm{equal}} = Ya_k \tag{6.16}$$

where

$$Y = \frac{1 - z^{-1/N}}{\ln z} \tag{6.17}$$

and

$$a_k = z^{(1-k)/N} \qquad k = 1, 2, \ldots, N-1$$

$$a_N = z^{+1/N} \tag{6.18}$$

In theoretical studies, we may be interested in getting the z-domain transfer function. In such a case we solve the system with the right-hand-side vector (6.14) and obtain the output of the discrete system

$$\mathbf{\Phi}_{\mathrm{discrete}} = \sum_{k=1}^{N} a_k \mathbf{d}_k{}^t \mathbf{V}_k \tag{6.19}$$

7 SOLUTION OF THE SYSTEM MATRIX

All types of frequency domain problems call for an efficient solution of the system (5.6). We will give now a method which, in addition to the compressions already achieved by the application of the two-graph method, further compresses the system matrix to a size equal to that of the system matrix of the last phase, $\mathbf{A}_N$. To simplify notation, let (6.14) be the right-hand-side vector.

We wish to reduce the matrix in (5.6) to upper block diagonal form and make the blocks below the main diagonal zero. To this purpose premultiply the first row by $\mathbf{B}_2\mathbf{A}_1{}^{-1}$ and add to the second row. A zero matrix is created in the position where we had $-\mathbf{B}_2$ but a new entry is created in the last column of the second row, namely $-\mathbf{B}_2\mathbf{A}_1{}^{-1}\mathbf{B}_1$, and the product $\mathbf{B}_2\mathbf{A}_1{}^{-1}\mathbf{g}_1 z^{0/N}$ is added to the second row of the right-hand-side vector. We can now proceed similarly by premultiplying the second row by $\mathbf{B}_3\mathbf{A}_2{}^{-1}$ and adding to the third row. This changes the second entry of the third row to a zero matrix, but we create a new entry $-\mathbf{B}_3\mathbf{A}_2{}^{-1}\mathbf{B}_2\mathbf{A}_1{}^{-1}\mathbf{B}_1$ in the last column; in addition, the same row of the right side changes to $\mathbf{g}_3 z^{2/N} + \mathbf{B}_3\mathbf{A}_2{}^{-1}\mathbf{g}_2 z^{1/N} + \mathbf{B}_3\mathbf{A}_2{}^{-1}\mathbf{B}_2\mathbf{A}_1{}^{-1}\mathbf{g}_1 z^{0/N}$. Continuing similarly, we obtain as a result in the Nth row

$$(z\mathbf{A}_N - \mathbf{E})\mathbf{V}_N = \sum_{k=1}^{n} \mathbf{g}_k{}^P z^{(k-1)/N} \tag{7.1}$$

where

$$\mathbf{E} = \mathbf{B}_N \mathbf{A}_{N-1}{}^{-1} \mathbf{B}_{N-1} \mathbf{A}_{N-2}{}^{-1} \cdots \mathbf{B}_3 \mathbf{A}_2{}^{-1} \mathbf{B}_2 \mathbf{A}_1{}^{-1} \mathbf{B}_1 \tag{7.2}$$

and

$$\mathbf{g}_k{}^P = \mathbf{B}_N \mathbf{A}_{N-1}{}^{-1} \mathbf{B}_{N-1} \mathbf{A}_{N-2}{}^{-1} \cdots \mathbf{B}_{k+1} \mathbf{A}_k{}^{-1} \mathbf{g}_k \qquad k \neq N$$

$$\mathbf{g}_N{}^P = \mathbf{g}_N \tag{7.3}$$

Since $\mathbf{E}$ and $\mathbf{g}_k{}^P$ are independent of frequency, they can be precomputed and stored. What is even more important, the fills we discussed above in the explanation *are not stored*. When (7.1) has been solved, we go back to the original system and solve, in sequence,

$$\mathbf{A}_1 \mathbf{V}_1 = \mathbf{B}_1 \mathbf{V}_N + \mathbf{g}_1 z^{0/N}$$

$$\mathbf{A}_k \mathbf{V}_k = \mathbf{B}_k \mathbf{V}_{k-1} + \mathbf{g}_k z^{(k-1)/N} \qquad k = 2, 3, \ldots, N-1 \tag{7.4}$$

In fact, we can use definitions (4.2) and (4.3) and reduce the computational effort by solving instead

$$\mathbf{V}_1 = \mathbf{B}_1^* \mathbf{V}_N + \mathbf{g}_1^* z^{0/N}$$

$$\mathbf{V}_k = \mathbf{B}_k^* \mathbf{V}_{k-1} + \mathbf{g}_k^* z^{(k-1)/N} \qquad k = 2, 3, \ldots, N-1 \tag{7.5}$$

Most important about this preprocessing is the fact that the final system matrix $(z\mathbf{A}_N - \mathbf{E})$ is so compressed that there is no need to use sparse matrix solvers. This opens the way for the use of all the highly efficient and available programs dealing with full matrices, for instance, the QZ algorithm for finding the system poles.

8 SENSITIVITIES IN THE FREQUENCY DOMAIN

Sensitivity analysis in the frequency domain has two important applications. First, it gives the researcher an idea how much the network performance is influenced by small changes of the network elements. It is clearly desirable to have small sensitivity to changes of elements. The other reason for calculating sensitivities lies in design by optimization. Efficient optimization programs require gradients of the objective functions, and these, in turn, are determined by the sensitivities of the network.

We will simplify the derivations by assuming that the signal was sampled and held before it was applied to the network. Derivations for full signal can be found in Refs. [1, 3]. We start with (6.13)

$$\Phi_{SH} = \sum_{k=1}^{N} d_k{}^t D_k \mathbf{V}_k$$

but for sensitivity calculations it is better to avoid the sum and instead define a new vector

$$\boldsymbol{\delta}^t = [\mathbf{d}_1{}^t D_1, \mathbf{d}_2{}^t D_2, \ldots, \mathbf{d}_N{}^t D_N] \tag{8.1}$$

and, as in (5.7),

$$\mathbf{V}^t = [\mathbf{V}_1{}^t, \mathbf{V}_2{}^t, \ldots, \mathbf{V}_N{}^t] \tag{8.2}$$

Then the output is

$$\Phi_{SH} = \boldsymbol{\delta}^t \mathbf{V} \tag{8.3}$$

Let any capacitor or amplifier gain be denoted by the letter h. We wish to derive a method by which we can obtain the derivative of the output with respect to the element. We recall from mathematics that the derivative of a matrix with respect to h is taken by differentiating each entry with respect to h and that the usual rules for differentiation apply. Thus

$$\frac{\partial \Phi}{\partial h} = \boldsymbol{\delta}^t \frac{\partial \mathbf{V}}{\partial h} \tag{8.4}$$

since $\boldsymbol{\delta}$ does not depend on the elements. In order to obtain $\partial \mathbf{V}/\partial h$ we differentiate (5.7) with respect to h

$$\frac{\partial \mathbf{M}}{\partial h}\mathbf{V} + \mathbf{M}\frac{\partial \mathbf{V}}{\partial h} = 0$$

or

$$\frac{\partial \mathbf{V}}{\partial h} = -\mathbf{M}^{-1}\frac{\partial \mathbf{M}}{\partial h}\mathbf{V} \tag{8.5}$$

Inserting into (8.4)

$$\frac{\partial \Phi}{\partial h} = -\boldsymbol{\delta}^t \mathbf{M}^{-1}\frac{\partial \mathbf{M}}{\partial h}\mathbf{V} \tag{8.6}$$

Now consider the term $-\boldsymbol{\delta}^t\mathbf{M}^{-1}$. The product is some transpose vector to which we can give the name $\mathbf{V}^a$

$$(\mathbf{V}^a)^t = -\boldsymbol{\delta}^t \mathbf{M}^{-1}$$

Postmultiply by $\mathbf{M}$ and transpose; the result is

$$\mathbf{M}^t \mathbf{V}^a = -\boldsymbol{\delta} \tag{8.7}$$

Now suppose that we have solved the original system (5.7) with the appropriate right-hand-side vector and the transpose system (8.7). Inserting

$\mathbf{V}$ and $\mathbf{V}^a$ into (8.6), we get the final result

$$\frac{\partial \Phi}{\partial h} = (\mathbf{V}^a)^t \frac{\partial \mathbf{M}}{\partial h} \mathbf{V} \tag{8.8}$$

We must still find an efficient way to solve (8.7) but the reader should note here that (5.7) and (8.7) *do not* depend on the element we consider for sensitivity. The elements appear only in the matrix $\mathbf{M}$, which we know and which we can easily differentiate. As an example, consider the network in Figure 6.4 and the derivative of the output with respect to C_2. The matrix was given in (5.16), and (8.8) becomes

$$\frac{\partial \Phi}{\partial C_2} = [V_{1,1}{}^a \quad V_{1,2}{}^a \quad V_{2,1}{}^a] \begin{bmatrix} 0 & -1 & 1 \\ 0 & 0 & 0 \\ 0 & 1 & -z \end{bmatrix} \begin{bmatrix} V_{1,1} \\ V_{1,2} \\ V_{2,1} \end{bmatrix}$$

The matrix-vector product is in fact *never* programmed. All we have to know are the *positions* in which the element appears in the matrix and the *sign*. For the example we have

$$\frac{\partial \Phi}{\partial C_2} = V_{1,1}{}^a(-V_{1,2} + V_{2,1}) + V_{2,1}{}^a(V_{1,2} - zV_{2,1})$$

Sensitivity with respect to C_1 will be $-V_{2,1}{}^a V_{1,1}$.

9 SOLUTION OF THE TRANSPOSE SYSTEM

We must still provide an efficient method for the solution of the transpose problem (8.7). Rewriting in expanded form

$$\begin{bmatrix} \mathbf{A}_1{}^t & -\mathbf{B}_2{}^t & 0 & \cdots & 0 & 0 \\ 0 & \mathbf{A}_2{}^t & -\mathbf{B}_3{}^t & \cdots & 0 & 0 \\ 0 & 0 & \mathbf{A}_3{}^t & \cdots & 0 & 0 \\ \cdots & \cdots & \cdots & \cdots & \cdots & \cdots \\ 0 & 0 & 0 & \cdots & \mathbf{A}_{N-1}{}^t & -\mathbf{B}_N{}^t \\ -\mathbf{B}_1{}^t & 0 & 0 & \cdots & 0 & z\mathbf{A}_N{}^t \end{bmatrix} \begin{bmatrix} \mathbf{V}_1{}^1 \\ \mathbf{V}_2{}^a \\ \mathbf{V}_3{}^a \\ \cdots \\ \mathbf{V}_{N-1}{}^a \\ \mathbf{V}_N{}^a \end{bmatrix} = \begin{bmatrix} \mathbf{d}_1 D_1 \\ \mathbf{d}_2 D_2 \\ \mathbf{d}_3 D_3 \\ \cdots \\ \mathbf{d}_{N-1} D_{N-1} \\ \mathbf{d}_N D_N \end{bmatrix} \tag{9.1}$$

We wish to reduce the matrix to upper block diagonal form. To this purpose we premultiply the first row by $\mathbf{B}_1{}^t(\mathbf{A}_1{}^t)^{-1}$ and add to the *last* row. This creates a zero matrix in the left bottom corner but $-\mathbf{B}_1{}^t(\mathbf{A}_1{}^t)^{-1}\mathbf{B}_2{}^t$ appears in the last entry of the second column, and $\mathbf{B}_1{}^t(\mathbf{A}_1{}^t)^{-1}\mathbf{d}_1 D_1$ is added to the last entry of the right-hand-side vector. We can now proceed similarly through the rest of the matrix. At the end we arrive at the system

$$(z\mathbf{A}_N{}^t - \mathbf{E}^t)\mathbf{V}_N{}^a = \sum_{k=1}^{N} \mathbf{d}_k{}^P D_k \tag{9.2}$$

where

$$\mathbf{d}_k{}^P = \mathbf{B}_1{}^t(\mathbf{A}_1{}^t)^{-1}\mathbf{B}_2{}^t(\mathbf{A}_2{}^t)^{-1} \cdots \mathbf{B}_k{}^t(\mathbf{A}_k{}^t)^{-1}\mathbf{d}_k \qquad k = 1, 2, \ldots, N-1$$

$$\mathbf{d}_N{}^P = \mathbf{d}_N \tag{9.3}$$

The system matrix in (9.2) is the transpose of the system matrix in (7.1) and the LU decomposition, performed there, need not be repeated. The vectors $\mathbf{d}_k{}^P$ are independent of frequency and can be precomputed and stored. Again, the fills during the above process *are not stored*. Once (9.2) has been solved, we go back to the original system (9.1) and solve, in sequence,

$$\mathbf{A}_k{}^t\mathbf{V}_k{}^a = \mathbf{B}_{k+1}{}^t\mathbf{V}_{k+1}{}^a + \mathbf{d}_k D_k \qquad k = N-1, N-2, \ldots, 1 \tag{9.4}$$

As before, we can remove the $\mathbf{A}_k{}^t$ matrix by defining

$$\mathbf{B}_k{}^{\#} = (\mathbf{A}_k{}^t)^{-1}\mathbf{B}_{k+1}{}^t \tag{9.5}$$

$$\mathbf{d}_k{}^{\#} = (\mathbf{A}_k{}^t)^{-1}\mathbf{d}_k \tag{9.6}$$

This simplifies (9.4) to

$$\mathbf{V}_k{}^a = \mathbf{B}_{k+1}{}^{\#}\mathbf{V}_{k+1}{}^a + \mathbf{d}_k{}^{\#} D_k \qquad k = N-1, N-2, \ldots, 1 \tag{9.7}$$

10 GROUP DELAY

Computerized evaluation of the group delay will be explained for the case of a sampled and held signal. The interested reader can find formulas for a full signal in Ref. [1]; this reference also derives the sensitivity of the group delay with respect to the network elements.

In equation (8.3) we derived the expression for one output. Since it is a complex function, we can write

$$\Phi = |\Phi| e^{j\phi(\omega)} \tag{10.1}$$

First taking the logarithm and then differentiating with respect to ω,

$$\frac{1}{\Phi}\frac{d\Phi}{d\omega} = \frac{1}{|\Phi|}\frac{d|\Phi|}{d\omega} + j\frac{d\phi(\omega)}{d\omega} \tag{10.2}$$

The group delay is defined as the negatively taken derivative of the phase with respect to omega:

$$\tau(\omega) = -\frac{d\phi(\omega)}{d\omega} = -\mathrm{Im}\left[\frac{1}{\Phi}\frac{d\Phi}{d\omega}\right] \tag{10.3}$$

The output, Φ, was already obtained in (8.3),

$$\Phi_{SH} = \boldsymbol{\delta}^t \mathbf{V}$$

and this provides the denominator in the square brackets of (10.3). We still need

$$\frac{d\Phi}{d\omega} = \frac{d\boldsymbol{\delta}^t}{d\omega}\mathbf{V} + \boldsymbol{\delta}^t \frac{d\mathbf{V}}{d\omega} \tag{10.4}$$

The vector $\boldsymbol{\delta}$ was defined in (8.1) and the frequency-dependent terms in it are D_k; see (6.4). Since this involves primitive differentiation, we leave the details to the reader. We still need $d\mathbf{V}/d\omega$. Proceeding as in Section 8, we obtain it by differentiating (5.7) and realizing that now the right-hand-side vector is also a function of the frequency.

$$\frac{d\mathbf{M}}{d\omega}\mathbf{V} + \mathbf{M}\frac{d\mathbf{V}}{d\omega} = \frac{d\mathbf{H}}{d\omega} \tag{10.5}$$

or

$$\frac{d\mathbf{V}}{d\omega} = \mathbf{M}^{-1}\left[\frac{d\mathbf{H}}{d\omega} - \frac{d\mathbf{M}}{d\omega}\mathbf{V}\right] \tag{10.6}$$

Inserting into (10.4),

$$\frac{d\Phi}{d\omega} = \frac{d\boldsymbol{\delta}^t}{d\omega}\mathbf{V} + \boldsymbol{\delta}^t\mathbf{M}^{-1}\left[\frac{d\mathbf{H}}{d\omega} - \frac{d\mathbf{M}}{d\omega}\mathbf{V}\right]$$

At this point we realize that $-\boldsymbol{\delta}^t\mathbf{M}^{-1} = (\mathbf{V}^a)^t$ [see the discussion under (8.6)] and obtain

$$\frac{d\Phi}{d\omega} = \frac{d\boldsymbol{\delta}^t}{d\omega}\mathbf{V} - (\mathbf{V}^a)^t\frac{d\mathbf{H}}{d\omega} + (\mathbf{V}^a)^t\frac{d\mathbf{M}}{d\omega}\mathbf{V} \tag{10.7}$$

Straightforward differentiation of the right-hand-side vector (5.14) provides $d\mathbf{H}/d\omega$ but we still need a few steps for the last term in (10.7). Consider the system matrix in (5.6) and use for differentiation the chain rule

$$\frac{d\mathbf{M}}{d\omega} = \frac{d\mathbf{M}}{dz}\frac{dz}{d\omega} = jTe^{j\omega T}\frac{d\mathbf{M}}{dz} = jTz\frac{d\mathbf{M}}{dz}$$

The derivative of $\mathbf{M}$ with respect to z is a matrix which has zeros everywhere except in the bottom right corner, where we have A_N; (10.7) can be simplified to

$$\frac{d\Phi}{d\omega} = \frac{d\boldsymbol{\delta}^t}{d\omega}\mathbf{V} - (\mathbf{V}^a)^t\frac{d\mathbf{H}}{d\omega} + jTz(\mathbf{V}_N{}^a)^t\mathbf{A}_N\mathbf{V} \tag{10.8}$$

In summary, calculation of the group delay is similar to the calculation of the sensitivities. Once we have obtained the vectors **V** and $\mathbf{V}^a$, all the computational effort to get the group delay is reduced to programming the derivatives of D_k and the derivatives of the right-hand-side vector **H**.

11 SUMMARY OF COMPUTATIONAL STEPS

We will now summarize the steps needed for the various analyses. Although the algebra in deriving the formulas was considerable, it is surprising how simple the actual programming is since most of the computations can be transferred into frequency-independent preprocessing.

1. *Preprocessing*:
   a. Formulate the matrices $\mathbf{A}_k$, $\mathbf{B}_k$ and the vectors $\mathbf{g}_k$ and $\mathbf{d}_k$.
   b. Calculate **E**, $\mathbf{g}_k{}^P$, and $\mathbf{d}_k{}^P$ using (7.2), (7.3), and (9.3).
   c. Calculate $\mathbf{B}_k^*$ and $\mathbf{g}_k^*$ using (4.2) and (4.3). Also obtain $\mathbf{B}_k{}^\#$ and $\mathbf{d}_k{}^\#$ using (9.5) and (9.6).
2. *Time domain*: Use (4.4) for any input signal $w(t)$.
3. *Frequency domain*: Define $\mathbf{H}_{FS}$ or $\mathbf{H}_{SH}$ using (5.13) or (5.14). Solve (7.1) and (7.5) and insert into (6.12) or (6.13).
4. *Sensitivities*: In addition to the steps from point 3, solve (9.2) and (9.7).
5. *Group delay*: Use **V** and $\mathbf{V}^a$ obtained in steps 3 and 4. Obtain $d\boldsymbol{\delta}^t/d\omega$ and $d\mathbf{H}/d\omega$ and insert into (10.8).

12 CONCLUSION

This chapter summarized all the important steps needed for computerized analysis of switched-capacitor networks. Many methods have been proposed in the literature and we decided to present one which automatically reduces the matrices to the minimum and makes it possible to prepare many of the steps in a preprocessing, done only once. Emphasis in this chapter was placed on the way how the various matrices and vectors are formulated. The reader can find many other details in the references given below.

REFERENCES

1. J. Vlach, K. Singhal, and M. Vlach, Computer oriented formulation of equations and analysis of switched capacitor networks, *IEEE Trans. Circuits Syst.*, vol. CAS-31, pp. 753–765, Sept. 1984.
2. J. Vlach and E. Christen, Poles, zeros and their sensitivities in switched capacitor networks, *IEEE Trans. Circuits Syst.*, vol. CAS-32, pp. 279–284, March 1985.
3. J. Vlach and K. Singhal, *Computer Methods for Circuit Analysis and Design*, Van Nostrand-Reinhold, New York, N.Y., 1983.
4. K. Singhal and J. Vlach, Two-graph tableau and mixed nodal tableau formulation on networks with ideal elements, *1978 European Conf. Circuit Theory and Design*, Lausanne, pp. 553–557, 1978.
5. P. E. Allen and E. Sanchez-Sinencio, *Switched Capacitor Circuits*, Van Nostrand-Reinhold, New York, N.Y., 1984.
6. M. Vlach, J. Vlach, K. Singhal, and R. Chadha, WATSCAD User's Manual, Faculty of Engineering, Univ. of Waterloo, Feb. 1986.
7. J. Vlach, M. Vlach, and K. Singhal, WATSCAD Tutorial, Faculty of Engineering, Univ. of Waterloo, Feb. 1986.

7

Techniques for Finding the Periodic Steady-State Response of Circuits

Kenneth S. Kundert and Alberto Sangiovanni-Vincentelli

University of California, Berkeley, California

Tsutomu Sugawara

Toshiba Corporation
Kawasaki, Japan

1 INTRODUCTION

Often, when simulating analog and microwave circuits, the steady-state behavior of the circuit is of primary interest. This is not necessarily because it is expected that the circuit will spend most of its life in steady state, but rather because the steady-state response contains important information that is obscured by any transient behavior. For example, the most common method used to measure the linearity of an amplifier is to apply a pure sinusoid to the input, allow the transient to decay, and then determine how much the output deviates from a pure sinusoid. Any transient that is present when the purity of the output is measured will be confused with nonlinear distortion.

There are many qualities of a circuit that can or should only be measured when the circuit is in steady state. Examples include distortion, power level, noise, and transfer characteristics such as gain and impedance. Therefore, a circuit simulator that is destined to be used for analog and microwave circuits should be able to calculate the steady-state response of a circuit efficiently and accurately.

One approach to calculating the steady-state response is to integrate the differential equations that describe the circuit from some chosen initial state until any transient behavior dies out—an approach that suffers from two basic drawbacks. First, it can be quite difficult to determine when the transient has died out. If the time constants involved in the transient are large, the circuit may erroneously be declared to be in steady state when in reality it is quite far from it. Second, even if it is possible to correctly detect that steady state has been achieved, it may take a long time for the transients to decay, and thus this approach would involve an expensive calculation. These problems can be greatly reduced by using customized integration methods to accelerate the process of reaching steady state. For example, if the circuit exhibits lightly damped oscillations, it is possible to have the integration method follow the envelope of the solution rather than the solution itself [20].

Another approach is to calculate the steady-state behavior directly. The problem of finding the periodic steady-state solution of a system of ordinary differential equations can be posed as a two-point boundary-value problem. There is a considerable amount of literature available on the numerical solution of these problems, of which a good cross section is given by Refs. [3, 7, 11, 14, 15, 21, 25]. The two-point boundary-value problem is fundamentally different from the initial-value problem and substantially more difficult to solve. The crucial difference is that in the latter case one starts from a known state and progresses forward in time with no constraints placed on the final state. Attention is focused locally; when finding the solution at a particular time point only the current time point and a few previous time points are of interest. In the former case, there is a known relationship between the initial state and the final state, but neither is known. Hence, a critical aspect of this case is that it is necessary to devise a numerical algorithm that finds a solution such that the initial and final states satisfy the given requirements.

There are many ways to find the periodic solution of a set of ordinary differential equations. In general, it is possible to classify these into three basic categories: shooting methods, finite-difference methods, and expansion methods. Shooting methods treat the problem as an initial-value problem to be evaluated over one period. They try to find an initial state that eliminates any transient behavior and results immediately in periodicity. Finite-difference methods replace the differential equations with finite-difference equations on a mesh of points that cover one period. Trial solutions consist of discrete values, one for each point on the mesh, that do not necessarily satisfy the difference equations but do satisfy the boundary conditions. The trial solution at each point is adjusted until it also satisfies the difference equations. Expansion methods start with a collection of linearly independent functions that form a basis for an appropriate function space and then represent the solution as a linear combination of those functions. The process of finding a solution is viewed as one of simply finding the coefficients of the basis functions. Since we are finding the solution numerically, it is necessary to use a finite number of basis functions. Thus, in general, the exact solution cannot be found. The desired approximate solution is one that minimizes some error function. There are several ways to define the error function, and each generates a method with a different name. If by residual we mean the amount by which the differential equation is not satisfied, then collocation methods force the residual to zero, and so satisfy the differential equation exactly, at a finite number of "collocation points." Least-squares methods minimize the integral of the residual squared. Galerkin methods force the residual to be orthogonal to the basis functions. Of all these methods, only one has gained popularity for use in circuit simulation; this is a Galerkin method referred to as harmonic balance, a method characterized by the use of trigonometric polynomials as basis functions.

The shooting, finite-difference, and expansion methods are introduced and contrasted in a unified mathematical framework. The emphasis is on presenting methods that are suitable for forced periodic systems, though methods for solving autonomous systems are discussed briefly. We start in Section 2 with the shooting methods, covering both the Newton-Raphson and extrapolation approaches. The parallel shooting method is also discussed as it acts as a bridge between the shooting methods and the finite-difference methods. Section 3 covers the finite-difference method. In Section 4 harmonic balance, an expansion method, is addressed. Last, the shooting method and harmonic balance are modified to handle autonomous circuits in Section 5.

1.1 Problem Formulation

In the interest of keeping notation simple we consider only nonlinear time-invariant circuits consisting of independent current sources and voltage-controlled resistors and capacitors. These restrictions are just cosmetic; they allow the use of simple nodal analysis to formulate the circuit equations. All the results in this chapter can be applied to circuits containing inductors, voltage sources, and current-controlled components if a more general equation formulation method such as modified nodal analysis is used [22]. Initially we also consider only nonautonomous (or forced) lumped circuits, that is, circuits with at least one periodic input source and no distributed components.

Define $P^N(T)$ as the space of all T-periodic functions of bounded variation that map into $\mathbf{R}^N$, where N is the number of nodes in the circuit (excluding ground). Assume that the current source waveforms belong to $P^N(T)$, that the circuit has an isolated asymptotically stable periodic solution $\hat{v} \in P^N(T)$ and that all device constitutive equations are differentiable when written as a function of voltage. Now the circuit can be described by

$$f(v, t) = \dot{q}(v(t)) + i(v(t)) + u(t) = \mathbf{0} \tag{1}$$

where $t \in \mathbf{R}$ is time; $\mathbf{0} \in \mathbf{R}^N$ is the zero vector; v is the vector of node voltage waveforms; u is the vector of source current waveforms; i, q: $\mathbf{R}^N \to \mathbf{R}^N$ are differentiable functions representing respectively the sum of the currents entering the nodes from the conductors and the sum of the charge entering the nodes from the capacitors; and f is the function that maps the node voltage waveforms into the sum of the currents entering each node.

1.2 Initial-Value Problems

Circuits are modeled using a system of nonlinear differential equations. Before the system can be solved it is necessary to specify the boundary conditions. Traditionally, circuit simulators treat only initial-value problems, so the initial state (the node voltages) is specified at $t = 0$ and the equations are integrated forward in time. Equation (1) can be written as an initial-value problem if the periodicity constraint on v is lifted and an initial state is specified.

$$\dot{q}(v(t)) + i(v(t)) + u(t) = \mathbf{0} \qquad v(0) = v_0 \tag{2}$$

It is not possible to numerically solve systems of nonlinear differential equations directly; first they must be discretized.

Discretization approximates a system of differential equations with a system of difference equations. In other words, the time interval of interest $[0, T]$ is divided into a finite number of possibly nonuniform subintervals with a monotonically increasing sequence of time points $\{t_0, t_1, \ldots, t_M\}$ where $t_0 = 0$ and $t_M = T$. The subintervals are called time steps and denoted by $h_m = t_m - t_{m-1}$. At t_m the solution of the discretized system v_m is an approximation to $v(t_m)$, the solution of the original differential equation (2). At each time point, an algebraic system of equations must be solved; thus discretization converts a differential equation into a sequence of algebraic equations that can be solved numerically.

To discretize a system of differential equations it is necessary to have a discrete approximation to $\dot{q}$. A set of approximations commonly used in circuit simulation are the backward difference formulas [4], which are defined by

$$\dot{q}_{m+1} = \frac{1}{bh_{m+1}} \sum_{n=-1}^{p} a_n q_{m-n} \qquad a_{-1} = -1 \tag{3}$$

The simplest of the backward difference formulas are the one-step methods

$$\text{Explicit Euler:} \qquad \dot{q}_m = \frac{q_{m+1} - q_m}{h_m} \tag{4}$$

Implicit Euler: $$\dot{q}_{m+1} = \frac{q_{m+1} - q_m}{h_{m+1}} \qquad (5)$$

Of these two methods, implicit Euler has the desirable property of being stiffly stable, which means that it is well behaved even if the differential equations being solved have widely separated time constants. This is not true for explicit Euler [8].

It is natural to apply backward difference formulas to initial-value problems because, when computing the solution at t_m, it is only necessary to know the solution at previous values of time. The integration is conveniently carried out by starting at t_0 and progressing forward in time forward t_M.

The algebraic equations generated by discretization are nonlinear and so are not directly solvable. Linearization is the process of converting an implicit nonlinear equation into a sequence of implicit linear equations. The sequence of linear equations is constructed such that, if a limit point exists, its solution is the solution of the nonlinear problem. Usually, the Newton-Raphson algorithm or one of its variants is used to construct the sequence of linear problems. For example, consider the implicit nonlinear system of equations

$$g(\hat{x}) = \mathbf{0}$$

where $\hat{x} \in \mathbf{R}^N$ and $g\colon \mathbf{R}^N \to \mathbf{R}^N$. The Newton-Raphson algorithm needs an initial guess $x^{(0)}$ of the solution $\hat{x}$ to start. It then linearizes $g(x)$ about $x^{(0)}$ by using the Taylor expansion while neglecting the higher-order terms.

$$g(x^{(1)}) = g(x^{(0)}) + \frac{dg(x^{(0)})}{dx}(x^{(1)} - x^{(0)}) + O((x^{(1)} - x^{(0)})^2)$$

where $dg(x)/dx$ is the Frechet derivative of g with respect to x [19] and is such that

$$\frac{dg(x)}{dx} = J_g(x) = \left[\frac{\partial g_i(x)}{\partial x_j}\right] \qquad i, j = 1, 2, \ldots, N$$

$J_g(x)$ is called the Jacobian of g, and $O(\cdot)$ is a function that represents the higher-order terms and is such that $\lim_{\alpha \to 0}(\|O(\alpha)\|/\alpha)$ is bounded. Let

$$g_L{}^{(0)}(x^{(1)}) = g(x^{(0)}) + J_g(x^{(0)})(x^{(1)} - x^{(0)})$$

where $g_L{}^{(0)}(x)$ is the linearized approximation to $g(x)$. It is the hyperplane that is tangent to $g(x)$ at $x^{(0)}$. An improved approximation to $\hat{x}$ is now found by solving for the root of the linearized approximation to $g(x)$, that is, finding the value of x, denoted by $x^{(1)}$, that satisfies $g_L{}^{(0)}(x) = 0$.

$$x^{(1)} = x^{(0)} - J_g{}^{-1}(x^{(0)})g(x^{(0)})$$

If $g_L{}^{(0)}$ is a good approximation to g near $\hat{x}$, then $x^{(1)}$ will be closer to $\hat{x}$ than was $x^{(0)}$. This procedure is repeated by replacing the initial guess $x^{(0)}$ with $x^{(1)}$.

The iteration is repeated until some convergence criterion is satisfied.

$$x^{(j+1)} = x^{(j)} - J_g^{-1}(x^{(j)})g(x^{(j)}) \tag{6}$$

The sequence generated by (6) will converge to $\hat{x}$ if g is continuously differentiable, $J_g(\hat{x})$ is nonsingular, and $x^{(0)}$ is sufficiently close to $\hat{x}$. Furthermore, if $dg(x)/dx$ is Lipschitz-continuous,† the asymptotic rate of convergence will be at least quadratic. More explicitly. let $\varepsilon^{(j)} = \|x^{(j)} - \hat{x}\|$ be the error of the jth iterate. If there exist constants p and $\alpha \neq 0$ such that

$$\lim_{j \to \infty} \frac{\varepsilon^{(j+1)}}{(\varepsilon^{(j)})^p} = \alpha$$

then p is called the rate (or order) of convergence. For Newton's method, $p \geqslant 2$. In general, there is no way to ensure that the initial guess $x^{(0)}$ is sufficiently close to the solution $\hat{x}$, so convergence can be elusive.

Newton's method requires that the Jacobian be constructed and factored on each iteration, an expensive series of operations that, under certain circumstances, can be avoided. In a variation on Newton's method attributed to Šamanskii [19], the factored Jacobian from one iteration is used for several subsequent iterations. If the changes in the Jacobian from iteration to iteration are sufficiently small, then the old Jacobian being used closely approximates the true Jacobian and this new method should converge to the correct solution. The Jacobian is used only to generate new iterates and is not used when confirming convergence, so errors resulting from approximations in the Jacobian affect only the rate and region of convergence, not the accuracy of the final solution. With large systems of equations Šamanskii's variation can be considerably faster than the standard Newton's method, even though it usually requires a greater number of iterations, because each iteration is less expensive. However, the region of convergence is often smaller than with the standard Newton's method. Therefore, progress toward convergence should be monitored and the true Jacobian used if the sequence $\{\|f(x^{(j)})\|\}$ begins to diverge.

1.3 Boundary-Value Problems

A boundary-value problem for a system of differential equations is obtained by requiring that the solution satisfy subsidiary conditions at two or more distinct points. For example, finding the solution to

$$\dot{x}(t) = f(x(t), t)$$

†A function f is Lipschitz-continuous if $\|f(x) - f(y)\| \leqslant K\|x - y\|$ for all x and y in the domain of f, where K is a fixed positive number.

over the interval $[0, T]$ is a two-point boundary-value problem if the solution is required to satisfy

$$g(x(0), x(T)) = \mathbf{0}$$

In order to write the circuit equation (1) as a two-point boundary-value problem it is necessary to formulate the periodicity requirement as a two-point constraint on the solution. For v to be T-periodic, it must satisfy $v(t) = v(t + T)$ for all t. Fixing $t = 0$ makes (1) a two-point boundary-value problem.

$$f(v, t) = \dot{q}(v(t)) + i(v(t)) + u(t) = \mathbf{0} \tag{7}$$

where

$$v(0) - v(T) = \mathbf{0} \tag{8}$$

Clearly, any T-periodic solution of (7) satisfies (8), but since the periodicity constraint was weakened by fixing $t = 0$, it is possible for a function that is not T-periodic to satisfy both (7) and (8). This can be troublesome in the shooting methods, but the finite-difference method and the expansion methods place additional constraints on $\dot{v}(0)$ and $\dot{v}(T)$ and thus do not suffer from this problem. If for every initial state in (2) there is a unique solution, then (8) is sufficient to guarantee that the solution of (7) is T-periodic. The uniqueness of the solution is ensured if i is Lipschitz-continuous, u is bounded, and the capacitance matrix $C(v(t)) = dq(v(t))/dv(t)$ is nonsingular and $\|C^{-1}(\cdot)\|$ is bounded [10].

It is not always possible to cast the problem of finding the steady-state response of a circuit as a two-point boundary-value problem. If the circuit is autonomous, the period is unknown, which violates the strict definition of a two-point boundary-value problem and increases the difficulty of finding the solution. More troublesome are circuits with two or more input signals at incommensurable frequencies. The response of these circuits is not periodic and steady state cannot be verified using only two points. Another problem with the two-point boundary-value problem approach is that it does not differentiate between stable and unstable solutions.

Define $\phi_t(v_0)$ as the solution to (2) at time t given the initial condition $v(0) = v_0$. Now the two-point periodicity constraint (8) can be rewritten

$$\hat{v}(0) = \phi_T(\hat{v}(0)) \tag{9}$$

Thus $\hat{v}(0)$ is a fixed point of ϕ_T and can be found with the fixed-point iteration

$$v^{(j+1)}(0) = \phi_T(v^{(j)}(0)) \tag{10}$$

if ϕ_T is a contraction map [19]. Solving for $\hat{v}(0)$ using (10) is equivalent to integrating (7) until the transient decays. Since the transient may decay very slowly, solving for the steady-state solution by applying straight fixed-point iteration can be very inefficient.

2 SHOOTING METHODS

Shooting methods attack boundary-value problems by converting them into a sequence of initial-value problems. The limit of the sequence of solution waveforms generated by the initial-value problems is the solution to the boundary-value problem. Shooting methods vary as to how the solution of the preceding initial-value problem is used to start the next in the sequence. It is possible to cast the obvious process of integrating (7) until the transient decays to an acceptably small level as a shooting method by using a fixed point iteration. Each initial-value problem in the sequence takes as its initial state the final state from the previous initial-value problem. Each waveform in the sequence represents a one period interval in the waveform that results if f is integrated normally from v_0 and the one-period intervals are adjacent.

There are two ways to accelerate the convergence to the desired solution. The first is by use of so-called extrapolation methods. The other approach is to use the Newton-Raphson method.

In extrapolation methods, the circuit is simulated for several periods and the progress toward steady state is monitored. The sequence constructed from the state of the circuit at the end of each period is extrapolated to what it would be at steady state. This extrapolated state, for various reasons, may not be the one that results in steady state, but it should be close and can be improved by repeating the extrapolation procedure starting with the new extrapolated state. Use of the extrapolation shooting methods in circuit simulation was championed by Skelboe [23].

The Newton-Raphson method simulates the circuit for one period and then compares the final state to the initial state. Any difference between the two implies that periodic steady state has not been reached. The derivative of the final state with respect to changes in the initial state is computed and used to determine how to change the initial state to achieve steady state. The combination of Newton-Raphson and the shooting method has long been used by mathematicians to solve the two-point boundary-value problem; it was first used to find the periodic-steady-state response of circuits by Aprille and Trick [1, 2].

2.1 Shooting by Extrapolation

Construct a sequence $\{v_j\}$ by letting $v_0 = v(0)$ and using

$$v_{j+1} = \phi_T(v_j) \tag{11}$$

Convergence of this sequence can be accelerated by extrapolation. Though several extrapolation techniques can be used [23], the one based on minimum polynomials is presented here. It is normally the most efficient because it requires fewer periods to perform an extrapolation.

The extrapolation is made by assuming that the sequence $\{v_j\}$ is generated by a linear finite-dimensional system of the form

$$v_{j+1} = Av_j + b \tag{12}$$

where $A \in \mathbf{R}^{N \times N}$ and $b \in \mathbf{R}^N$. By just observing $\{v_j\}$ and without explicitly calculating A and b, the fixed point v^* of this linear model can be found. If ϕ_T is linear, then (12) models ϕ_T exactly, $v^* = \hat{v}$, and the solution is found in one iteration. However, if ϕ_T is nonlinear, then more than one iteration is usually needed. Expand ϕ_T about its fixed point $\hat{v}$:

$$\begin{aligned}\phi_T(\hat{v} + \delta v) &= \phi_T(\hat{v}) + J_\phi(\hat{v})\delta v + O(\delta v^2) \\ &= \phi_T(\hat{v}) - J_\phi(\hat{v})\hat{v} + J_\phi(\hat{v})(\hat{v} + \delta v) + O(\delta v^2) \\ &= b + A(\hat{v} + \delta v) + O(\delta v^2)\end{aligned}$$

If δv is large, then $O(\delta v^2)$ is large and the extrapolated value v^* is different from $\hat{v}$. Presumably, though, v^* is closer to $\hat{v}$ than was the initial guess v_0 and the extrapolation process can be repeated until it converges to $\hat{v}$. Convergence is achieved if v_0 is close enough to $\hat{v}$ and if $J_\phi(\hat{v})$ is nonsingular, and it is quadratic if ϕ_T is sufficiently smooth [24].

Now the extrapolation algorithm is presented. Consider the sequence $\{\delta v_j\}$ generated by (12) where $\delta v_j = v_j - v^*$. Since $\delta v_j \in \mathbf{R}^N$, there are at most N vectors in the sequence that are linearly independent. It may happen that A is not of full rank, either because of algebraic constraints on (1) or because of time constants that are very short compared to T. These short time constants correspond to eigenvalues of A that are small and can be ignored for the purposes of the following calculations. Let the resulting rank of A be $r \leqslant N$; then A has a null space of dimension $N - r$. None of the vectors in $\{\delta v_j\}$ lies in the null space of A, so there are at most r linearly independent vectors in the sequence $\{\delta v_j\}$. If some of the eigenvalues of A have a multiplicity greater than one, then it is possible that even fewer than r of the vectors in the sequence are independent. In fact, the number of independent vectors in the sequence cannot be greater than the degree of the minimum polynomial of A. This conclusion, however, is only of theoretical interest. The important point is that there exists a number $p \leqslant r \leqslant N$ such that there are at most p linearly independent vectors in the sequence $\{\delta v_j\}$. Hence, there exists a set of $p + 1$ nonzero coefficients $\{c_j\}$, $j = 0, 1, \ldots, p$, such that

$$\sum_{j=0}^{p} c_j \delta v_j = \mathbf{0} \tag{13}$$

If the coefficients c_j are found, then it is possible to compute the fixed point v^* for (12) from (13) and the fact that $\delta v_j = v_j - v^*$.

$$v^* = \frac{\sum_{j=0}^{p} c_j v_j}{\sum_{j=0}^{p} c_j} \tag{14}$$

In order to find the coefficients c_j, define $\Delta v_j = v_{j+1} - v_j$ and recall that $v_{j+1} = Av_j + b$ and $v^* = Av^* + b$ so that $v_{j+1} = Av_j + v^* - Av^*$. Then

$$\sum_{j=0}^{p} c_j \Delta v_j = \sum_{j=0}^{p} c_j (A - \mathbf{1})(v_j - v^*) = \mathbf{0} \tag{15}$$

We can solve this equation to find the coefficients c_j. Let $V = [\Delta v_0, \Delta v_1, \ldots, \Delta v_{p-1}]$, $c = [c_0, c_1, \ldots, c_{p-1}]^T$, and $c_p = -1$. Then (15) becomes

$$Vc = \Delta v_p \tag{16}$$

If $p < N$, the problem is overdetermined and so cannot be solved using LU factorization. Even if $p = N$, for reasons given above, one or more of the eigenvalues of A may be very small, which results in V being ill-conditioned and makes LU factorization risky. Thus (16) is treated as a least-squares problem and is solved using QR factirization [5]. In other words, the coefficient vector c is chosen by the QR algorithm to minimize ε, where

$$\varepsilon = \| Vc - \Delta v_p \|_2^2 \tag{17}$$

Since A and its eigenvalues are unknown, there is no way to explicitly compute p. Instead, its value is estimated by monitoring ε as the number of periods in the computed response is increased. The value of p is taken as the smaller of either N or the number of periods used for the computation of c when ε drops below some small threshold. Once p has been determined, the extrapolation should be performed using (14) and (16).

The calculation of v^* represents one iterate of the extrapolation process. The iteration is continued until the sequence of v^*'s converges. Each iterate requires simulating the circuit for at least p iterations. The value of p is roughly equal to the number of independent slowly decaying states in the circuit, so if there are few, the extrapolation version of the shooting method should be efficient. In order to eliminate any effect of the short-lived time constants, it is a good idea to discard the first period of the circuit response waveform in each extrapolation iterate.

2.2 Shooting with Newton-Raphson

Newton-Raphson methods calculate the response of the circuit over one period. Also calculated is the sensitivity of the final state with respect to changes in the initial state. The sensitivity is used to determine how to correct the initial state once the difference between the achieved and the desired final state is found. Perhaps conceptually the easiest way to determine the sensitivity of the final state to the initial state is to use finite differences. In this case, the circuit equations are solved N times, each time perturbing slightly a different entry in the v_0 vector. The approach taken when using Newton's method is similar except that the circuit is linearized about the v_0 solution trajectory and the resulting linear time-varying system is solved for its zero-input response with N different initial conditions. The N initial conditions are normally taken to be the N unit vectors that span $\mathbf{R}^N$.

At this point it is important to realize that we are not solving the original circuit equation (1), but rather a discretized approximation. This distinction is important to achieving quadratic convergence in the Newton-Raphson iteration [24]. The notation needed to perform the derivation for the general backward difference discretization is complex enough to obscure the basic concepts behind the derivation, so for simplicity and clarity (1) is discretized using implicit Euler (6), though any discretization formula could have been used instead.

$$\frac{1}{h_m}[q(v_m) - q(v_{m-1})] + i(v_m) + u_m = \mathbf{0} \qquad m = 1, 2, \ldots, M \tag{18}$$

Applying Newton's method to

$$\phi_T(\hat{v}_0) - \hat{v}_0 = \mathbf{0} \tag{19}$$

results in the iteration

$$v_0^{(j+1)} = v_0^{(j)} - [J_\phi(v_0^{(j)}) - \mathbf{1}]^{-1}[\phi_T(v_0^{(j)}) - v_0^{(j)}] \tag{20}$$

where $\mathbf{1}$ is the identity matrix and

$$[J_\phi(v_0) - \mathbf{1}] = \frac{d}{dv_0}(\phi_T(v_0) - v_0) = \frac{dv_M}{dv_0} - \mathbf{1} \tag{21}$$

The derivative dv_M/dv_0 is taken to be the final value of the dv_m/dv_0 trajectory, which is found by differentiating both sides of (18) with respect to v_0:

$$\frac{1}{h_m}\frac{d}{dv_0}[q(v_m) - q(v_{m-1})] + \frac{d}{dv_0}i(v_m) = \mathbf{0} \tag{22}$$

Applying the chain rule

$$\frac{1}{h_m}\left[\frac{dq(v_m)}{dv_m}\frac{dv_m}{dv_0} - \frac{dq(v_{m-1})}{dv_{m-1}}\frac{dv_{m-1}}{dv_0}\right] + \frac{di(v_m)}{dv_m}\frac{dv_m}{dv_0} = \mathbf{0}$$

Let $di(v)/dv = g(v)$ and $dq(v)/dv = c(v)$.

$$\left[\frac{c(v_m)}{h_m} + g(v_m)\right]\frac{dv_m}{dv_0} - \frac{c(v_{m-1})}{h_m}\frac{dv_{m-1}}{dv_0} = \mathbf{0}$$

$$\frac{dv_m}{dv_0} = J_f^{-1}(v_m)\frac{c(v_{m-1})}{h_m}\frac{dv_{m-1}}{dv_0} \tag{23}$$

where $J_f(v_m) = c(v_m)/h_m + g(v_m)$.

The Jacobian $J_\phi(v_0) = dv_M/dv_0$ is computed by repeated application of (23) starting from the initial condition $dv_0/dv_0 = \mathbf{1}$. Note that for each time step the derivatives $J_f(v_m)$ and $c(v_{m-1})$ were previously computed during the application of the Newton-Raphson method to (18). In fact, $J_f(v_m)$ is available in LU decomposed form. Thus, applying (23) to compute $J_\phi(v_0)$ is relatively efficient despite the fact that $J_\phi(v_0)$ is an $N \times N$ matrix. However, this matrix is not sparse. Hence, it requires a great deal of memory to store and is expensive to LU factor.

The size of $J_\phi(v_0)$ can be reduced somewhat by eliminating from consideration entries in v that result from algebraic constraints or from quickly decaying states. This approach has also been found to aid convergence [13].

Since (19) is being solved using Newton-Raphson, it is necessary to ensure that $\phi_T(v_0)$ is continuously differentiable with respect to v_0. Sufficient conditions for this to be true before time has been discretized are that i, q, and u satisfy the conditions imposed in Section 1.3 to ensure that a unique solution to (2) exists for every initial state, as well as the additional conditions that i and q are continuously differentiable with respect to v [10]. These conditions are also sufficient to ensure that $\phi_T(v_0)$ is continuously differentiable with respect to v_0 when time has been discretized with a fixed discretization mesh. However, $\phi_T(v_0)$ is not guaranteed to vary smoothly with changes in the mesh. Indeed, insertion or deletion of points is inherently a discontinuous operation that is likely to introduce convergence problems unless care is taken. It is possible to avoid this problem by simply using the same mesh on each iteration; however, this may result in unacceptable constraints on the time step selection algorithm and therefore either excessive truncation error† or an excessively fine mesh. To avoid these problems, a mesh is chosen to achieve the desired accuracy and used on successive iterations for as long as that accuracy can be maintained. Once it is no longer maintainable, the Newton iteration is restarted with a new mesh and using the final iterate from the previous mesh as the starting point. It may happen that when far from the solution the mesh will be changed often, perhaps on

†Truncation error is the error generated in discretizing a differential equation [8]. The truncation error is normally reduced by reducing the size of the time steps.

each iteration. Once near the solution, however, the mesh should stabilize and allow the Newton iteration to converge.

Like any Newton-Raphson-based method, the shooting method will converge if the function (19) varies smoothly in the neighborhood of the solution and if the initial guess is given sufficiently close to the solution. Thus, an important part of the shooting method is the selection of a good initial guess for the solution. A reasonable start is to set the time-varying input sources to their average value and use the resulting DC operating point for $v_0^{(0)}$. An improvement on this procedure is to linearize the circuit about the DC operating point, convert the input source waveforms into the frequency domain using the discrete Fourier transform, and perform a phasor analysis [6] to find the periodic steady-state response of the linearized circuit. From this response, determine $v_0^{(0)}$ (this only requires the inverse discrete Fourier transform to be evaluated at $t = 0$), and use this initial guess to start the shooting method. The initial guess can be further improved by integrating the circuit for several periods before applying the shooting method to allow any rapid time constants to decay. When generating the initial guess the truncation error criteria can be relaxed and larger time steps taken to reduce the computational cost.

It is still possible for the shooting method to have convergence problems. As always with Newton's method, damping can be used to improve convergence. A damping factor α is introduced into (20) so that

$$v_0^{(j+1)} = v_0^{(j)} + [\alpha J_\phi(v_0^{(j)}) - \mathbf{1}]^{-1}[v_0^{(j)} - \phi_T(v_0^{(j)})] \tag{24}$$

where $0 \leqslant \alpha \leqslant 1$. With $\alpha = 1$, (24) reverts to undamped Newton-Raphson; if $\alpha = 0$ then (24) becomes the fixed-point iteration $v_0^{(j+1)} = \phi_T(v_0^{(j)})$. The damping parameter should be automatically controlled on each iteration, with α close to zero when ϕ_T is strongly nonlinear over the size of a step $v_0^{(j+1)} - v_0^{(j)}$ and with α close to one when ϕ_T is almost linear over the step. To achieve quadratic convergence, α must go to one as the solution is approached. See Refs. [9, 13] for specific algorithms to control α. Note that for this damped shooting method to work it is necessary for $v_0^{(j)}$ to be within the region of attraction for an asymptotically stable limit cycle of period T, otherwise the fixed point iteration that results when $\alpha = 0$ will not converge.

2.3 Parallel Shooting

Shooting methods can have convergence and overflow problems when applied to circuits with unstable modes. For each iteration, only the initial state is specified; therefore any unstable modes may cause the trajectory to grow exponentially and leave the vicinity of the desired solution. The likelihood of this occurring decreases if the shooting interval T is reduced.

Parallel, or multiple, shooting methods [14, 15, 25] effectively reduce the shooting interval by dividing it into several subintervals. For example, if the shooting interval is divided into two equally sized subintervals, shooting is performed twice per iteration, once for each subinterval. Thus, the problem is restructured into another two-point boundary-value problem with twice as many unknowns (two sets of initial conditions, one set per subinterval) but with the shooting interval halved.

Divide the interval $[0, T]$ into K subintervals defined by the mesh $\{\tau_0, \tau_1, \tau_2, \ldots, \tau_K\}$ where $\tau_0 = 0$, $\tau_K = T$, and $\tau_k < \tau_{k+1}$. Let $v_k = v(\tau_k)$ and define $\phi_k(v_k) = v_{k+1}$. Since v is T-periodic, $v_0 = v_K$, and by forcing v to be continuous at each τ_k

$$\begin{aligned} \phi_0(v_0) - v_1 &= \mathbf{0} \\ \phi_1(v_1) - v_2 &= \mathbf{0} \\ \vdots \qquad & \quad \vdots \\ \phi_{K-1}(v_{K-1}) - v_0 &= \mathbf{0} \end{aligned} \tag{25}$$

This is a system of nonlinear algebraic equations that is solved using Newton-Raphson.

$$\begin{bmatrix} J_{\phi_0}(v_0^{(j)}) & -I & & \\ & J_{\phi_1}(v_1^{(j)}) & \ddots & \\ & & \ddots & -I \\ -I & & & J_{\phi_{K-1}}(v_{K-1}^{(j)}) \end{bmatrix} \begin{bmatrix} v_0^{(j+1)} - v_0^{(j)} \\ v_1^{(j+1)} - v_1^{(j)} \\ \vdots \\ v_{K-1}^{(j+1)} - v_{K-1}^{(j)} \end{bmatrix} = \begin{bmatrix} v_1^{(j)} - \phi_0(v_0^{(j)}) \\ v_2^{(j)} - \phi_1(v_1^{(j)}) \\ \vdots \\ v_0^{(j)} - \phi_{K-1}(v_{K-1}^{(j)}) \end{bmatrix} \tag{26}$$

By taking this iteration to convergence the value of the solution waveform is found at each of the points of the mesh. Both $\phi_k(v_k)$ and $J_{\phi_k}(v_k)$ are evaluated by integrating the circuit equations as in the previous subsection.

The computational complexity of the parallel shooting method is higher than that of the standard shooting method because the Jacobian in (26) has much larger dimension than the one in (20). The Jacobian is treated as a sparse block matrix and is efficiently factored by simply avoiding operations on zero blocks [17] and possibly applying the Sherman-Morrison-Woodbury formula [12] to convert it into a banded matrix. Besides the disadvantage of increased computational complexity, parallel shooting methods are also more difficult to program and require considerably more memory. These disadvantages, however, are offset by an advantage alluded to earlier. Parallel shooting methods have better convergence properties. In particular, the region of convergence is larger for the parallel shooting methods and increases in size as the number of subintervals increases [15]. This is primarily of importance when the circuit exhibits unstable modes. Also, the parallel shooting methods are more suitable for implementation on parallel processing computers, a feature that should grow in importance in the future.

In the parallel shooting method, the circuit equations must be integrated over each subinterval individually. Thus each subinterval is further subdivided to perform the numerical integration of the differential equations. As the number of shooting subintervals increases, the number of subdivisions per interval decreases. This causes a problem if it has been deemed desirable to use a high-order integration method. At each step a high-order integration method needs to know the history of the solution over several past time steps. This history cannot extend beyond a shooting interval boundary. Thus it is necessary to build up to higher-order integration methods by taking several steps of a low-order method at the beginning of each interval. When an interval contains only a few time points, high-order methods lose their advantage because of the large percentage of time steps taken with the low-order methods.

3 FINITE-DIFFERENCE METHODS

Like almost all approaches to solving differential equations numerically, the finite-difference methods approximate the original system with a set of difference equations. Thus a mesh $\{t_m\}$, $m = 0, 1, \ldots, M$, is chosen and the finite sequence $\{v_m\}$ is computed as an approximation to $v(t)$ on the mesh. The difference equations are formed by using a discrete time approximation to the time derivative, such as one of those presented in Section 1.2. For example, implicit Euler could be applied to

$$f(v, t) = \dot{q}(v) + i(v) + u(t) = \mathbf{0} \tag{27}$$

to generate

$$\frac{1}{h_{m+1}}(q(v_{m+1}) - q(v_m)) + i(v_{m+1}) + u_{m+1} = \mathbf{0} \qquad m = 0, \ldots, M-1 \tag{28}$$

As v is T-periodic, setting $v_0 = v_M$ results in the following system of nonlinear algebraic equations:

$$
\begin{aligned}
q(v_1) - q(v_M) + h_1 i(v_1) + h_1 u_1 &= \mathbf{0} \\
q(v_2) - q(v_1) + h_2 i(v_2) + h_2 u_2 &= \mathbf{0} \\
\vdots \qquad \vdots \qquad\qquad \vdots \qquad & \quad \vdots \\
q(v_M) - q(v_{M-1}) + h_M i(v_M) + h_M u_M &= \mathbf{0}
\end{aligned}
$$

As usual, the system is solved using Newton-Raphson.

$$
\begin{bmatrix}
c(v_1^{(j)}) + h_1 g(v_1^{(j)}) & & & -c(v_M^{(j)}) \\
-c(v_1^{(j)}) & c(v_2^{(j)}) + h_2 g(v_2^{(j)}) & & \\
& \ddots & \ddots & \\
& & -c(v_{M-1}^{(j)}) & c(v_M^{(j)}) + h_M g(v_M^{(j)})
\end{bmatrix}
$$

$$
\times \begin{bmatrix} v_1^{(j+1)} - v_1^{(j)} \\ v_2^{(j+1)} - v_2^{(j)} \\ \vdots \\ v_M^{(j+1)} - v_M^{(j)} \end{bmatrix}
= - \begin{bmatrix} q(v_1^{(j)}) - q(v_M^{(j)}) + h_1 i(v_1^{(j)}) + h_1 u_1 \\ q(v_2^{(j)}) - q(v_1^{(j)}) + h_2 i(v_2^{(j)}) + h_2 u_2 \\ \vdots \\ q(v_M^{(j)}) - q(v_{M-1}^{(j)}) + h_M i(v_M^{(j)}) + h_M u_M \end{bmatrix} \tag{29}
$$

The solution waveform $\{v_m\}$ is found by taking this iteration to convergence.

It is not necessary to use implicit Euler to discretize the differential equations; any valid discrete approximation to a time derivative will do. In fact, finite-difference methods, when applied to finding the periodic solution, are more flexible in this regard than difference methods for initial-value problems because the discrete differentiation operator need not be causal. It is possible to use future time points as well as past time points in the approximate derivative. For example, though not recommended because of inherent accuracy problems, it is possible to use $\dot{v}_m = (1/2h_m)(v_{m+1} - v_{m-1})$, in which case (29) would become

$$
\begin{bmatrix}
h_1 g(v_1^{(j)}) & c(v_2^{(j)}) & & -c(v_M^{(j)}) \\
-c(v_1^{(j)}) & h_2 g(v_2^{(j)}) & \ddots & \\
& \ddots & \ddots & c(v_M^{(j)}) \\
c(v_1^{(j)}) & & -c(v_{M-1}^{(j)}) & h_M g(v_M^{(j)})
\end{bmatrix}
\begin{bmatrix} v_1^{(j+1)} - v_1^{(j)} \\ v_2^{(j+1)} - v_2^{(j)} \\ \vdots \\ v_M^{(j+1)} - v_M^{(j)} \end{bmatrix}
$$

$$
= - \begin{bmatrix} q(v_1^{(j)}) - q(v_M^{(j)}) + h_1 i(v_1^{(j)}) + h_1 u_1 \\ q(v_2^{(j)}) - q(v_1^{(j)}) + h_2 i(v_2^{(j)}) + h_2 u_2 \\ \vdots \\ q(v_M^{(j)}) - q(v_{M-1}^{(j)}) + h_M i(v_M^{(j)}) + h_M u_M \end{bmatrix}
$$

In addition, the finite-difference methods when applied to find periodic solutions do not have start-up problems with high-order methods. These advantages accrue from calculating the entire solution waveform at once.

The finite-difference methods are elegant and simple. When applied to two-point boundary-value problems with linear boundary constraints, such as the periodicity constraint, they have the characteristic that each iterate generated by the Newton-Raphson method satisfies the boundary condition, though it may not satisfy the difference equation. This contrasts with shooting methods, for which each iterate satisfies the difference equation but not the boundary conditions.

The finite-difference methods can generate large systems of equations, especially if either the number of unknown waveforms or the number of time points is large. The systems are sparse and hence not overly expensive to solve. The benefit of the finite-difference methods is their robustness, which results from iterating on waveforms rather than initial conditions. By iterating on initial conditions, the shooting methods are susceptible to exploding waveforms due to unstable modes. Once the initial condition has been chosen, the trajectory is free to wander as it will and can stray quite far, even if there are no unstable modes. With the finite-difference methods, the trajectory is constrained to satisfy the boundary conditions and so is less likely to go astray. The finite-difference methods are like the parallel shooting methods in this regard. In fact, a parallel shooting method, when the shooting intervals are taken to be so small that there is one time step per interval, becomes a finite-difference method. This is easily seen by using the one step approximation $\phi_k(t_{k-1}) = x_k + (1/h_k)\dot{x}_k$ in equations (25), which becomes a finite-difference method with explicit Euler used to form the difference equations. The convergence properties of parallel shooting improve as the size of the shooting intervals decreases, so it is expected that the finite-difference methods should have convergence properties at least as good as those of any shooting method.

It is possible to reduce the time required for the finite-difference methods by carefully choosing the time steps to achieve a desired accuracy, clustering them in troublesome spots to reduce error while spreading them out in quiescent areas to reduce computer resource usage. If the solution is expected to be smooth, it is possible to use high-order integration methods to achieve low truncation error using widely separated time points. Lastly, it is possible to use Šamanskii's method [19] to reduce execution time further. The possible efficiency gain for Šamanskii's method is considerable if a high-order integration method is used (and so the bandwidth of the Jacobian is large and therefore expensive to factor) or if the Jacobian is expensive to construct.

4 EXPANSION METHODS

In Section 1.1 it was assumed that the solution $\hat{v}$ of (1) was a member of the linear space of T-periodic functions $P^N(T)$. This is an infinite-dimensional space and so it is impossible to represent exactly an arbitrary element of the space with a finite set of numbers. If we wish to solve (1) numerically, it is necessary to limit our attention to some subspace of $P^N(T)$ that has reasonably small dimension. This subspace is referred to as the *reduced* space and $P^N(T)$ is referred to as the *original* space. A normed linear space is completely defined by its norm [we use the L_2 norm to make $P^N(T)$ a Hilbert space] and its basis functions. Thus, the reduced space is constructed by choosing a set of basis functions. Normally, we choose a set of orthogonal basis functions $\{\psi_1, \psi_2, \ldots, \psi_K\}$ so that in the limit, as $K \to \infty$, the set spans a dense subset of the original space. The approximate numerical solution always lies in the finite-dimensional reduced space and so can be represented as a linear combination of the basis functions

$$v^* = \alpha_1\psi_1 + \alpha_2\psi_2 + \cdots + \alpha_K\psi_K$$

where the α_i are scalars and v^* approximates the true solution $\hat{v}$. If $\hat{v}$ happens to lie inside the reduced space, then the approximate solution v^* is exact.

By viewing the solution of (1) as an element of a function space, we have converted the problem of finding the solution of differential equations into an approximation problem. That is, we want to find the element in the reduced space that is in some sense closest to the true solution, which may well lie outside the reduced space. Since the reduced space has smaller dimension than the original space, we have no hope of accurately approximating any arbitrary element of the original space. Some *a priori* information about the form of the expected solutions is needed so that the reduced space can be constructed in such a way that it is "near" the expected solutions. Clearly, the choice of basis functions has a profound influence on the accuracy of the approximate solution. A good measure of performance for a basis is how large K must be to approximate a range of typical solutions to some given accuracy. If K is small, then the numerical solution procedure should be efficient. Of course, the ease of manipulation of the basis functions influences the efficiency as well, so a basis should be chosen taking this into consideration. Examples of possible bases include collections of polynomials, piecewise polynomials, trigonometric polynomials, piecewise exponentials, and splines.

Once the basis of the reduced space has been selected, there are two ways to approach the problem of finding the solution of (1). One is to discretize the functions in the reduced space and evaluate (1) at only a finite number of time points. The number of time points used is chosen equal to the dimension of the reduced space. The fact that the basis functions are actually defined for all $[0, T]$ is exploited to compute the time derivatives at the time points. For example, consider the basis and time points shown in Figure 7.1. The time derivative of the basis functions is not defined for the given time points, but it is possible to skirt this problem by using either the right or left derivative. For the right derivative

$$\dot{v}_{m-1} = \frac{K}{T}(v_m - v_{m-1})$$

which is, of course, explicit Euler. The left derivative

$$\dot{v}_m = \frac{K}{T}(v_m - v_{m-1})$$

results in implicit Euler. By discretizing the basis functions, we have rederived the finite-difference methods.

The other approach is to work with the coefficients of the basis functions directly. Methods that do this are referred to as expansion methods. This name is not at all standard; these methods are also referred to as variational methods, function-space methods, projection methods, and semianalytical methods. Expansion methods are analogous to finite-element methods for partial differential equations. As an example of how expansion methods might be applied, consider a linear version of (1)

$$C\dot{v}(t) + Gv(t) + \cos(\omega t) = 0 \tag{30}$$

and choose the basis for the reduced space as $\psi_1 = \cos(\omega t)$ and $\psi_2 = \sin(\omega t)$. Then

$$v^* = \alpha_1 \cos(\omega t) + \alpha_2 \sin(\omega t) \tag{31}$$

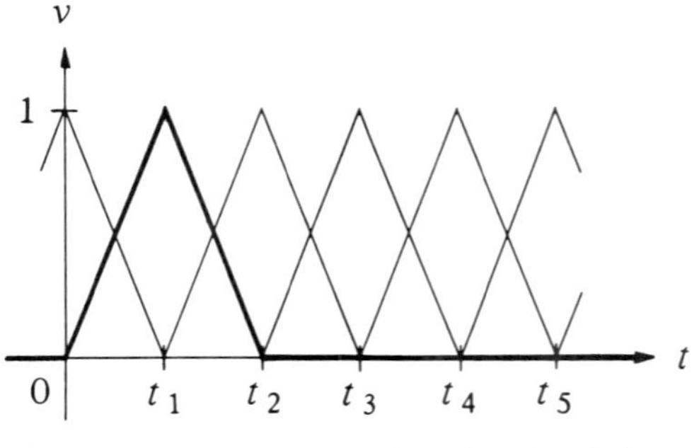

Figure 7.1 The basis for the fixed-time explicit and implicit Euler integration methods; zero order piecewise polynomials.

Substituting (31) into (30) results in

$$C\omega[-\alpha_1 \sin(\omega t) + \alpha_2 \cos(\omega t)] + G[\alpha_1 \cos(\omega t) + \alpha_2 \sin(\omega t)] + \cos(\omega t) = 0$$

which is satisfied when

$$G\alpha_1 + C\omega\alpha_2 = -1$$

$$-C\omega\alpha_1 + G\alpha_2 = 0$$

It happens that the solution of (30) lies in the reduced space, so it is found exactly. Notice that by working with functions we were able to evaluate the time derivatives and convert the differential equation to an algebraic equation.

It was mentioned previously that we are seeking the element in the reduced space that is closest to the solution. That is, we want to minimize $\|v^* - \hat{v}\|$. It is in general not possible to find a method that does this. Instead, we minimize the residual of (1), which is defined as

$$r(t) = f(v^*, t) \qquad 0 \leqslant t \leqslant T$$

There are many ways in which the residual can be minimized. If the residual is minimized in the least-squares sense,

$$\text{minimize} \int_0^T r(t)^T r(t)\, dt$$

then it is called a *least-squares* method. Another approach, referred to as *collocation*, forces the residual to zero at K disjoint time points:

$$r(t_k) = \mathbf{0} \qquad k = 1, 2, \ldots, K$$

Galerkin methods force the residual to be orthogonal to the basis functions:

$$\int_0^T r(t)\psi_k(t)\, dt = \mathbf{0} \qquad k = 1, 2, \ldots, K$$

It may seem that forcing the residual to be orthogonal to the basis functions used to represent the solution is arbitrary. Under certain hypotheses,† however, it is provably (i.e., can be proved) the most accurate method in the sense that $\|v^* - \hat{v}\|$ is minimized [5]. Even when those hypotheses are not satisfied, Galerkin methods still work well if the basis functions are chosen to accurately represent the various contributions to the residual, as well as the solution.

It happens that for a large class of circuits for which the periodic solution

---

†The required hypotheses are that (1) can be written in the form $Av - u = 0$ and that A is a linear symmetric and positive-definite operator. A is symmetric if $(x, Ay) = (Ax, y)$ for all $x, y \in P^N(T)$ where $(\cdot, \cdot)$ is the inner product. A is positive-definite if $(x, Ax) > 0$ for all $x \neq 0$.

is desired, the solutions are nearly sinusoidal. For problems of this class, it is desirable to have a basis that approximates sinusoids accurately with only a few elements. An obvious choice is the set of sinusoids $\cos(k\omega t)$ and $\sin(k\omega t)$ for $k = 0, 1, \ldots, K - 1$. Using this basis and the Galerkin error criterion results in the harmonic balance method.

4.1 Harmonic Balance

Harmonic balance has been of interest for many years to people who work with microwave circuits because it easily handles distributed devices. For this reason, we generalize (1) to include linear distributed devices. Let

$$f(v, t) = \dot{q}(v(t)) + i(v(t)) + \int_{-\infty}^{\infty} y(t - \tau)v(\tau)\, d\tau + u(t) = \mathbf{0} \tag{32}$$

where i, q: $\mathbf{R}^N \to \mathbf{R}^N$ are differentiable functions representing, respectively, the sum of the currents entering the nodes from the nonlinear conductors and the sum of the charge entering the nodes from the nonlinear capacitors, and y is the matrix-valued impulse response of the circuit with the nonlinear devices removed. By using the impulse response to represent the linear portion of the circuit, we have gained the generality needed to include distributed devices in the circuit.

Harmonic balance can use either $\cos(k\omega t)$ and $\sin(k\omega t)$ or $e^{jk\omega t}$ as the basis functions. We use the exponential form because of the simplicity it brings to the notation. If the complex exponential form is used, the coefficients are complex numbers and the functions constructed from this basis are complex-valued. There are two approaches to making the functions constructed with this basis real-valued. The first is simply to ignore the imaginary part

$$x(t) = \operatorname{Re}\left\{\sum_{k=0}^{\infty} X_k e^{jk\omega t}\right\}$$

The other approach is to have k take on both negative and positive values and force the sequence of coefficients to be conjugate symmetric (i.e., $X_k = \bar{X}_{-k}$ for all k, where the bar denotes the complex conjugate). A periodic function can be written

$$x(t) = \sum_{k=-\infty}^{\infty} X_k e^{jk\omega t} \tag{33a}$$

The conjugate symmetry constraint on $\{X_k\}$ is assumed for the remainder of this chapter. The inverse of (33a) is

$$X(k) = \int_0^T x(t) e^{-jk\omega t}\, dt \tag{33b}$$

Together these two equations are called the Fourier series pair. Individually the $X(k)$ are referred to as Fourier coefficients, whereas the sequence $\{X(k)\}$ is called the spectrum of $x(t)$. In shorthand, the Fourier series pair is written $X = \mathscr{F}x$ and $x = \mathscr{F}^{-1}X$.

The fact that v is periodic implies that both $i(v)$ and $q(v)$ are periodic and so all three of these quantities can be written in terms of their Fourier coefficients $\mathscr{F}v = V$, $\mathscr{F}i(v) = \mathscr{F}i(\mathscr{F}^{-1}V) = I(V)$, and $\mathscr{F}q(v) = \mathscr{F}q(\mathscr{F}^{-1}V) = Q(V)$. The Fourier coefficients of the convolution integral are computed by exploiting its linearity. If y satisfies

$$\int_{-\infty}^{\infty} y(t)^T y(t)\, dt < \infty$$

and $y(t) = 0$ for all $t < 0$, that is, if y is causal and has finite energy (or if the circuit with all nonlinear devices removed is causal and asymptotically stable), then

$$\mathscr{F}\int_{-\infty}^{\infty} y(t-\tau)v(\tau)\, d\tau = YV$$

where

$$Y = [Y_{rs}] \qquad r, s \in \{1, 2, \ldots, N\}$$
$$Y_{rs} = [Y_{rs}(k, l)]$$

where r, s are the node indices; k, l are the frequency indices, and

$$Y_{rs}(k, l) = \begin{cases} \Upsilon_{rs}(\mathbf{j}k\omega) & \text{if } k = l \\ \mathbf{0} & \text{if } k \neq l \end{cases}$$

where Υ is the Laplace transform of y [6], $\mathbf{j} = \sqrt{-1}$, and $\omega = 2\pi/T$. Now (32) can be rewritten in terms of Fourier coefficients, which are the basis coefficients, as

$$F(V) = I(V) + \mathbf{j}\Omega Q(V) + YV + U = \mathbf{0} \tag{34}$$

where

$$\Omega = [\Omega_{rs}] \qquad r, s \in \{1, 2, \ldots, N\}$$

$$\Omega_{rs} = \begin{cases} \text{diag}\{\ldots, -2\omega, -\omega, 0, \omega, 2\omega, \ldots\} & \text{if } r = s \\ \mathbf{0} & \text{if } r \neq s \end{cases}$$

That $\mathscr{F}\dot{q}(v) = \mathbf{j}\Omega Q(V)$ follows from the differentiation rule of the Fourier series.

It is important to realize that the nonlinear device equations are not explicitly formulated in terms of Fourier coefficients; instead, the voltage spectra V is converted to v using (33a), and then the waveforms $i(v)$ and $q(v)$ are computed and converted into the spectra $I(V)$ and $Q(V)$ using (33b).

To make (34) tractable, it is necessary to truncate the number of harmonics to some finite number. The Nyquist sampling theorem indicates that this truncation is analogous to the discretization of time when using numerical integration and it is theoretically not a limitation because, for all realizable circuits, there exists a frequency beyond which there is negligible power. Truncating the number of harmonics requires that the Fourier series pair of (33) be replaced with the discrete Fourier transform pair

$$X(k) = \frac{1}{M} \sum_{m=0}^{M-1} x(mh) \exp\left(-\mathbf{j} \frac{2\pi km}{M} \right) \tag{35a}$$

$$x(mh) = \sum_{k=1-K}^{K-1} X(k) \exp\left(\mathbf{j} \frac{2\pi km}{M} \right) \tag{35b}$$

where K is the number of harmonics, M the number of time points, $M = 2K - 1$, and $h = T/M$. Now (34) is replaced with a finite-dimensional approximation

$$F(V) = I(V) + \mathbf{j}\Omega Q(V) + YV + U = \mathbf{0} \tag{36}$$

where $V, U, F(V), I(V), Q(V) \in \mathbb{C}^{(2K-1)N}$ and $\Omega \in \mathbb{C}^{(2K-1)N \times (2K-1)N}$

Applying Newton's method to (36) results in the iteration

$$V^{(j+1)} = V^{(j)} - J_F^{-1}(V^{(j)}) F(V^{(j)}) \tag{37}$$

where $J_F(V) \in \mathbb{C}^{(2K-1)N \times (2K-1)N}$ is the harmonic Jacobian

$$J_F(V) = \frac{\partial F(V)}{\partial V} = \frac{\partial I(V)}{\partial V} + \mathbf{j}\Omega \frac{\partial Q(V)}{\partial V} + Y$$

The harmonic Jacobian is organized as a block node admittance matrix of the form

$$J_F(V) = \left[\frac{\partial F_r(V)}{\partial V_s} \right] \qquad r, s \in \{1, 2, \ldots, N\} \tag{38}$$

where $F_r(V), V_s \in \mathbb{C}^{2K-1}$. The blocks of the harmonic Jacobian are referred to as conversion matrices (as in frequency conversion); they have the form

$$\frac{\partial F_r(V)}{\partial V_s} = \left[\frac{\partial F_r(V, k)}{\partial V_s(l)} \right] \tag{39}$$

where

$$k, l \in \{1 - K, \ldots, -1, 0, 1, \ldots, K - 1\}$$

$$\frac{\partial F_r(V, k)}{\partial V_s(l)} \in \mathbb{C}$$

and

$$J_{F,rs}(V, k, l) = \frac{\partial F_r(V, k)}{\partial V_s(l)}$$
$$= \frac{\partial I_r(V, k)}{\partial V_s(l)} + \mathbf{j}k\omega \frac{\partial Q_r(V, k)}{\partial V_s(l)} + Y_{rs}(k, l) \tag{40}$$

Only the derivation of $\partial I_r(V, k)/\partial V_s(l)$ is given; the derivation of $\partial Q_r(V, k)/\partial V_s(l)$ is identical. From (35a),

$$I_r(V, k) = \frac{1}{M} \sum_{m=0}^{M-1} i_r(v(mh)) \exp\left(-\mathbf{j}\frac{2\pi km}{M}\right)$$

Differentiating and applying the chain rule,

$$\frac{\partial I_r(V, k)}{\partial V_s(l)} = \frac{1}{M} \sum_{m=0}^{M-1} \frac{\partial i_r(v(mh))}{\partial V_s(l)} \exp\left(-\mathbf{j}\frac{2\pi km}{M}\right)$$
$$= \frac{1}{M} \sum_{m=0}^{M-1} \frac{\partial i_r(v(mh))}{\partial v_s(mh)} \frac{\partial v_s(mh)}{\partial V_s(l)} \exp\left(-\mathbf{j}\frac{2\pi km}{M}\right) \tag{41}$$

Now the derivative of v_s is calculated. For simplicity, $v(t)$ is considered complex, thus eliminating the constraint that $V_s(k) = \bar{V}_s(-k)$, which is a nonanalytic relationship that results in $\partial v_s(t)/\partial V_s(l)$ being unrepresentable as a complex number. In removing the conjugate symmetry relationship between the positive and negative harmonics of the solution, the number of unknowns has been doubled. The derivation has been simplified at the expense of a factor of two reduction in efficiency of the method. The derivation for the more efficient approach where only nonnegative harmonics are considered is presented in Ref. [16]. Even though v_s is being treated as complex-valued, if the Newton iteration is primed with a conjugate symmetric initial guess, it will naturally find a real-valued v_s. Round-off errors may cause Newton's method to deviate from conjugate symmetry, so this is normally corrected on each iteration.

From (35b)

$$v_s(mh) = \sum_{k=1-K}^{K-1} V_s(k) \exp\left(\mathbf{j}\frac{2\pi km}{M}\right)$$

Differentiating [it is here that $V_s(k) = \bar{V}_s(-k)$ must be avoided]

$$\frac{\partial v_s(mh)}{\partial V_s(l)} = \exp\left(\mathbf{j}\frac{2\pi lm}{M}\right) \tag{42}$$

Substituting (42) into (41),

$$\frac{\partial I_r(V,k)}{\partial V_s(l)} = \frac{1}{M}\sum_{m=0}^{M-1} \frac{\partial i_r(v(mh))}{\partial v_s(mh)} \exp\left(\mathbf{j}\frac{2\pi lm}{M}\right)\exp\left(-\mathbf{j}\frac{2\pi km}{M}\right)$$
$$= \frac{1}{M}\sum_{m=0}^{M-1} \frac{\partial i_r(v(mh))}{\partial v_s(mh)} \exp\left(-\mathbf{j}\frac{2\pi(k-l)m}{M}\right) \tag{43}$$

Let $g_{rs}(mh) = \partial i_r(v(mh))/\partial v_s(mh)$ and

$$G_{rs}(k) = \frac{1}{M}\sum_{m=0}^{M-1} g_{rs}(mh)\exp\left(-\mathbf{j}\frac{2\pi km}{M}\right) \tag{44}$$

Then clearly

$$\frac{\partial I_r(V,k)}{\partial V_s(l)} = G_{rs}(k-l) \tag{45}$$

In other words, if g_{rs} is the waveform that results when the voltage waveform is applied to the nonlinear conductor's derivative equation, then $\partial I_r(V,k)/\partial V_s(l)$ is the $(k-l)$th harmonic of that conductance waveform. Similarly,

$$\frac{\partial Q_r(V,k)}{\partial V_s(l)} = C_{rs}(k-l)$$

where $c_{rs}(mh) = \partial q_r(v(mh))/\partial v_s(mh)$ and

$$C_{rs}(k) = \frac{1}{M}\sum_{m=0}^{M-1} c_{rs}(mh)\exp\left(-\mathbf{j}\frac{2\pi km}{M}\right)$$

Thus

$$\frac{\partial I_r(V)}{\partial V_s} = \begin{bmatrix} G_{rs}(0) & G_{rs}(-1) & G_{rs}(-2) & \cdots \\ G_{rs}(1) & G_{rs}(0) & G_{rs}(-1) & \cdots \\ G_{rs}(2) & G_{rs}(1) & G_{rs}(0) & \cdots \\ \vdots & \vdots & \vdots & \ddots \end{bmatrix}$$

The cyclic nature of the discrete Fourier transform [i.e., that $G_{rs}(k) = G_{rs}(k+M)$] is used to form the upper right and lower left corners of the conversion matrices.

For a one-node circuit at three frequencies, the complete harmonic Jacobian is

$$J_F(V) = \frac{\partial I(V)}{\partial V} + \mathbf{j}\Omega\frac{\partial Q(V)}{\partial V} + Y$$

where

$$\frac{\partial I(V)}{\partial V} = \begin{bmatrix} G(0) & G(-1) & G(-2) & G(2) & G(1) \\ G(1) & G(0) & G(-1) & G(-2) & G(2) \\ G(2) & G(1) & G(0) & G(-1) & G(-2) \\ G(-2) & G(2) & G(1) & G(0) & G(-1) \\ G(-1) & G(-2) & G(2) & G(1) & G(0) \end{bmatrix}$$

$\partial Q(V)/\partial V$ is similar, with G replaced everywhere with C.

$$\mathbf{j}\Omega = \begin{bmatrix} -2\mathbf{j}\omega & & & & \\ & -\mathbf{j}\omega & & & \\ & & 0 & & \\ & & & \mathbf{j}\omega & \\ & & & & 2\mathbf{j}\omega \end{bmatrix}$$

and

$$Y = \begin{bmatrix} Y(-2\mathbf{j}\omega) & & & & \\ & Y(-\mathbf{j}\omega) & & & \\ & & Y(0) & & \\ & & & Y(\mathbf{j}\omega) & \\ & & & & Y(2\mathbf{j}\omega) \end{bmatrix}$$

The harmonic Jacobian is organized as a block node admittance matrix. Each block is a complex conversion matrix that is full if it is associated with a node that has a nonlinear device attached, otherwise it is diagonal. The size of the conversion matrix is proportional to the number of harmonics being computed. If the circuit being analyzed has few nonlinear devices and if few harmonics are being computed, then harmonic balance is efficient. The number of harmonics chosen is based on the input signals and the nonlinearity of the circuit, not on the stiffness or Q of the circuit. Thus harmonic balance is a good choice when few nonlinear devices are present, input waveforms are sinusoidal, and the circuit is behaving almost linearly. It is particularly appealing when distributed devices are also present.

Of the time spent performing harmonic balance, most is spent constructing and factoring the harmonic Jacobian. Two things can be done to reduce this time. The first is to employ Šamanskii's method (Section 1.2); simply reuse the factored harmonic Jacobian from the previous iteration. If the circuit is nearly linear, then a Jacobian may be used many times. If, however, the Jacobian is varying appreciably on each step, then using Šamanskii's method can result in a bad step being taken, which leads to nonconvergence. To alleviate this problem and decide how many times to use an old Jacobian, $\|F(V)\|$ should be monitored and a new Jacobian computed if the norm is not sufficiently reduced at each step.

The second way to improve the harmonic Newton algorithm is to exploit the natural characteristics of the conversion matrices. Equation (45) shows that the lower harmonics of the derivative spectrum lie close to the diagonal and the upper harmonics lie far away. If all the nonlinear devices associated with a particular derivative spectrum are behaving nearly linearly, then the upper harmonics are small, which implies that the resulting conversion matrix has large elements only near the diagonal. It is possible to exploit this characteristic to speed the factorization [16]. To do so, two approximations are made. First, in conversion matrices that have contributions only from devices behaving linearly or almost linearly, the small elements far from the diagonal are set to zero and the operations that would normally be performed on these elements are avoided. The decision on which elements are small enough to ignore is made by comparing the magnitude of the upper harmonics of the derivative spectrum to some small fraction of the DC component. The value $10^{-4}G_{rs}(0)$ [or $10^{-4}Q_{rs}(0)$ if the device is capacitive] seems to work well. Of the harmonics smaller than the cutoff criterion, only the first is kept; all others are set to zero. This last nonzero harmonic is called the *guard harmonic*. Second, all nonzero fill-ins† that result during LU factorization from operations involving the guard harmonic are ignored. This prevents the bandwidth of the blocks from growing unnecessarily during the factorization.

5 OSCILLATORS

A circuit is said to be autonomous if all its elements do not vary with time. That is, the relationship between voltage and current for a resistor, voltage and charge for a capacitor, and flux and current for an inductor is time-invariant. Independent sources can be thought of as resistors, and so in autonomous circuits all sources are constant-valued. Oscillators are autonomous circuits that have nonconstant periodic solutions. The problem of finding the steady-state solution of an oscillator does not fit into the standard form for two-point boundary-value problems because the period of oscillation is unknown. It is possible to adapt each of the methods previously presented for two-point boundary-value problems to the oscillator problem.

†A fill-in is an element in a matrix that is initially zero but becomes nonzero during an LU factorization.

Only the application of shooting methods and harmonic balance is discussed here. The adaptation of finite-difference methods to the oscillator problem follows naturally from the discussion of shooting methods.

Oscillators present two problems not previously faced. The first, as pointed out above, is that the period of the oscillation is unknown and must be determined. The second is that the time origin is arbitrary, and thus if one solution exists, an infinite continuum of solutions exists. In other words, if v is a solution, then so is any time-shifted version of v. The problem is that all the methods presented fail if the solution is not isolated. It is necessary to modify either the methods for handling nonisolated solutions or the problem formulation to eliminate the nonisolated solutions.

There are two degenerate cases that cause any Newton-Raphson-based method to fail when applied to the oscillator problem. Surprisingly enough, linear problems are one such case. In linear autonomous circuits, the amplitude of the oscillation is not unique: if the circuit supports an undamped oscillation, then the oscillation may be of any amplitude. Thus, there is not only a continuum of solutions parameterized on t but also a continuum parameterized on the amplitude of the oscillation. A similar situation arises when a solution is a constant waveform. For this case, the additional continuum is parameterized in the period T.

5.1 Shooting Methods

It is possible to handle oscillators with extrapolation-based shooting methods [23]; however, there is no natural way to find T. It is necessary to look for the maxima or threshold crossings on the solution waveforms and estimate T. Other than the rather distasteful methods that must be employed to find T, extension of extrapolation to the oscillator problem is straightforward and well behaved.

When applying Newton-Raphson-based shooting methods to autonomous oscillators, T is added to the list of unknowns to be determined and an extra equation is added that addresses the problem of having a continuum of solutions. The added equation is constructed either to eliminate almost all solutions (with those that remain being isolated from each other) or to modify Newton's method so that it is capable of handling the continuum. One way to restrict the set of solutions such that each is isolated is to force $y(0)$ to lie on a hyperplane that has been carefully selected so that it intersects the solution trajectory. The resulting system of equations is

$$\begin{aligned} \phi_T(\hat{v}(0)) - \hat{v}(0) &= \mathbf{0} \\ \xi^T \hat{v}(0) &= \alpha \end{aligned} \tag{46}$$

where ξ is a constant vector that is normal to the hyperplane and α is a scalar.

Unfortunately, ξ and α cannot be chosen arbitrarily; they must satisfy

$$\max_t \xi^T \hat{v}(t) > \alpha$$

$$\min_t \xi^T \hat{v}(t) < \alpha$$

$$\xi^T \frac{d\hat{v}(0)}{dt} \neq 0$$

As shown in Figure 7.2, the first two constraints ensure that the hyperplane intersects the solution orbit. The last constraint is necessary to prevent the Jacobian from being singular, which results if the hyperplane is tangent to the solution trajectory at $\hat{v}(0)$. Initially, ξ and α are selected after integrating the circuit equations for a few cycles, as are the initial Newton guess of T and $v(0)$. It may be necessary to update α as the iteration progresses.

Newton's method can be modified [18] to handle nonisolated solutions by constraining the Newton step direction to be perpendicular to the trajectory, as shown in Figure 7.3. Thus if $\Delta v^{(j+1)}(0) = v^{(j+1)}(0) - v^{(j)}(0)$, then the equation $\dot{v}(0)^T \Delta v(0) = 0$ is added to the Newton update iteration for

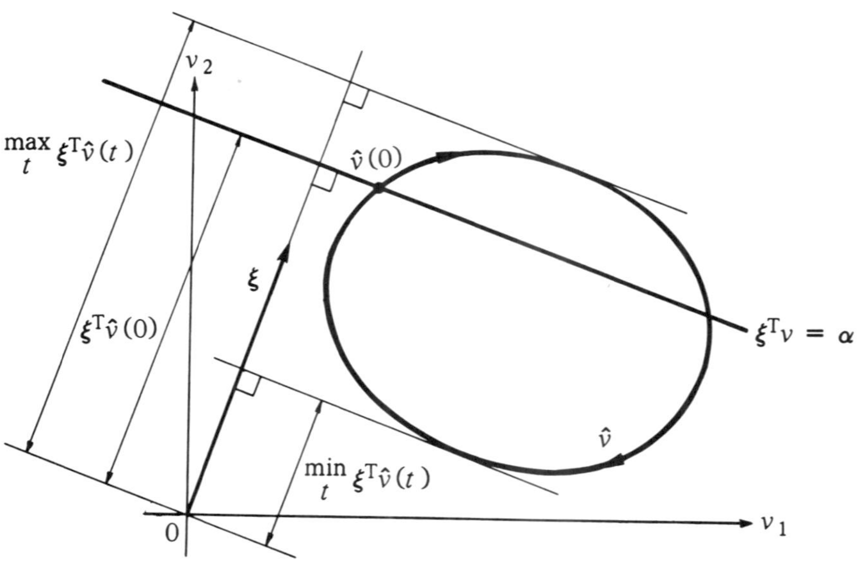

Figure 7.2 Orbit and hyperplane of Eq. 46, showing in two dimensions how $v(0)$ is selected by intersecting a hyperplane with the solution trajectory.

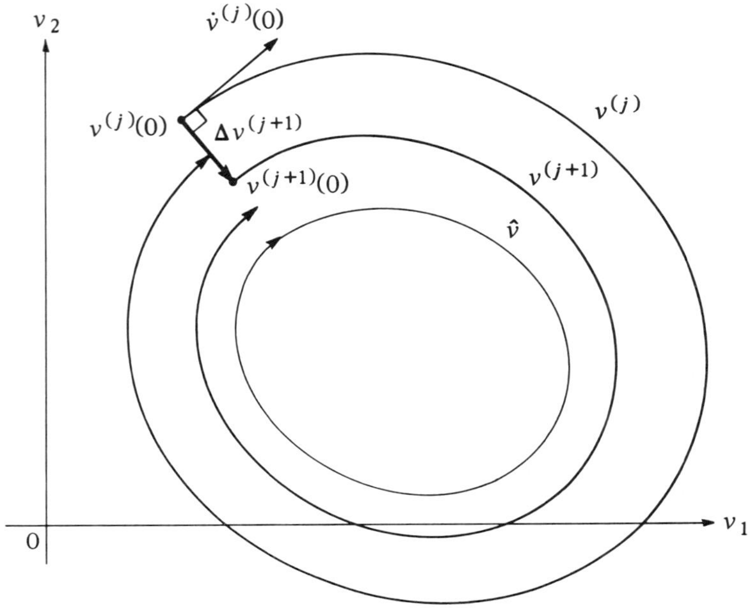

Figure 7.3 Two steps of the shooting method on a two-dimensional oscillator problem with $\Delta v^{(j+1)}$ constrained to be perpendicular to $\dot{v}^{(j)}(0)$.

$\phi_T(v(0)) - v(0) = \mathbf{0}$, where both $v(0)$ and T are considered unknown.

$$\begin{bmatrix} J_\phi(v^{(j)}(0), T^{(j)}) - \mathbf{1} & \dfrac{\partial \phi_T(v^{(j)}(0), T^{(j)})}{\partial T} \\ \dot{v}^{(j)}(0)^T & 0 \end{bmatrix} \begin{bmatrix} \Delta v^{(j+1)}(0) \\ \Delta T^{(j+1)} \end{bmatrix} = \begin{bmatrix} v^{(j)}(0) - \phi_T(v^{(j)}(0)) \\ \mathbf{0} \end{bmatrix} \tag{47}$$

where

$$J_\phi(v(0), T) = \frac{\partial \phi_T(v(0))}{\partial v(0)} \in \mathbf{R}^{N \times N}$$

$$\frac{\partial \phi_T(v(0))}{\partial T} \in \mathbf{R}^N$$

$$\Delta T^{(j+1)} = T^{(j+1)} - T^{(j)}$$

This approach does not require the selection parameters such as ξ and α, but a standard Newton-Raphson package cannot be used because the added equation is in terms of $\Delta v(0)$ rather than $v(0)$. Small errors in $\dot{v}^{(j)}(0)$ do not affect the accuracy of the solution, and so it can be calculated using the approximation $\dot{v}(0) \approx (v(t_1) - v(t_0))/h_1$. The computation of $\partial\phi_T/\partial T$ is more difficult. As in Section 2.2, the derivative must be derived from the discretized circuit equations. Equation (1) is discretized using implicit Euler and $\partial\phi_T/\partial T = \partial v_M/\partial T$ is computed by taking the final value of the $\partial v_m/\partial T$ trajectory. To compute $\partial v_m/\partial T$, it is necessary to specify how t_m, $m = 0, 1, \ldots, M$ vary with T. Let $t_m = \alpha_m T$ where $0 = \alpha_0 < \alpha_1 < \cdots < \alpha_M = 1$. From (18),

$$\frac{1}{h_m}[q(v_m) - q(v_{m-1})] + i(v_m) + u_m = \mathbf{0} \qquad m = 1, 2, \ldots, M$$

where $v_m = v(\alpha_m T)$ and $u_m = u(\alpha_m T)$. Differentiating with respect to T leads to

$$\frac{-1}{h_m T}[q(v_m) - q(v_{m-1})] + \frac{1}{h_m}\left[\frac{\partial q(v_m)}{\partial T} - \frac{\partial q(v_{m-1})}{\partial T}\right] + \frac{\partial i(v_m)}{\partial T} + \frac{\partial u_m}{\partial T} = \mathbf{0}$$

Applying the chain rule and recalling that u is constant gives

$$\frac{-1}{h_m T}[q(v_m) - q(v_{m-1})] + \frac{1}{h_m}\left[\frac{\partial q(v_m)}{\partial v_m}\frac{\partial v_m}{\partial T} - \frac{\partial q(v_{m-1})}{\partial v_{m-1}}\frac{\partial v_{m-1}}{\partial T}\right] + \frac{\partial i(v_m)}{\partial v_m}\frac{\partial v_m}{\partial T} = \mathbf{0}$$

Again let $g = \partial i/\partial v$ and $c = \partial q/\partial v$.

$$\left[g(v_m) + \frac{c(v_m)}{h_m}\right]\frac{\partial v_m}{\partial T} = c(v_{m-1})\frac{\partial v_{m-1}}{\partial T} + \frac{1}{h_m T}[q(v_m) - q(v_{m-1})]$$

$$\frac{\partial v_m}{\partial T} = J_f^{-1}(x_m)\left\{c(v_{m-1})\frac{\partial v_{m-1}}{\partial T} + \frac{1}{h_m T}[q(v_m) - q(v_{m-1})]\right\} \tag{48}$$

This difference equation is solved starting with the initial state $\partial v_0/\partial T = 0$.

It is important to realize that Newton's method has been applied to the set of finite-difference equations that approximate the original set of differential equations, and not directly to the differential equations. In computing the derivatives of v_M needed by Newton's method, it is therefore necessary to use the finite-difference equations. It is also important to notice that the time points are independent variables that affect the value of v_M. If the time points are not fixed, they must be included in the list of independent variables being solved for by the Newton iteration. This has been done in a manner that is at least tractable by allowing T to be independent and insisting that $t_m = \alpha_m T$, $m = 0, 1, \ldots, M$. However, this approach severely constrains the time steps and may result in excessive truncation error. If the truncation error becomes intolerable, a new mesh is chosen with both M and the α_m's changing in such a way that the error specification is satisfied. In doing so, the finite-difference equations are changed and Newton's method should be restarted. However, the last iterate from the previous mesh may be used as an initial guess for the iteration on the new mesh. Initially, the mesh may need to be changed often, but once near the solution the mesh should stabilize and allow the Newton iteration to converge.

It is possible to change the way in which $\partial v_M/\partial T$ is computed, which may result in some gain in efficiency. One way is to fix the time steps $t_0, t_1, \ldots, t_{M-1}$ and only allow $t_M = T$ to vary. This greatly simplifies (48) but requires that the mesh be updated more often. Another approach is to use the approximation $\partial v_M/\partial T \approx \dot{v}(T)$. Thus, in an interesting twist, the original continuous time solution is used as an approximation to the discrete time solution. When using this approach, it is necessary to use at least a second-order integration method and control the truncation error to ensure that $\dot{v}$ is sufficiently accurate to ensure convergence.

5.2 Harmonic Balance

Harmonic balance is modified to handle oscillators by adding the fundamental frequency ω to the list of unknowns and an equation to enforce the constraint that solutions be isolated from one another. Perhaps the easiest way to ensure isolated solutions is to choose some signal in the circuit and insist that the imaginary part of its fundamental is zero. This fixes the solution to within a sign change. For this approach to work it is necessary that the fundamental of the signal chosen have nonzero magnitude.

The harmonic balance equations modified for the oscillator problem are

$$\begin{aligned} &F(V, \omega) = I(V) + \mathbf{j}\Omega(\omega)Q(V) + Y(\omega)V + U = \mathbf{0} \\ &\operatorname{Im}\{V_r(1)\} = 0 \end{aligned} \tag{49}$$

Newton's method is now applied to these two equations,

$$\begin{bmatrix} J_F(V^{(j)}, \omega^{(j)}) & \dfrac{\partial F(v^{(j)}, \omega^{(j)})}{\partial \omega} \\ e_r(1)^T & 0 \end{bmatrix} \begin{bmatrix} \Delta V^{(j+1)} \\ \Delta \omega^{(j+1)} \end{bmatrix} = -\begin{bmatrix} F(V^{(j)}, \omega^{(j)}) \\ \operatorname{Im}\{V_r(1)\} \end{bmatrix} \tag{50}$$

where

$$\frac{\partial F(v, \omega)}{\partial \omega} = \frac{\mathbf{j}}{\omega}\,\Omega(\omega)Q(V) + \frac{\partial Y(\omega)}{\partial \omega}\,V$$

and $e_r(1)$ is the unit vector that selects the imaginary part of the first harmonic of the chosen node voltage.

The most difficult part of applying harmonic balance to the oscillator problem is determining a good initial guess for both V and ω. A good initial guess is required not only for the standard reason of ensuring convergence but also to avoid the valid but undesirable solution where all but the DC terms in V are zero. We know of no general algorithm for generating a good initial guess.

6 CONCLUSION

Several different methods for finding the steady-state solution of a circuit have been presented and analyzed. It is impossible to find an absolute rank for the methods. Given a particular problem, a method that performed poorly in one instance could give the best results in another. Shooting methods are generally fast and require little memory compared to the alternatives. They should not, however, be applied to circuits containing distributed devices. The problem is one of specifying the initial state. It is not enough to simply specify the terminal voltages or currents for a distributed device at one point in time; rather the terminal waveforms must be given over some, possibly infinite, interval. Shooting methods are also not applicable to the problem of finding the steady-state solution when two or more signals at incommensurable frequencies are applied to a circuit. They also have trouble on the admittedly rare circuit that has very fast unstable modes, though parallel shooting methods address this problem.

At the far end of the spectrum from the shooting methods lies harmonic balance. This method easily handles distributed devices and is naturally extended to handle circuits with two or more input signals at incommensurable frequencies. It is also not affected by unstable modes. However, it can require a great deal of memory and time when the circuit is acting strongly nonlinear or when input signals are not sinusoidal. Harmonic balance uses an interesting discrete time differentiation approximation that is exact for sinusoids. This makes harmonic balance very accurate when signals in the circuit are nearly sinusoidal and exact when the circuit is linear and input signals are sinusoidal. However, the approximation is also noncausal, a fact that is normally hidden when signals are smooth but becomes apparent on signals with sharp transitions, where it manifests itself as preshoot. This "feature" can be disconcerting to the uninitiated.

The finite-difference methods lie between the shooting methods and harmonic balance. These methods use the same integration methods as the shooting methods but are otherwise like harmonic balance. Though they iterate on whole waveforms, they can be made to be efficient by using one-step integration methods and sparse matrix techniques. With some difficulty, finite-difference methods can handle distributed devices and can be extended to handle multiple-input-frequency circuits. Unlike harmonic balance, they are not constrained to use equally spaced time points and can be efficient on strongly nonlinear circuits or on those with nonsinusoidal stimulus.

The determination of the steady-state response of a circuit is still an open research area, with many promising avenues to be explored. For example, very little work has been done on finding the steady-state response of a circuit with two or more incommensurable input frequencies. Such circuits form a very important class of circuits called mixers that are used extensively in communications. More work is also needed on finding the steady-state response of oscillators. In particular, a way to generate a good initial guess of the solution waveform and frequency would be a very nice contribution. Finally, an efficient way to determine whether a computed solution is stable is needed for all the methods presented.

REFERENCES

1. T. J. Aprille and T. N. Trick, Steady-state analysis of nonlinear circuits with periodic inputs, *Proc. IEEE*, vol. 60, pp. 108–114, Jan. 1972.
2. T. J. Aprille and T. N. Trick, A computer algorithm to determine the steady-state response of nonlinear oscillators, *IEEE Trans. Circuit Theory*, vol. CT-19, no. 4, pp. 354–360, 1972.
3. B. Childs, M. Scott, J. W. Daniel, E. Denman, and P. Nelson (eds.), *Codes for Boundary-Value Problems in Ordinary Differential Equations*, Springer-Verlag, New York, 1979.
4. L. O. Chua and P.-M. Lin, *Computer-Aided Analysis of Electronic Circuits: Algorithms and Computational Techniques*, Prentice-Hall, Englewood Cliffs, N.J., 1975.
5. G. Dahlquist and Å. Björck, *Numerical Methods*, Prentice-Hall, Englewood Cliffs, N.J., 1974.
6. C. A. Desoer and E. S. Kuh, *Basic Circuit Theory*, McGraw-Hill, New York, 1969.
7. L. Fox, *The Numerical Solution of Two-Point Boundary Value Problems in Ordinary Differential Equations*, Oxford University Press, London, 1957.
8. C. W. Gear, *Numerical Initial Value Problems in Ordinary Differential Equations*, Prentice-Hall, Englewood Cliffs, N.J., 1971.
9. F. B. Grosz and T. N. Trick, Some modifications to Newton's method for the determination of the steady-state response of nonlinear oscillatory circuits, *IEEE Trans. Computer-Aided Design of Integrated Circuits and Systems*, vol. CAD-1, no. 3, pp. 116–120, 1982.
10. J. K. Hale, *Ordinary Differential Equations*, Krieger, Malabar Florida, 1980.
11. G. Hall and J. M. Watt (eds.), *Modern Numerical Methods for Ordinary Differential Equations*, Oxford University Press, London, 1976.

12. A. S. Householder, *The Theory of Matrices in Numerical Analysis*, Dover, New York, 1975.
13. M. Kakizaki and T. Sugawara, A modified Newton method for the steady-state analysis, *IEEE Trans. Computer-Aided Design of Integrated Circuits and Systems*, vol. CAD-4, no. 4, pp. 662–667, 1985.
14. H. B. Keller, *Numerical Methods for Two-Point Boundary Value Problems*, Ginn-Blaisdell, Waltham, Mass., 1968.
15. H. B. Keller, *Numerical Solution of Two Point Boundary Value Problems*, Society for Industrial and Applied Mathematics, Philadelphia, 1976.
16. K. S. Kundert and A. Sangiovanni-Vincentelli, Simulation of nonlinear circuits in the frequency domain, *IEEE Trans. Computer-Aided Design of Integrated Circuits and Systems*, vol. CAD-5, no. 4, pp. 521–535, 1986.
17. K. S. Kundert, Sparse matrix techniques, in *Circuit Analysis, Simulation and Design*, vol. 3, part 1, A. E. Ruehli, ed., North-Holland, Amsterdam, 1986.
18. A. I. Mees, *Dynamics of Feedback Systems*, Wiley, New York, 1981.
19. J. M. Ortega and W. C. Rheinboldt, *Iterative Solution of Nonlinear Equations in Several Variables*, Academic Press, New York, 1970.
20. L. R. Petzold, An efficient numerical method for highly oscillatory ordinary differential equations, *SIAM J. Numer. Anal.*, vol. 18, no. 3, pp. 455–479, 1981.
21. W. H. Press, B. P. Flannery, S. A. Teukolsky, and W. T. Vetterling, *Numerical Recipes: The Art of Scientific Computing*, Cambridge Univ. Press, London, 1986.
22. A. L. Sangiovanni-Vincentelli, Circuit simulation, in *Computer Design Aids for VLSI Circuits*, P. Antognetti, D. O. Pederson, and H. DeMan, eds., pp. 19–112, Sijthoff & Noordhoff, 1981.
23. S. Skelboe, Computation of the periodic steady-state response of nonlinear networks by extrapolation methods, *IEEE Trans. Circuits Syst.*, vol. CAS-27, no. 3, pp. 161–175, 1980.
24. S. Skelboe, Conditions for quadratic convergence of quick periodic steady-state methods, *IEEE Trans. Circuits Syst.*, vol. CAS-29, no. 4, pp. 234–239, 1982.
25. J. Stoer and R. Bulirsch, *Introduction to Numerical Analysis*, Springer-Verlag, New York, 1980.

8
Symbolic Network Analysis

Tadashi Matsumoto

Department of Electrical Engineering, Faculty of Engineering, Fukui University, Fukui, Japan

1 INTRODUCTION

1.1 Overview of Symbolic Network Analysis

Symbolic network analysis is a process by which we generate a function either of the form

$$H(s) = \frac{N(s)}{D(s)} \tag{1}$$

when all network elements are considered as known and numerically given, or of the form

$$H(s, p_1, p_2, \ldots, p_m) = \frac{N(s, p_1, p_2, \ldots, p_m)}{D(s, p_1, p_2, \ldots, p_m)} \tag{2}$$

where some or all elements (besides the complex frequency s) of the network are kept as variables.

The advantages offered by symbolic network analysis compared with purely numerical analysis are as follows [9, 18, 30, 36, 59]:

1. It provides insight into the behavior of the network.
2. It can be used for optimization of network performance [28, 29].
3. It can be used for error control in numerical calculations.

4. It can be used for small and large sensitivity evaluation [6, 21, 24, 36, 49, 59, 64].
5. It can be used for tolerance analysis.
6. It can be used for pole zero calculation [13, 41].
7. It can be used for other calculations of rational matrices [2, 7, 20, 25, 27, 39].

The methods used in symbolic network analysis programs may be classified as follows [9, 18, 30, 36, 59]:

1. Tree enumeration methods [1, 8, 10, 21, 30, 33, 54, 55, 63, 67, 68]
2. Numerical interpolation methods [11, 19, 22, 23, 28, 29, 31, 32, 34, 37, 39, 49, 51, 53, 59, 60, 64]
3. Nodal analysis eigenvalue methods (or parameter extraction methods) [12, 14, 18, 30, 45]
4. Signal flow graph methods [30, 38, 42, 58, 62, 65]
5. Algebraic methods [36, 44, 46, 57]
6. State variable eigenvalue methods [14, 18]
7. Iterative methods [18]
8. Others [40, 66]

Besides the references given above, lists of complete references before 1973 are available in Refs. [9, 18], which were surveys of existing symbolic methods and applications at that time.

Early works on symbolic network analysis are primarily concerned with obtaining $H(s)$ of Eq. (1), in which s is the only variable and all coefficients are real numbers. Many programs with the capability of finding $H(s)$ were available in 1972, and applications of those programs were intensively investigated and reported in the literature (see also the references in [9, 18]).

In the more general sense of symbolic network analysis, some or all of the network elements are allowed to be represented by variables (besides the complex frequency s) shown in Eq. (2). Before 1973 only a few programs were available for producing symbolic network functions in the general sense. The methods used in those programs were the tree enumeration method [18, 30], the signal flow graph method [18, 30], and the parameter extraction method [12, 30]. See the references in [18] in more detail.

Since 1973 there has been considerable and growing interest in developing computer-aided procedures capable of symbolic analysis. Several such procedures in categories 1 to 8 above are already available, but the methods in 1 to 5 are prominent in this regard. In this chapter only the methods in items 2 and 4 are discussed.

1.2 Linear Networks

In this chapter, we consider almost lumped linear time-invariant analog networks, but we will also refer to digital networks [28, 29, 34, 53, 59, 64, 66], some kinds of distributed circuits [22, 34, 53], and switched capacitor networks [47, 50, 52, 53, 64, 69] as an example of time-varying networks.

The network functions for lumped linear finite networks are rational functions of complex frequency s and have the following basic property with respect to a specific network element.

Theorem 1 [18] Let a lumped linear time-invariant network consist of impedances, admittances, and all four types of controlled sources (VCCS, VCVS, CCCS, and CCVS). Let some or all of these network elements be characterized by distinct variables $(p_1, \ldots, p_m)$, while the remaining elements are assigned numerical values. Then any network function H that is V_o/V_i, V_o/I_i, I_o/V_i, or I_o/I_i may be expressed as the ratio of two polynomials of degree 1 in each variable p_i.

According to the theorem, any network function H is given by $H(s, p_1, \ldots, p_m)$ of Eq. (2), where N and D are polynomials of degree 1 in each p_i. Sensitivity functions can, of course, be obtained by direct differentiation of Eq. (2), once the symbolic network function H has been obtained by any suitable symbolic programs. However, for digital computer solution of the problem, it is more convenient to work with the closed system defined in the next subsection and see more details of [18, 59]. It is noted that Theorem 1 is not valid in general for distributed networks [22, 34, 53] and switched capacitor networks [47, 50, 52, 53, 64, 69].

1.3 Closed System [18]

Let us consider here only lumped linear time-invariant networks. Assume that only one independent source U_1 is present. Then the equilibrium equations for the network can always be expressed in the frequency domain in the following form:

$$\mathbf{A}\mathbf{x} = \mathbf{b}U_1 = (b_1, b_2, \ldots, b_n)^T U_1 \tag{3}$$

where $\mathbf{A}$ is $n \times n$ and $\mathbf{b}$ is $n \times 1$, all with constant entries. Here, $\mathbf{x}$ is the $n \times 1$ unknown vector. Suppose that x_i is the desired output. Then the transfer function $H = x_i/U_1$ may be expressed by using Cramer's rule as

$$H = \frac{x_i}{U_1} = \frac{b_1\Delta_{1i} + \cdots + b_n\Delta_{ni}}{\Delta} = \frac{N}{D} \tag{4}$$

where Δ and Δ_{ij} are usual notations for the determinant of $\mathbf{A}$ and the cofactor of a_{ij}, respectively.

In all existing methods such as the generalized eigenvalue problem [3, 14, 18], some topological methods [8, 10], or signal flow graph methods [10], different rules or formulas are given for Δ and Δ_{ij}. It is highly desirable, especially from a computer-programming point of view, that both the numerator N and denominator D of Eq. (4) can be obtained in a single analysis, eliminating the need for the formulas of Δ_{ij}. This objective may be achieved by using the closed system for the given system of Eq. (3).

Let the signal source U_1 in the network be changed from an independent source into a source that is controlled by the variable x_i in a linear fashion. That is,

$$U_1 = Px_i \tag{5}$$

where P is a variable distinct from all other variables in the network. We say that we have formed a closed system, implying that there are no longer any independent sources in the network. For the closed system, we have

$$\mathbf{A}'\mathbf{x} = \mathbf{0} \tag{6}$$

where

$$\mathbf{A}' = \begin{bmatrix} a_{11} & \cdots & (a_{1i} - b_1 P) & \cdots & a_{1n} \\ a_{21} & \cdots & (a_{2i} - b_2 P) & \cdots & a_{2n} \\ & & \cdots & & \\ & & \cdots & & \\ a_{n1} & \cdots & (a_{ni} - b_n P) & \cdots & a_{nn} \end{bmatrix} \tag{7}$$

The determinant of $\mathbf{A}'$ in Eq. (7) for the closed system, denoted by Δ_c, may be found by applying a Laplace expansion to the ith column. Then we have

$$\Delta_c = \Delta - P(b_1\Delta_{1i} + \cdots + b_n\Delta_{ni}) = D - PN \tag{8}$$

The above equation shows that both N and D of the transfer function $H = N/D$ may be found in one analysis.

If the oscillation condition on Eq. (6) or Eq. (8) is satisfied, that is,

$$\Delta_c = D - PN = 0 \tag{9}$$

then we have

$$H = \frac{N}{D} = \frac{1}{P} \tag{10}$$

and the process for sorting the terms of Δ_c with respect to P is called a "sorting scheme."

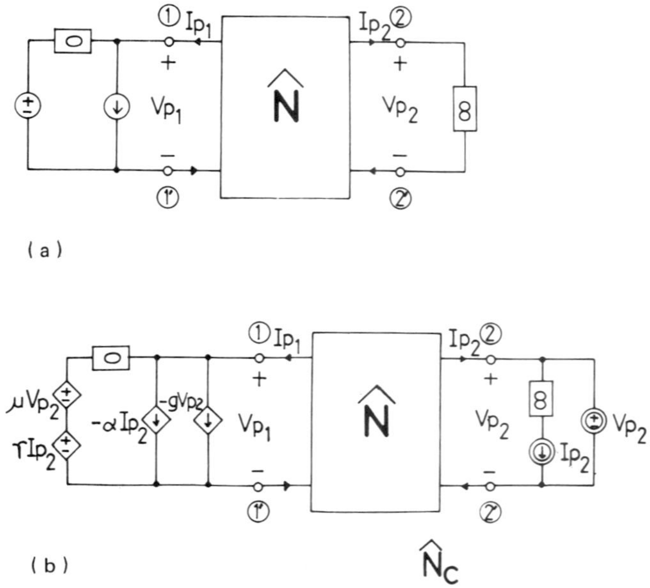

Figure 8.1 (a) Two-port $\hat{N}$ excited by a bigenerator and terminated by a norator. (b) Generalized closed system $\hat{N}_c$ derived from (a).

Now let us apply the above concept of closed system to the 2-port $\hat{N}$ (shown in Figure 8.1a) excited by a bigenerator [5] at port 1 and terminated by a norator at port 2 as a typical example. Assume also that 2-port $\hat{N}$ is the linear time-invariant circuit. Then it is expressed uniquely by the transmission parameters A', B', C', and D' as follows:

$$\begin{bmatrix} V_{p2} \\ -I_{p2} \end{bmatrix} = \begin{bmatrix} A'B' \\ C'D' \end{bmatrix} \begin{bmatrix} V_{p1} \\ I_{p1} \end{bmatrix} \tag{11}$$

Therefore, we have the generalized closed system $\hat{N}_c$ shown in Figure 8.1b for two-port $\hat{N}$ of Figure 8.1a, where μ, r, g, and α are defined by $V_{p_2} = \mu V_{p_1} + r(-I_{p_1})$, $I_{p_2} = gV_{p_1} + \alpha(-I_{p_1})$, and the notation used is defined in Figure 8.3. This generalized closed system $\hat{N}_c$ will be used effectively in Section 3.

The network $\hat{N}_c$ of Figure 8.1b is also the "augmented network" of Figure 8.1a, for the transmission two-port in this case. If we calculate Δ_c for Figure 8.1b and find the coefficients of possible combinations of the augmented variables r, g, μ, and α, then all symbolic network functions of Figure 8.1a are obtained.

2 NUMERICAL INTERPOLATION USING FFT ALGORITHMS

2.1 Interpolation Using the FFT Algorithm [11, 22]

Consider a polynomial scalar

$$Q(s) = \sum_{i=0}^{\mu} q_i s^i \tag{12}$$

with real coefficients q_i. If it is possible to evaluate Q at any desired value of s, then, from values at $\mu + 1$ distinct points $s_0, s_1, \ldots, s_\mu$, one can generate the coefficients q_i by solving the set of algebraic equations

$$\begin{bmatrix} 1 & s_0 & s_0^{\,2} & \cdots & s_0^{\,\mu} \\ 1 & s_1 & s_1^{\,2} & \cdots & s_1^{\,\mu} \\ \vdots & & & & \\ 1 & s_\mu & s_\mu^{\,2} & \cdots & s_\mu^{\,\mu} \end{bmatrix} \begin{bmatrix} q_0 \\ q_1 \\ \vdots \\ q_\mu \end{bmatrix} = \begin{bmatrix} Q(s_0) \\ Q(s_1) \\ \vdots \\ Q(s_\mu) \end{bmatrix} \tag{13}$$

In the past, numerical interpolation was carried out by selecting points on the real axis, and it is well known that such a procedure is numerically ill-conditioned [2]. In 1972 a method for carrying out interpolation in the complex plane by selecting points equally spaced on the unit circle was proposed [11]. It proceeds as described briefly below [22].

Let K be an integer greater than μ, the degree of the polynomial Q in Eq. (12). If K equally spaced points are selected on the unit circle in the s-plane, then at each of these points Eq. (12) has the form

$$Q(s_k) = Q\left[\exp\left(\frac{2\pi jk}{K}\right)\right] = \sum_{i=0}^{K-1} \hat{q}_i \exp\left(\frac{2\pi ijk}{K}\right) \qquad k = 0, 1, \ldots, K-1 \tag{14a}$$

where $j = \sqrt{-1}$, $\hat{q}_i = q_i$ for $i \leqq \mu$, and $\hat{q}_i = 0$ otherwise.

Equation (14a) is the standard form of the "finite Fourier transform" [26], and in terms of the values $Q(s_k)$ the coefficients $\hat{q}_i$ are given as

$$\hat{q}_i = \frac{1}{K} \sum_{k=0}^{K-1} Q(s_k) \exp\left(\frac{-2\pi ijk}{K}\right) \qquad i = 0, 1, \ldots, K-1 \tag{14b}$$

When the number K is selected to be a power of 2, Eq. (14b) can be solved in only $K \log_2 K$ complex operations (multiplication-additions) using the fast Fourier transform (FFT) algorithm [26]. Most of the computation time is spent in evaluating Q at various points, and the FFT takes only a very small fraction of the overall time.

Stability considerations, the influence of various numerical errors, and ways to reduce them can be found in Ref. [22].

2.2 Partially or Fully Symbolic Network Functions Using the FFT Algorithm

Multidimensional FFT method [37, 51]

For simplicity, we use the closed system given by Eq. (10) instead of Cramer's rule, Eq. (4), to get the partially or fully symbolic network function $H(s, p_1, p_2, \ldots, p_m)$. Therefore, we should consider $\Delta_c(\mathbf{x})$ given by Eq. (8) with $\mathbf{x} = (x_1, x_2, \ldots, x_\alpha)$ denoting the vector of variables to be left in symbolic form, in which the complex frequency s and some symbols for the closed system are also contained, and we have

$$\Delta_c(\mathbf{x}) = \det \mathbf{A}' = \sum_{q_1=0}^{J_1-1} \cdots \sum_{q_\alpha=0}^{J_\alpha-1} \Delta_{q_1\cdots q_\alpha} x_1^{q_1} \cdots x_\alpha^{q_\alpha} \tag{15}$$

where $J_i - 1$ is the order of the x_i in $\Delta_c(\mathbf{x})$, $i = 1, \ldots, \alpha$, and $\mathbf{A}'$ is defined by Eq. (7). The desired symbolic network function $H(s, p_1, \ldots, p_m)$ is obtained by applying the oscillation condition $\Delta_c = 0$ to Eq. (15), once $\Delta_{q_1\cdots q_\alpha}$ is found by any other procedure.

We now show how $\Delta_{q_1\cdots q_\alpha}$ ($q_i = 0, 1, \ldots, J_i - 1$, $i = 1, 2, \ldots, \alpha$) can be obtained by using the multidimensional FFT algorithm, where the interpolation points for symbols, $x_1, \ldots, x_\alpha$, are selected on the unit circle in the s-plane as shown in the following:

$$w_i^{-n_i} = \exp\left(\frac{-j2\pi n_i}{J_i}\right) \qquad n_i = 0, 1, \ldots, J_i - 1,\ i = 1, 2, \ldots, \alpha \tag{16}$$

Let $\Delta^{[n_1,\ldots,n_\alpha]}$ be the value of $\Delta_c(\mathbf{x}) = \Delta_c(x_1, \ldots, x_\alpha)$ in the interpolation point $(w_1^{-n_1}, \ldots, w_\alpha^{-n_\alpha})$. That is,

$$\Delta^{[n_1,\ldots,n_\alpha]} = \Delta_c(w_1^{-n_1}, \ldots, w_\alpha^{-n_\alpha}) \tag{17}$$

which can be calculated efficiently by using the matrix partition method based on the hierarchical decomposition of symbols for the matrix $\mathbf{A}'$ [51]. Then, by applying the inverse α-dimensional discrete Fourier transform to Eq. (15), we have

$$\Delta_{q_1\cdots q_\alpha} = \frac{1}{J_1 J_2 \cdots J_\alpha} \sum_{n_1=0}^{J_1-1} \cdots \sum_{n_\alpha=0}^{J_\alpha-1} \Delta^{[n_1,\ldots,n_\alpha]} w_1^{-n_1 q_1} w_2^{-n_2 q_2} \cdots w_\alpha^{-n_\alpha q_\alpha} \tag{18}$$

It is noted that this multidimensional FFT method is applicable to any type of formulation and any class of linear circuit, that is, lumped circuits or some kinds of distributed circuits, analog or digital circuits, and time-invariant circuits or some kinds of time-varying circuits, because the order $(J_i - 1)$ of the x_i in Eqs. (15) and (18) is arbitrary.

One-dimensional FFT and partial derivative method [22, 34, 59]

Let there be m unspecified elements shown in Eq. (2), and let

$$H(s, p_1, \ldots, p_m) = H(s, \mathbf{p}) = \frac{N(s, \mathbf{p})}{D(s, \mathbf{p})} \tag{19}$$

be the immittance function, with $\mathbf{p}$ denoting the vector of elements to be left in symbolic form, for the class of network under consideration, N and D are bilinear in each of the p_i as shown by Theorem 1, and if Q is used to represent either N or D, then

$$Q(s, \mathbf{p}) = \sum_{j_1=0}^{1} \sum_{j_2=0}^{1} \cdots \sum_{j_m=0}^{1} p_1^{j_1} p_2^{j_2} \cdots p_m^{j_m} Q_{j_1 j_2 \cdots j_m}(s) \tag{20}$$

with $Q_{j_1 j_2 \cdots j_m}(s)$ being polynomials in s. There are 2^m terms on the right-hand side of Eq. (20). If all possible partial derivatives of Q with respect to the p_i are taken, only $2^m - 1$ of them are nonzero.

The various polynomials $Q_{j_1 j_2 \cdots j_m}(s)$ in (20) can be obtained from Q and its partial derivatives by the solution of a triangular system of linear equations, and then the FFT algorithm can be used to generate $Q_{j_1 j_2 \cdots j_m}(s)$, once values of the various partial derivatives of $Q(s, \mathbf{p})$ with respect to the p_i are found for values s on the unit circle in the s-plane.

How to obtain these partial derivatives was shown by using the adjoint network approach and sparse matrix methods in Ref. [22] and by using the tableau formulation and the theory of compound matrices in Ref. [34] but the results are applicable to any formulation.

It is noted that this method is applicable to the class of networks in which N and D are bilinear in each of the p_i. However, it is also shown in Refs. [22, 34] how the symbolic function for lumped distributed active networks can be generated. When distributed elements are present, straightforward interpolation fails because the immittance functions are meromorphic rather than rational functions. Then new variables are introduced and the multidimensional version of the FFT (described in Section 2.2) is used to generate $H(s, \mathbf{p}, \boldsymbol{\eta})$ by using multinomial interpolation, where the η's are some transcendental functions of s of the uniform lossy transmission lines.

Extended one-dimensional FFT method [53]

In Ref. [53], an extension of the one-dimensional FFT algorithm to obtain $H(s, p_1, \ldots, p_m)$ is proposed by arranging variable symbols including s in the special dictionary fashion. It is stressed that this method is effectively applicable to distributed circuits, digital circuits, and switched capacitor circuits as well as lumped linear time-invariant networks, because there is no restriction on the order of the network element p_i.

2.3 Inversion of Rational Matrices by Using the FFT Algorithm [39]

Introduction

Inversion of rational and/or polynomial matrices arises in many fields of engineering such as the analysis and synthesis of passive and active *RLC* networks, the analysis of power systems, and the analysis and design of multivariable control systems.

With respect to this problem, many methods have been proposed [16, 20, 25, 27, 31, 32, 39]. These methods are based on finding the coefficients of the determinantal polynomial $\det[\mathbf{A}(s)]$ and the coefficient matrices of the adjoint polynomial matrix $\mathrm{adj}[\mathbf{A}(s)]$ of a polynomial matrix $\mathbf{A}(s)$. The techniques for finding them can be classified into two groups: the method of undetermined coefficients [7, 16, 20, 25, 27] and the method of interpolation [31, 32, 39]. Here we use the latter method.

Inversion of a rational matrix

In this section, we shall propose a method for calculating the inverse of an $M \times M$ rational matrix $\mathbf{R}(s)$.

Let $r(s)$ be the least common polynomial of all the denominators of the elements of $\mathbf{R}(s)$. Then $\mathbf{R}(s)$ is given by

$$\mathbf{R}(s) = \frac{\mathbf{A}(s)}{r(s)} \tag{21}$$

where $\mathbf{A}(s)$ is a polynomial matrix.

Let $\det[\mathbf{A}(s)]$ and $\mathbf{B}(s)$ be the determinant and the adjoint matrix of $\mathbf{A}(s)$, respectively. Then the inverse of $\mathbf{A}(s)$ is given by

$$[\mathbf{A}(s)]^{-1} = \frac{\mathbf{B}(s)}{\det[\mathbf{A}(s)]} \tag{22}$$

From Eqs. (21) and (22), the inverse of $\mathbf{R}(s)$ is easily found as

$$[\mathbf{R}(s)]^{-1} = r(s)[\mathbf{A}(s)]^{-1} = \frac{r(s)\mathbf{B}(s)}{\det[\mathbf{A}(s)]} \tag{23}$$

Therefore, we shall consider the problem of determining the adjoint matrix $\mathbf{B}(s)$ and the determinant $\det[\mathbf{A}(s)]$ of the polynomial matrix $\mathbf{A}(s)$.

Suppose that each element of $\mathbf{A}(s)$ is a polynomial in s, whose degree is at most L; that is, $\mathbf{A}(s)$ is given by

$$\mathbf{A}(s) = \mathbf{A}_0 + \mathbf{A}_1 s + \cdots + \mathbf{A}_L s^L \tag{24}$$

where $\mathbf{A}_i \in C^{M \times M}$, $i = 0, 1, \ldots, L$.

Let $\beta_{km}(s)$ be the (k, m)th element of $\mathbf{B}(s)$:

$$\beta_{km}(s) \triangleq \mathbf{B}(s) = \det[\mathbf{A}(s)][\mathbf{A}(s)]^{-1} \tag{25}$$

Since the adjoint matrix $\mathbf{B}(s)$ of a polynomial matrix $\mathbf{A}(s)$ is also a polynomial matrix, $\beta_{km}(s)$ is given by

$$\beta_{km}(s) = \sum_{q=0}^{K-1} b_{km}{}^{[q]} s^q \qquad k, m = 1, 2, \ldots, M \tag{26}$$

where $K - 1 \leqq (M - 1)L$.

Let $j \triangleq \sqrt{-1}$ and $\hat{w} = \exp(j2\pi/K)$, and suppose that we have

$$\hat{\boldsymbol{\beta}}^{[n]} = (\hat{\beta}_{km}{}^{[n]}) \triangleq \det[\mathbf{A}(\hat{w}^{-n})][\mathbf{A}(\hat{w}^{-n})]^{-1} \tag{27}$$

for K values of $\hat{w}^{-n} = \exp(-j2\pi n/K)$, $n = 0, 1, \ldots, K-1$. Then from Eqs. (26) and (27) we obtain a system of simultaneous linear equations with the unknown variables $\{b_{km}{}^{[q]}\}$:

$$\hat{\beta}_{km}{}^{[n]} = \sum_{q=0}^{K-1} b_{km}{}^{[q]} \hat{w}^{-nq} \qquad n = 0, 1, \ldots, K-1,\ k, m = 1, 2, \ldots, M \tag{28}$$

Note that, for each k, $m \in \{1, 2, \ldots, M\}$, Eq. (28) implies that the sequences $\{\hat{\beta}_{km}{}^{[0]}, \hat{\beta}_{km}{}^{[1]}, \ldots, \hat{\beta}_{km}{}^{[K-1]}\}$ and $\{b_{km}{}^{[0]}, b_{km}{}^{[1]}, \ldots, b_{km}{}^{[K-1]}\}$ form the discrete Fourier transform pair. Therefore, $\{b_{km}{}^{[q]}\}$ is given as the inverse discrete Fourier transform of $\{\hat{\beta}_{km}{}^{[n]}\}$:

$$b_{km}{}^{[q]} = \frac{1}{K} \sum_{n=0}^{K-1} \hat{\beta}_{km}{}^{[n]} \hat{w}^{nq} \qquad q = 0, 1, \ldots, K-1 \tag{29}$$

Moreover, $\{b_{km}{}^{[q]}\}$ is effectively calculated by using the FFT algorithm [26].

In the same way as Eq. (29), the coefficients d_q $(q = 0, 1, \ldots, N-1)$ of $\Delta(s) = \sum_{q=0}^{N-1} d_q s^q$, the determinant of $\mathbf{A}(s)$, are given by

$$d_q = \frac{1}{N} \sum_{n=0}^{N-1} \Delta_n w^{nq} \qquad q = 0, 1, \ldots, N-1 \tag{30}$$

where

$$w \triangleq \exp\left(\frac{j2\pi}{N}\right)$$

$$\Delta_n \triangleq \det[\mathbf{A}(w^{-n})] \qquad n = 0, 1, \ldots, N-1 \tag{31}$$

and

$$N - 1 \leqq ML$$

Generally speaking, the maximal order $K-1$ of the adjoint matrix $\mathbf{B}(s)$ is not equal to the maximal order $N-1$ of the determinant $\Delta(s)$; more precisely, $K \leqq N$. Therefore, $\{\hat{\beta}_{km}{}^{[n]}\}$ in Eq. (29) and $\{\Delta_n\}$ in Eq. (30) are evaluated at the different interpolation points $\{\hat{w}^{-n}\}$ and $\{w^{-n}\}$, respectively. However, it is desirable to evaluate these numbers at the same interpolation points $\{w^{-n}\}$. If $K < N$, let

$$b_{km}{}^{[q]} = 0 \qquad q = K, K+1, \ldots, N-1,\ k, m = 1, 2, \ldots, M$$

Then from Eq. (26), $\beta_{km}(s)$ can be rewritten as

$$\beta_{km}(s) = \sum_{q=0}^{N-1} b_{km}{}^{[q]} s^q$$

Suppose that we have

$$\boldsymbol{\beta}^{[n]} \triangleq (\beta_{km}{}^{[n]}) = \det[\mathbf{A}(w^{-n})]\cdot[\mathbf{A}(w^{-n})]^{-1}$$

Then, in the same way as Eq. (29), $\{b_{km}{}^{[q]}\}$ is determined by

$$b_{km}{}^{[q]} = \begin{cases} \dfrac{1}{N}\displaystyle\sum_{n=0}^{N-1} \beta_{km}{}^{[n]} w^{nq} & q = 0, 1, \ldots, K-1,\ k, m = 1, 2, \ldots, \mathrm{M} \\ 0 & q = K, K+1, \ldots, N-1,\ k, m = 1, 2, \ldots, M \end{cases} \tag{32}$$

The flowchart for finding $\mathbf{B}(s) = \operatorname{adj}[\mathbf{A}(s)]$ and $\Delta(s) = \det[\mathbf{A}(s)]$ is shown in Figure 8.2.

Example

In this section, we shall give a simple example to illustrate the proposed method. Let

$$\mathbf{A}(s) = \begin{bmatrix} 1+3s & 5+2s \\ s & 4+s \end{bmatrix} = \begin{bmatrix} 1 & 5 \\ 0 & 4 \end{bmatrix} + \begin{bmatrix} 3 & 2 \\ 1 & 1 \end{bmatrix} s$$

be given. It follows that $M = 2$ and $L = 1$, therefore $N = 3$ and $K = 2$.

Now, let $w \triangleq \exp(j2\pi/3)$. Then by step 1, we have

$$w^{-0} = 1.0000000$$

$$w^{-1} = -0.5000000 - j0.8660260$$

$$w^{-2} = -0.5000000 + j0.8660260$$

$$\Delta_0 = \det \mathbf{A}(W^{-0}) = 13.000000\pi$$

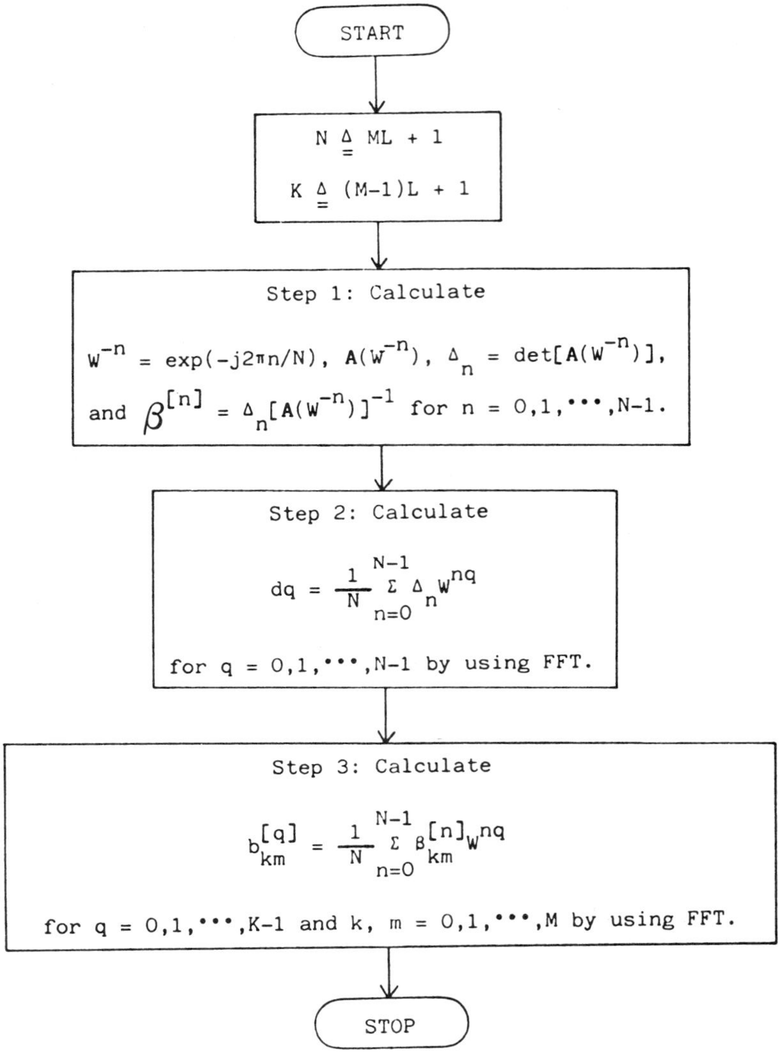

Figure 8.2 Procedure for finding **B**(s) and $\Delta(s)$.

$$\Delta_1 = \det \mathbf{A}(w^{-1}) = -0.5000010 - j6.0621820$$

$$\Delta_2 = \det \mathbf{A}(w^{-2}) = -0.5000010 + j6.0621820$$

$$\boldsymbol{\beta}^{[0]} = \begin{bmatrix} \beta_{11}{}^{[0]} & \beta_{12}{}^{[0]} \\ \beta_{21}{}^{[0]} & \beta_{22}{}^{[0]} \end{bmatrix}$$

$$= \begin{bmatrix} 5.0000000 & -7.0000000 \\ -1.0000000 & 4.0000000 \end{bmatrix}$$

$$\boldsymbol{\beta}^{[1]} = \begin{bmatrix} \beta_{11}{}^{[1]} & \beta_{12}{}^{[1]} \\ \beta_{21}{}^{[1]} & \beta_{22}{}^{[1]} \end{bmatrix}$$

$$= \begin{bmatrix} 3.5000000 - j0.8660260 & -4.0000000 + j1.7320520 \\ 0.5000000 + j0.8660260 & -0.5000000 - j2.5980780 \end{bmatrix}$$

and

$$\boldsymbol{\beta}^{[2]} = \begin{bmatrix} \beta_{11}{}^{[2]} & \beta_{12}{}^{[2]} \\ \beta_{21}{}^{[2]} & \beta_{22}{}^{[2]} \end{bmatrix}$$

$$= \begin{bmatrix} 3.5000000 + j0.8660260 & -4.0000000 - j1.7320520 \\ 0.5000000 - j0.8660260 & -0.5000000 + j2.5980780 \end{bmatrix}$$

Next, by step 2, we have

$$d_0 = 3.9999993 \simeq 4$$

$$d_1 = 8.0000046 \simeq 8$$

$$d_2 = 0.9999954 \simeq 1$$

Then we have

$$\Delta(s) \triangleq \det[\mathbf{A}(s)] = d_0 + d_1 s + d_2 s^2 = 4 + 8s + s^2$$

Finally, by step 3, we have

$$\beta_{11}(s) = \sum_{q=0}^{1} b_{11}{}^{[q]} s^q = 4.0000000 + 1.0000006s \simeq 4 + s$$

$$\beta_{12}(s) = \sum_{q=0}^{1} b_{12}{}^{[q]} s^q = -5.0000000 - 2.0000013s \simeq -5 - 2s$$

$$\beta_{21}(s) = \sum_{q=0}^{1} b_{21}{}^{[q]} s^q = 0.0000000 - 1.0000006s \simeq -s$$

$$\beta_{22}(s) = \sum_{q=0}^{1} b_{22}{}^{[q]} s^q = 1.0000000 + 3.0000020s \simeq 1 + 3s$$

Then we have

$$\mathbf{B}(s) = \begin{bmatrix} \beta_{11}(s) & \beta_{12}(s) \\ \beta_{21}(s) & \beta_{22}(s) \end{bmatrix} = \begin{bmatrix} 4+s & -5-2s \\ -s & 1+3s \end{bmatrix}$$

Therefore, the inverse of $\mathbf{A}(s)$ is given by

$$\mathbf{A}(s)^{-1} = \frac{\mathbf{B}(s)}{\Delta(s)} = \frac{1}{4+8s+s^2} \times \begin{bmatrix} 4+s & -5-2s \\ -s & 1+3s \end{bmatrix}$$

Conclusion

Here, an algorithm using the FFT algorithm for the calculation of the inverse of rational matrices is presented. Although this method requires complex arithmetic, the total computational time is significantly reduced in comparison to the conventional method [25] because the FFT algorithm is used in the proposed method [39].

2.4 Remarks on Interpolation Methods

These three types of methods, the multidimensional FFT method [37, 51], one-dimensional FFT and partial derivative method [22, 34, 59], and extended one-dimensional FFT method [53], are applicable to both partially and fully symbolic network functions. It is clear from Sections 2.1–2.3 above that these interpolation methods are based on the theory and implementation of numerical methods for generating symbolic functions for analog, digital, distributed, or switched capacitor networks and seem to have a lower computational cost than other well-known symbolic analysis algorithms such as parameter extraction methods [12, 30].

The upper limits to problems to be solved in symbolic form by using direct interpolation methods are a system matrix size of 30, number of variable elements of 10, and maximum degree of the polynomials of 20 [34], but it is possible to overcome these upper limits to some extent by using matrix partition methods [51].

It is noted that descriptions of interpolation methods have also been given in Refs. [19, 23, 31, 32, 37, 60] as well as Ref. [11].

In Refs. [49, 59] an entirely new and considerably simplified approach to the generation of symbolic functions, in which interpolation methods using the FFT algorithm were also effectively used, was proposed. Instead of giving the symbolic function in terms of element values, arbitrary increments, including zero and infinity, to the nominal values are used in the symbolic function. The steps are based on the generation of a special matrix, which, for

m variable elements (R, L, C elements, the four transducers, and the inverse gain of the operational amplifier are examples of variables), is of dimension $(m + 1)$. All information about the symbolic function is contained in this matrix.

If we use the interpolation methods described in Section 2.2 to derive the symbolic network function from the above $(m + 1) \times (m + 1)$ matrix, the complex frequency s can be retained as a variable as well [22, 34]. The theory of Ref. [49] has many applications in calculating large-change sensitivity, generating fault directories needed in fault analysis of networks, extending a zero pivot in sparse matrix solutions to several zero pivots, and so forth (see [59] for more details).

3 SIGNAL FLOW GRAPH METHODS [58, 62]

3.1 Introduction

The signal flow graph method based on Mason's gain formula has received attention from many researchers [10, 18, 30, 36]. However, the method has been considered inefficient because of the cancellation of terms in the expansion formula. To overcome this inefficiency, Mielke [38] established a new signal flow graph topological formula, in which no term cancellation occurs, by evaluating the topological formula in terms of tree admittance products on the corresponding primitive signal flow graph.

In this section we extend the formula to the most general networks (shown in Figure 8.3 and Table 8.1), which contain two-terminal regular elements

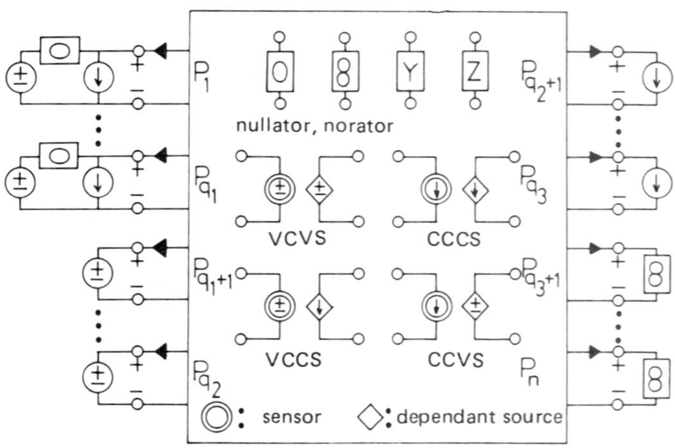

Figure 8.3 General linear n-port $\hat{N}$, $q_1 = n - q_3$.

Table 8.1 Network Function X_{ij} of n-port $\hat{N}$ Shown in Figure 8.3[a]

Network functions X_{ij}	i	j
$\mu_{ij} = \dfrac{V_{P_i}}{V_{P_j}}$	$q_2 + 1 \leqslant i \leqslant n$	$1 \leqslant j \leqslant q_2$
$-Y_{ij} = \dfrac{I_{P_i}}{V_{P_j}}$	$q_1 + 1 \leqslant i \leqslant q_2$ or $q_3 + 1 \leqslant i \leqslant n$	
$\alpha_{ij} = \dfrac{I_{P_i}}{I_{P_j}}$		$1 \leqslant j \leqslant q_1$ or $q_2 + 1 \leqslant j \leqslant q_3$
$-Z_{ij} = \dfrac{V_{P_i}}{I_{P_j}}$	$q_2 + 1 \leqslant i \leqslant n$	

[a] X_{ij} is defined as $X_{ij} = y_{P_i}/x_{P_j}|_{x_{P_k}=0}, j \neq k, k = 1, 2, \ldots, q_3$, and x_{P_j} (y_{P_i}, respectively) is an exciting (measuring, resp.) voltage variable or current variable of the port P_j (P_i, resp.).

(i.e., admittance elements and impedance elements), any type of controlled sources (i.e., VCVS, VCCS, CCCS, and CCVS), and two-terminal singular elements (i.e., norators and nullators) and are terminated by norators, independent sources, and bigenerators [5].

First, we derive the equation for a given network for a generalized common tree-cotree pair in the voltage and current graphs and then draw a chain path graph [35], which is also called a primitive signal flow graph [38]; in this chain path graph the network topology is expressed best. After these preliminaries, the general signal flow graph topological formulas are derived [58, 62].

3.2 Chain Path Graph for Closed System

For simplicity, let $\hat{N}_c$ be a closed system corresponding to a desired network function, which can be a transmission parameter. In $\hat{N}_c$ it is assumed that an independent source corresponding to a desired network function has been replaced by a dependent source controlled by the specified output variables, and the other independent voltage sources and current sources have been contracted and removed from the original network (see Figure 8.1).

The system $\hat{N}_c$ can be represented topologically by a linear graph G

consisting of a voltage graph G_V and a current graph G_I, which are defined by Eqs. (33) and (34):

$$G_V = G(E_0 \cup E_\alpha \cup E_r : E_\infty \cup E_{\hat{\alpha}} \cup E_{\hat{g}}) \tag{33}$$

$$G_I = G(E_\infty \cup E_{\hat{\mu}} \cup E_{\hat{r}} : E_0 \cup E_\mu \cup E_g) \tag{34}$$

The notation $G(E_1 : E_2)$ represents the graph derived from G by contracting all edges of E_1 and removing all edges of E_2, where E_1 and E_2 are the subsets of the edge set of G and $E_1 \cap E_2 = \phi$, and E_0 and E_∞ are the edge sets of nullators and norators. Furthermore, E_μ and $E_{\hat{\mu}}$ (or E_g and $E_{\hat{g}}$, E_r and $E_{\hat{r}}$, E_α and $E_{\hat{\alpha}}$) are respectively the edge set of sensors and that of dependent sources of VCVS (or VCCS, CCVS, and CCCS).

A generalized common tree-cotree pair for G_V and G_I is defined as follows, and guarantees the existence of a topological unique solution.

Definition 1 Let t_V and $\bar{t}_V$ (or t_I and $\bar{t}_I$) be, respectively, a tree and a cotree of G_V (or G_I) and let them be defined by Eq. (35), in which conditions (I) and (II) are satisfied:

$$\begin{aligned}
t_V &= E'_\mu \cup E''_{\hat{\mu}} \cup E'_g \cup E'_{\hat{r}} \cup E'_z \cup E'_y \\
\bar{t}_V &= E''_\mu \cup E'_{\hat{\mu}} \cup E''_g \cup E''_{\hat{r}} \cup E''_z \cup E''_y \\
t_I &= E'_\alpha \cup E''_{\hat{\alpha}} \cup E'_{\hat{g}} \cup E'_r \cup E'_z \cup E'_y \\
\bar{t}_I &= E''_\alpha \cup E'_{\hat{\alpha}} \cup E''_{\hat{g}} \cup E''_r \cup E''_z \cup E''_y
\end{aligned} \tag{35}$$

Condition (I):

$$E'_x \cup E''_x = E_x, \qquad E'_x \cap E''_x = \phi, \qquad x = \mu, \alpha, g, r, y, z$$

$$E'_{\hat{x}} \cup E''_{\hat{x}} = E_{\hat{x}}, \qquad E'_{\hat{x}} \cap E''_{\hat{x}} = \varnothing, \qquad x = \mu, \alpha, g, r$$

Condition (II):

$$e_x \in E'_x \ (\text{or } e_x \in E''_x) \rightleftarrows e_{\hat{x}} \in E'_{\hat{x}} \ (\text{or } e_{\hat{x}} \in E''_{\hat{x}}), \qquad x = \mu, \alpha, g, r$$

From now on we call this tree-cotree pair $[t_I; \bar{t}_V]$ the generalized common tree-cotree pair for G_V and G_I.

The standard network equation for $\hat{N}_c$ for a generalized common tree-cotree pair $[t_I; \bar{t}_V]$ is given by Figure 8.4, where (1) $\mathbf{B}_p$ (or $\mathbf{Q}_p$) is the principal part of the fundamental tieset (or cutset) matrix for G_V (or G_I) for $[t_V; \bar{t}_V]$ (or $[t_I; \bar{t}_I]$), (2) $\boldsymbol{\mu}_*$ ($\boldsymbol{\alpha}_*$, $\mathbf{Z}_*^{-1}$, $\mathbf{Y}_*^{-1}$) is a diagonal matrix of order n_μ (n_α, n_z, n_y), (3) $E_{\mu*} = E''_\mu \cup E'_{\hat{\mu}}$, $E_{z*} = E''_g \cup E''_{\hat{r}} \cup E''_y \cup E''_z$, $E_{\hat{\mu}*} = E''_{\hat{\mu}} \cup E'_\mu$, $E_{\hat{y}*} = E'_g \cup E'_{\hat{r}} \cup E'_y \cup E'_z$, $E_{\hat{z}*} = E''_{\hat{g}} \cup E''_{\hat{r}} \cup E''_y \cup E''_z$, $E_{\hat{\alpha}*} = E''_\alpha \cup E'_{\hat{\alpha}}$, $E_{y*} = E'_{\hat{g}} \cup E'_r \cup E'_y \cup E'_z$, and $E_{\alpha*} = E'_\alpha \cup E''_{\hat{\alpha}}$, (4) "**1**" is the identity matrix and the entries in blank

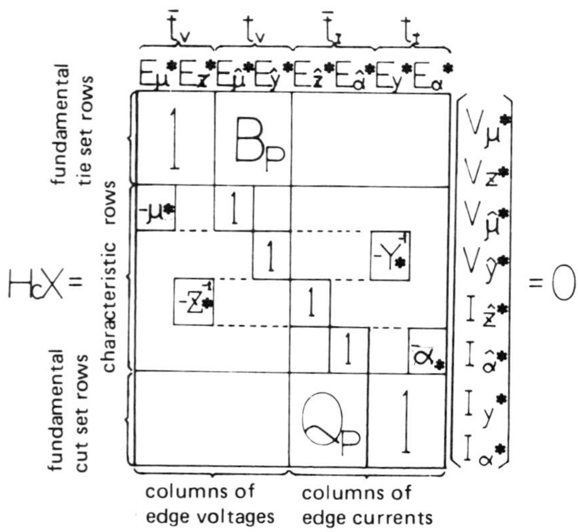

Figure 8.4 Network equation for the closed system $\hat{N}_c$ derived from n-port $\hat{N}$ in Figure 8.3.

submatrices are zeros, and (5) $\mathbf{V}_x$ ($\mathbf{I}_x$) is the vector of voltages (currents) of elements E_x, where $x = \mu^*, \hat{\mu}^*, z^*, \hat{y}^*$ ($x = \hat{z}^*, y^*, \alpha^*, \hat{\alpha}^*$).

The following definitions are useful for introducing a chain path graph [35, 38].

Definition 2 Suppose $\hat{G}$ is a weighted and directed graph with m vertices X_i, $i = 1, 2, \ldots, m$. The weight matrix $\mathbf{W} = [w_{ij}]$ of $\hat{G}$ is of order m, where the rows and columns correspond to the vertices of $\hat{G}$, and w_{ij} is the weight associated with the edge in $\hat{G}$ directed from X_j to X_i; if $w_{ij} = 0$, there is no edge from X_j to X_i in $\hat{G}$ [38].

Definition 3 The weighted and directed graph $\hat{G}[H_c]$ corresponding to the standard network equation for $\hat{N}_c$ is called the chain path graph if $\hat{G}[H_c]$ has the weight matrix $\mathbf{W} = -\mathbf{H}_c + \mathbf{1}$; the vertex label of $\hat{G}[H_c]$ associated with the i-row of $\mathbf{W}$ is the i-entry in $\mathbf{X}$ and with the j-column of $\mathbf{W}$ is the j-entry in $\mathbf{X}$ [35, 38].

It is convenient in the following discussion to refer to the different edge types in $\hat{G}[H_c]$ depending on the submatrix in $\mathbf{W}$ on which the corresponding edge weight appears. The following notation will be used: (1) a μ-edge (Z-edge, Y-edge, α-edge) corresponds to a nonzero entry in $\boldsymbol{\mu}_*$ ($\mathbf{Z}_*^{-1}$, $\mathbf{Y}_*^{-1}$, $\boldsymbol{\alpha}_*$) and (2) a B-edge (Q-edge) corresponds to a nonzero entry in $-\mathbf{B}_p$ ($-\mathbf{Q}_p$). Let the μ-, Z-, Y-, and α-edges all together be called a C-edge and, in $\hat{G}[H_c]$, denote a B-edge (Q-edge, C-edge) by a solid line (dashed line, dot-dashed line).

Example 1 Consider the closed system $\hat{N}_c$ shown in Figure 8.5, where we want to derive the transfer function $\alpha = I_\alpha / I_{\hat{\alpha}}$. In this figure the independent current source and voltage source, which form a bigenerator, have been replaced by a dependent current source controlled by the output variable I_α

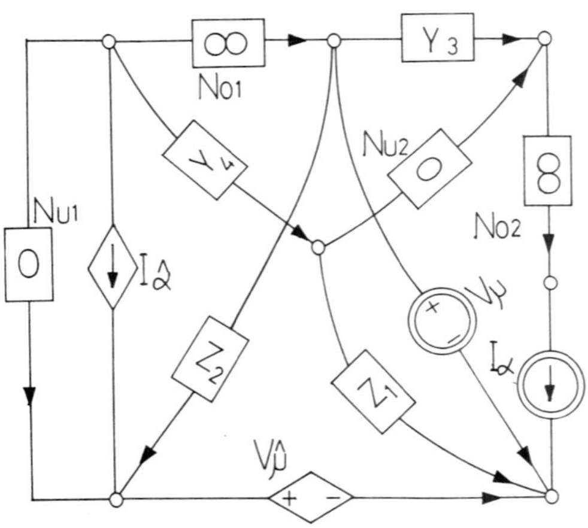

Figure 8.5 Example demonstrating how to derive the transfer function $\alpha = I_\alpha / I_{\hat{\alpha}}$, where $I_{\hat{\alpha}} = \alpha I_\alpha$ and $V_{\hat{\mu}} = \mu V_\mu$.

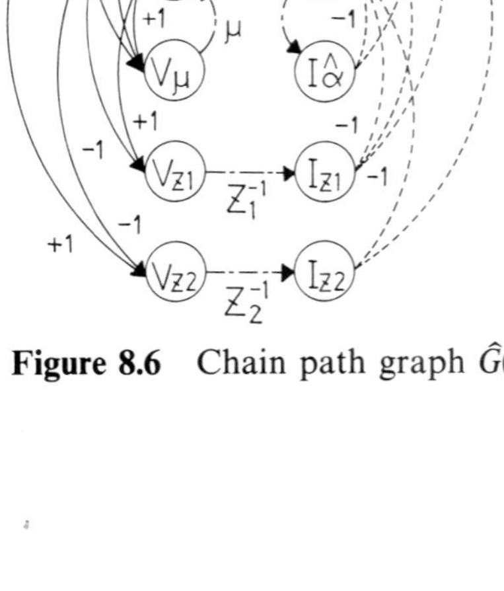

Figure 8.6 Chain path graph $\hat{G}(H_c)$ of Figure 8.5.

and contracted, respectively, and the current sensor is also connected in series with the norator N_{02}, as shown generally in Figure 8.1. The chain path graph $\hat{G}[H_c]$ for a generalized common tree-cotree pair $[t_I; \bar{t}_V] = [\alpha, y_3, y_4; \hat{\mu}, z_1, z_2]$ of the corresponding two-graph G_V and G_I can be given by Figure 8.6.

3.3 Modification of Mason's Gain Formula

In this section, by using the following two properties of $\hat{G}[H_c]$, Mason's gain formula will be converted into a semifinal form, which can be used for both evaluating noncanceling terms of $\det \mathbf{H}_c$ and deriving the final formula.

Property 1 Each directed loop in $\hat{G}[H_c]$ satisfies one of the following three statements: (1) it contains only μ-edges and B-edges, (2) it contains only α-edges and Q-edges, and (3) it contains B-edges, Q-edges, and C-edges.

Property 2 Each weight of C-edges is symbolized and assumed to be positive. On the other hand, each weight of the other edges is either $+1$ or -1.

The following definitions of various kinds of subgraphs of $\hat{G}[H_c]$ are useful for converting Mason's gain formula into the modified one.

Definition 4 (1) Let C_k be the kth subgraph of $\hat{G}[H_c]$ consisting of (n'_μ) μ-edges, (n'_α) α-edges, (l) Y-edges, and (l) Z-edges, where $0 \leqq n'_\mu \leqq n_\mu$, $0 \leqq n'_\alpha \leqq n_\alpha$, $0 \leqq l \leqq \min\{n_z, n_y\}$, and $n'_\mu + n'_\alpha + l \geqq 1$. (2) Let $\hat{g}(C_k)$ be the vertex section graph of $\hat{G}[H_c]$ with all vertices in C_k.

Definition 5 A spanning loop set of $\hat{g}(C_k)$ is the union of node disjoint loops of $\hat{g}(C_k)$ that contains all vertices of $\hat{g}(C_k)$. Let $n(C_k)$ be the total number of distinct spanning loop sets in $\hat{g}(C_k)$, and let $L_u(C_k)$ be the uth spanning loop set of $\hat{g}(C_k)$, if $n(C_k) \neq 0$.

Remark Let $f(C_k)$ be the product of the weights of all edges in C_k. Now the following facts are well known: If $n(C_k)$ is not zero, then the terms with absolute value $f(C_k)$ in the primitive expansion of $\det \mathbf{H}_c$ are in one-to-one correspondence with the spanning loop sets of the subgraph $\hat{g}(C_k)$, and if $n(C_k)$ is zero, then each term with absolute value $f(C_k)$ does not appear in the expansion of $\det \mathbf{H}_c$.

With these preliminaries, the modified signal flow graph topological formula is obtained, as will be shown in Theorem 2, by appropriately sorting similar terms with the same absolute value in the expansion of Mason's gain formula and then deriving the sign expression of each set of the similar terms.

Theorem 2 Suppose $\hat{G}[H_c]$ is the chain path graph corresponding to the equation shown in Figure 8.4. Then

$$\det \mathbf{H}_c = 1 + \sum_{k=1}^{\sigma} \varepsilon_k \times f(\hat{C}_k) \tag{36}$$

and

$$\varepsilon_k = \sum_{u=1}^{n(\hat{C}_k)} (-1)^{\nu_u + \omega_u} \tag{37}$$

where (1) $\hat{C}_k$ is the kth subgraph of $\hat{G}[H_c]$ consisting of (n'_μ) μ-edges, (n'_α) α-edges, (l) Z-edges, and (l) Y-edges, such that $n(\hat{C}_k)$ is nonzero, (2) ν_u is the number of node disjoint directed loops in $L_u(\hat{C}_k)$, (3) ω_u is the number of B-edges and Q-edges with edge weight -1 in $L_u(\hat{C}_k)$, and (4) σ is the total number of all possible distinct subgraphs $\hat{C}_k$.

The proof is omitted owing to limited space.

It should be noted that Eq. (36) is not the formula that generates only the noncanceling terms in Mason's gain formula and Eq. (37) does not guarantee that ε_k is either 0 or ± 1. We will discuss these points in the next subsection.

Example 2 The chain path graph shown in Figure 8.6 contains a total of 23 distinct subgraphs $\hat{g}(C_k)$. Of these subgraphs, 17 subgraphs $\hat{g}(\hat{C}_k)$ have nonzero spanning loop set number $n(\hat{C}_k)$ as shown in Table 8.2. For example, the 10th subgraph $\hat{g}(\hat{C}_{10})$ contains two spanning loop sets, shown in Figure 8.7, where $\hat{C}_{10} = \{z_2^{-1}, y_3^{-1}, \alpha^{-1}\}$. Now, from Eq. (37) we have

$$\varepsilon_{10} = (-1)^{2+2} + (-1)^{1+2} = 0$$

Therefore, the term with absolute value $f(\hat{C}_{10}) = z_2^{-1} \cdot y_3^{-1} \cdot \alpha^{-1}$ cancels out itself in the final expansion of $\det \mathbf{H}_c$.

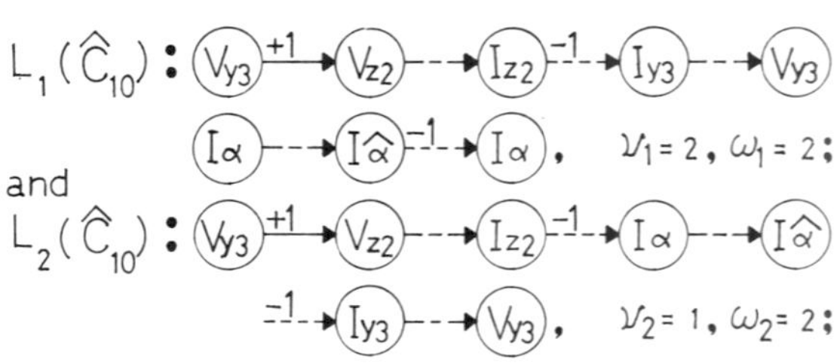

Figure 8.7 Two spanning loop sets in the 10th subgraph $\hat{g}(\hat{C}_{10})$.

Table 8.2 Complete Subgraphs of $\hat{G}(H_c)$; x Stands for $\hat{C}_x$ or $\tilde{C}_k$

k	k'	$f(x)$	$n_B(x)$	$n_Q(x)$	$n(x)$	$\varepsilon_K, \tilde{\varepsilon}'_K$
1	1	μ	1		1	-1
2	2	α^{-1}		1	1	$+1$
3	3	$\mu\alpha^{-1}$	1	1	1	-1
4	4	$Z_1^{-1}Y_4^{-1}$	1	1	1	$+1$
5	5	$Z_2^{-1}Y_3^{-1}$	1	1	1	$+1$
6	6	$\mu Z_1^{-1}Y_3^{-1}$	1	1	1	$+1$
7		$\mu Z_1^{-1}Y_4^{-1}$	2	1	2	0
8	7	$\mu Z_2^{-1}Y_3^{-1}$	1	1	1	-1
9	8	$Z_1^{-1}Y_4^{-1}\alpha^{-1}$	1	1	1	$+1$
10		$Z_2^{-1}Y_3^{-1}\alpha^{-1}$	1	2	2	0
11		$\mu Z_1^{-1}Y_3^{-1}\alpha^{-1}$	1	2	2	0
12		$\mu Z_1^{-1}Y_4^{-1}\alpha^{-1}$	2	1	2	0
13		$\mu Z_2^{-1}Y_3^{-1}\alpha^{-1}$	1	2	2	0
14	9	$Z_1^{-1}Z_2^{-1}Y_3^{-1}Y_4^{-1}$	1	1	1	$+1$
15	10	$\mu Z_1^{-1}Z_2^{-1}Y_3^{-1}Y_4^{-1}$	3	1	3	-1
16		$Z_1^{-1}Z_2^{-1}Y_3^{-1}Y_4^{-1}\alpha^{-1}$	1	2	2	0
17		$\mu Z_1^{-1}Z_2^{-1}Y_3^{-1}Y_4^{-1}\alpha^{-1}$	3	2	6	0

3.4 Evaluation of Noncanceling Terms

In this subsection, the relation between the structure of $\hat{g}(\hat{C}_k)$ and the noncanceling terms will be investigated.

Definition 6 Let $\hat{g}_B(\hat{C}_k)$ $[\hat{g}_Q(\hat{C}_k)]$ be the subgraph of $\hat{g}(\hat{C}_k)$ consisting of all voltage (current) vertices in $\hat{C}_k$ and all B-edges (Q-edges) in $\hat{g}(\hat{C}_k)$.

Definition 7 A spanning set of $\hat{g}_B(\hat{C}_k)$ $[\hat{g}_Q(\hat{C}_k)]$ is that union of node disjoint edges of $\hat{g}_B(\hat{C}_k)$ $[\hat{g}_Q(\hat{C}_k)]$ which contains all vertices of $\hat{g}_B(\hat{C}_k)$ $[\hat{g}_Q(\hat{C}_k)]$, and $n_B(\hat{C}_k)$ $[n_Q(\hat{C}_k)]$ denotes the total number of distinct spanning sets of $\hat{g}_B(\hat{C}_k)$ $[\hat{g}_Q(\hat{C}_k)]$.

First, let us examine the properties of the edge section graphs $\hat{g}_B(\hat{C}_k)$ and $\hat{g}_Q(\hat{C}_k)$ of $\hat{g}(\hat{C}_k)$.

Lemma 1 Let $V_V(\hat{C}_k)$ and $V_I(\hat{C}_k)$ be the sets consisting of all voltage vertices and all current vertices in $\hat{C}_k$, respectively. If $V_V(\hat{C}_k) \neq \phi$ and $V_I(\hat{C}_k) \neq \phi$, then

$$n(\hat{C}_k) = n_B(\hat{C}_k) \times n_Q(\hat{C}_k)$$

and if $V_I(\hat{C}_k) = \phi$ $[V_V(\hat{C}_k) = \phi]$, then

$$n(\hat{C}_k) = n_B(\hat{C}_k) \; [n(\hat{C}_k) = n_Q(\hat{C}_k)]$$

Proof. From Definitions 4 and 6, the conclusion follows directly.

Lemma 2 Let $\mathbf{b}_k$ $(\mathbf{q}_k)$ be the square submatrix of $\mathbf{B}_p$ $(\mathbf{Q}_p)$ whose rows and columns correspond to the vertices in $\hat{g}_B(\hat{C}_k)$ $[\hat{g}_Q(\hat{C}_k)]$. Then $\mathbf{b}_k$ $(\mathbf{q}_k)$ is nonsingular if and only if $n_B(\hat{C}_k)$ $[n_Q(\hat{C}_k)]$ is odd.

Lemma 3 (1) Both $\mathbf{b}_k$ amd $\mathbf{q}_k$ are nonsingular if and only if $n(\hat{C}_k)$ is odd, and (2)

$$\det \mathbf{b}_k \times \det \mathbf{q}_k = (-1)^l \times \varepsilon_k$$

where l is the number of Z-edges or Y-edges in $\hat{g}(\hat{C}_k)$.

The proofs of Lemmas 2 and 3 are essentially similar to those of Lemmas 1 and 2 in Ref. [38], respectively, and are omitted.

It is ensured that ε_k is either 0 or ± 1 by Lemma 3 and the unimodularity of $\mathbf{B}_p$ and $\mathbf{Q}_p$.

Theorem 3 The coefficient ε_k of Eq. (36) is not zero if and only if $n(\hat{C}_k)$ is odd.

Proof. It is clear from Lemma 3.

Corollary The term ε_k in Eq. (36) is zero if and only if $n_B(\hat{C}_k)$ and/or $n_Q(\hat{C}_k)$ are even.

3.5 Derivation of Formula with Only Noncanceling Terms

Lemma 4 Let T be the number of the generalized common tree-cotree pairs of G_V and G_I. Then $T - 1$ is equal to the number of such pairs of the corresponding nonsingular submatrices of $\mathbf{b}_k$ and $\mathbf{q}_k$ of all orders.

The proof is omitted for want of space.

By Lemma 3, Theorem 3, and Lemma 4, the number of noncanceling terms in Eq. (36) is equal to $T - 1$. Therefore, we have the following general formula, which generates only noncanceling terms.

Theorem 4 Suppose $\hat{G}[H_c]$ is the chain path graph corresponding to the equation shown in Figure 8.4. Then

$$\det \mathbf{H}_c = 1 + \sum_{k'=1}^{T-1} \tilde{\varepsilon}_{k'} \times f(\tilde{C}_{k'}) \tag{38}$$

and

$$\tilde{\varepsilon}_k = \sum_{u=1}^{n(\tilde{C}_{k'})} (-1)^{\nu_u + \omega_u} \tag{39}$$

where $\tilde{C}_{k'}$ is the k'th subgraph of $\hat{G}[H_c]$ consisting of (n'_μ) μ-edges, (n'_α) α-edges, (l) Z-edges, and (l) Y-edges, such that $n(\tilde{C}_{k'})$ is odd.

Proof. Theorem 4 follows from Theorems 2 and 3 and Lemma 4.

Example 3 In Table 8.2, among 17 subgraphs $\hat{g}(\hat{C}_k)$ with nonzero spanning loop sets, only 10 subgraphs $\hat{g}(\tilde{C}_{k'})$ have odd spanning loop set number $n(\tilde{C}_{k'})$. As a result, the final expansion of $\det \mathbf{H}_c$ using Eq. (38) yields 11 noncanceling terms, while use of Mason's gain formula yields a total of 31 terms. Now, it is easy to write down $\det \mathbf{H}_c$ from Table 8.2 and then to get $\alpha = I_\alpha / I_{\hat{\alpha}}$ by applying the oscillation condition to $\det \mathbf{H}_c$.

3.6 Conclusion and Remarks

The general signal flow graph topological formula that generates only noncanceling terms was presented by using generalized common tree-cotree pairs for a most general network. Any symbolic network function including a transmission parameter can be obtained directly by using the results of Theorem 4.

The present derivation of a topological formula in which no term cancelation occurs is more straightforward than that of Mielke [38]. Mielke's formula [38] was obtained by evaluating the topological formula in terms of tree admittance products on the corresponding primitive signal flow graph, whereas the formula of Eq. (38) was obtained directly by just converting Mason's gain formula into Eq. (36) and then evaluating the noncanceling terms in it.

Furthermore, in Section 3 there is no restriction on symbols, in number or type, and the results given by Mielke [38] are completely included in Theorem 4 as a special case.

For many years, topological methods have been used only for the analysis of very small networks. This is the result of the very fast rise of the number of terms in the topological formula expressing the determinant of the network matrix with the size of the network. This remark holds for both linear and flow graphs.

Direct application of topological formulas permits the analysis of networks with graphs having approximately 10 nodes [30]. Even if we could generate all terms in zero time, the time needed for weight evaluation would grow at least in proportion to the number of terms and, for relatively small networks with about 20 nodes, would attain enormous values. In any case, it is obvious that the application of topological formulas for networks having more than 10 nodes is much more time-consuming than the methods of symbolic analysis based on the numerical techniques of determinant evaluation [12, 22, 34, 37, 39, 51, 53, 59].

For these reasons the methods of topological analysis were judged completely inefficient [18]. Attempts to introduce methods of graph reduction or decomposition [21] in the analysis did not provide universally efficient programs and were deemed unacceptable [12] (see [65] and the references therein for more details).

An important development was the introduction of hierarchical decomposition [42, 43, 61, 65]. The methods for signal flow graph analysis were presented in Refs. [42, 65] and the hierarchical analysis of directed graphs was discussed in Refs. [43, 61]. The details of the upward hierarchical decomposition method were presented in [65], and the time consumption was reduced from involution dependence for the downward decomposition to linear dependence. These approaches will significantly affect the application of topological methods to the analysis of large networks, which was impossible even with the aid of the fastest computers. Hence, network design problems requiring topological analysis can be solved with the help of the symbolic form of the results. The method preserves the advantages of direct methods of topological analysis such as high accuracy of computations and possibility of generating fully symbolic results. As the method is based on hierarchical decomposition, different blocks can be analyzed independently. Thus the use of parallel processing techniques is feasible and further reduction in computation time is possible, as pointed out in Ref. [65].

4 OTHER METHODS AND REMARKS

In this section three other classes of typical methods for generating symbolic network functions are discussed very briefly. These are topological methods except the signal flow graph method, parameter extraction methods, and algebraic methods.

4.1 Topological Methods

Besides the signal flow graph method, which was described in Section 3, another widely known topological method is the tree enumeration method.

The essence of tree enumeration method is to represent a given network by a directed, weighted graph G_d constructed according to certain rules and then to evaluate any desired network function by listing trees (directed trees) of the graph [1, 8, 9, 10, 18, 30]. For the topological formulas to be of practical value, we must have efficient algorithms for enumerating directed trees; hopefully, the algorithm will not generate many directed-tree admittance products that will only be canceled in the final answer.

Unfortunately, topological formulas may have many term cancellations, where by topological formulas we mean the determinant and cofactors of a node admittance matrix of the linear active network when they are expressed in terms of directed-tree admittance products. A new step-by-step algorithm for the topological formulation of a symbolic network function for a general and a large linear network was presented in Ref. [21], and it has advantages such as overcoming the problem of sign evaluation and greatly reducing the number of term cancelations and the number of topological terms.

The most general topological formula without term cancelations would be the mixed-type one reported in Ref. [15]. Although its derivation is conceptually very straightforward, the practical procedures are rather complicated. Therefore, the simplified and useful formulas without term cancelations from Ref. [15] have been given by using the concepts of the "generalized tree-cotree pair" and "generalized common tree-cotree pair" (which is also defined in Definition 1 of Section 3) in Refs. [56] and [57], respectively.

In Refs. [33, 67, 68], the application of Feussner's principle to general linear active networks is discussed. It is noted that the generalized Feussner principle permits systematic and formal classification of all the common trees in a two-graph with respect to an arbitrary subset of edges [67, 68]. However, it should also be stressed that the basic concept of the generalized Feussner principle, a special case of which is the well-known parameter extraction process for the infinite admittance matrix [12, 45], is useful for graph reduction or decomposition rather than only tree enumeration.

It is also well known that tree enumeration methods have the same typical features as signal flow graph methods, as already discussed in Section 3.4. Therefore, it is hoped that the inefficiency of tree enumeration methods as well as signal flow graph methods can be overcome by using hierarchical decomposition [42, 43, 61, 65] or graph reduction such as the generalized Feussner principle [33, 67, 68] and the step-by-step procedure in Ref. [21].

A proposal for computer symbolic analysis of linear active circuits by the two-graph method was made in Refs. [54, 55], in which the operating principles and algorithms for the common tree generator and the tree and sign discriminators were also described by using parallel processing techniques. It was confirmed that the rational functions of complex frequency s

with numerical coefficients for circuits having fewer than 25 nodes can easily be generated.

4.2 Parameter Extraction Methods [12, 29, 45]

In symbolic network analysis, we often encounter a situation in which only a few elements of a large network are represented by symbolic parameters, whereas the remaining elements all have numerical values assigned. In such a case, it will be most advantageous to solve the problem by a combination of two methods: a parameter extraction process for removing symbolic parameters from a determinant, and various numerical methods for evaluating a determinant det **G** or det(s**C** + **G**), the entries of **G** and **C** being real constants [12, 30].

In Ref. [12], a new and useful method for the above parameter extraction process, using the infinite admittance matrix of the network consisting of R, L, C elements and VCCS only, was proposed and implemented in the computer program NAPPE. Although the procedure for evaluating det(s**C** + **G**) by converting det(s**C** + **G**) to det(s**I** + **A**) and the procedure for evaluating det(s**I** + **A**) in Refs. [2, 4] were used in Ref. [12], it is also very useful to apply directly the interpolation methods using the FFT algorithm, which was explained in Section 2 of this chapter, to obtain det(s**C** + **G**) [45]. Some extensions and improvements on the parameter extraction methods for obtaining network functions, in which some, none, or all of the elements are represented by symbolic variables, are given in Ref. [45].

It is stated in Ref. [30] that "In fact, a computer program using the parameter extraction approach has demonstrated that, with a comparable amount of computer storage, it is now possible to perform symbolic network analysis (provided that only a few, say 10, network elements are represented by symbols) on networks of an order that can be handled by a numerical program such as SPICE."

Therefore, if we use both the parameter extraction processes and the numerical interpolation methods employing the FFT algorithm, we can conclude that the parameter extraction method is very useful for obtaining network functions of a fairly large network with only a few variable elements in symbols.

4.3 Algebraic Methods [44, 46, 57]

Numerical interpolation methods [22, 34, 39, 51, 53] were shown in Section 2 to be computationally competitive with the parameter extraction method of Ref. [12]. Although it is possible to take advantage of powerful numerical techniques such as FFT algorithms, sparse matrix methods, and adjoint network methods to calculate the coefficients of possible symbol combinations [22, 34], numerical interpolation methods are still rather involved [44, 46].

In Ref. [46], a new algebraic method, based on exterior algebra [36], for generating symbolic network functions for linear active networks was described, and in Ref. [44] another algebraic method based on the product matrices was proposed. The foundation of both of the above methods is the diagonal expansion of the determinant of a matrix. Moreover, the general formula with no term cancelations for any type of symbolic network functions of the most general linear network shown in Figure 8.3 was described in Ref. [57] by using the generalized common tree-cotree pair in voltage and current graphs (see Definition 1 in Section 3). The results in Ref. [57] are an extension of Ref. [44] and completely correspond to those of the signal flow graph version of Refs. [58, 62].

Although those algebraic formulas are topological ones, procedures for their evaluation are quite systematic, completely indirect, and purely numerical, and no sign rule is required [44, 46, 57]. So the formulas in Ref. [57] are suitable for computer-aided symbolic network analysis without restriction on symbols, in number or type.

4.4 Large-Scale Networks

We have already referred to the problem of large-scale linear networks a few times. There are four typical approaches to this problem: (1) step-by-step or hierarchical decomposition algorithms for generation of k-trees [21, 43, 61], (2) the matrix partition method for calculating the coefficients of possible symbol combinations by numerical interpolation using FFT [51], (3) upward or downward hierarchical decomposition algorithms for generating k-connections (multiconnections) of the given signal flow graph or flow graph [42, 65], and (4) graph decomposition procedures for generating smaller trees or smaller common trees in a reduced graph or a reduced two-graph of the linear active network [33, 67, 68].

4.5 General Remarks on Various Applications

Digital circuits

Many results are available for automated equation formation, transfer function evaluation, transient response computation, sensitivity calculation, etc. in the area of computer-aided analysis and design of continuous-time networks. Although much of this information is of value for digital discrete-time networks, little attention had been paid to general-purpose computer algorithms to obtain it, as pointed out in 1975 [29]. There have been few publications about these topics since that time [28, 29, 34, 53, 59, 64, 66].

Distributed circuits [22, 34, 53]

When uniform lossy transmission lines are contained in a network, the interpolation technique used for linear lumped time-invariant networks fails, as the numerator and denominator of the immittance function are no longer polynomials of complex frequency s. To overcome this difficulty, a new variable η is introduced as a transcendental function of s,

$$\eta = y_0(s) \tanh \frac{\gamma(s)}{2} \tag{40}$$

where $y_0(s)$ and $\gamma(s)$ are the characteristic admittance and the propagation constant of the given line, respectively. Then the nodal equations for a lumped distributed active network are given by a matrix with three types of variables: complex frequency s, lumped variable elements p, and new variables η. Therefore, the multidimensional FFT algorithm is used to generate this new symbolic network function $H(s, \mathbf{p}, \boldsymbol{\eta})$ [22, 34].

In Ref. [53] another method for generating $H(s, \mathbf{p}, \boldsymbol{\eta})$ is described by using the extended one-dimensional FFT (see also Section 2.2).

Switched capacitor circuits

Since 1980, symbolic network analysis for switched capacitor circuits has appeared in the literature [47, 50, 52, 53, 59, 64, 69]. The most serious difficulty to be overcome was that the network function of switched capacitor networks did not satisfy Theorem 1 in Section 1. Therefore, numerical interpolation methods using multidimensional FFT algorithms [37, 51] and extended one-dimensional FFT algorithms [53] are employed to generate symbolic network functions of switched capacitor networks.

Sensitivity analysis [6, 18, 21, 24, 36, 49, 59, 64]

Interesting results are given in Refs. [49, 59] (see also Section 2.4). An extended version from Ref. [34] and its application to sensitivity analysis is described in Ref. [64].

Computer-aided design (CAD)

There have been few papers on this topic [18, 19, 28, 29, 48, 59]. In Ref. [29], digital filter design optimization with symbolic second-derivative information, using almost the same technique as the parameter extraction method [12], is discussed. Ref. [48] outlines a symbolic analysis computer program, TAPLAN, for active networks that is accurate, reliable, efficient, adaptable, and easy for a circuit designer to use. This program uses a topological analysis technique [17] in which the topological formulas are expressed entirely in terms of trees of the circuit graph and products of transmittances, thus avoiding the need to find k-trees. A detailed description of CAD and symbolic analysis may also be found in Ref. [59].

5 SUMMARY

During the 1950s research on topological network analysis using computers was reported for the first time, and many papers were concerned with $H(s)$ in Eq. (1) until about 1970.

Since about 1970, research on the principles, implementation, and applications of $H(s, p_1, \ldots, p_m)$ of Eq. (2) has been pursued actively and work on the large-scale network problem have continued [21, 41, 43, 51, 61, 65, 67].

In this chapter, an overview of symbolic network analysis emphasizing the main papers since 1970, numerical interpolation using the FFT with application to the inversion of rational matrices, most general signal flow graph methods, and brief descriptions of other methods and applications are presented. Implementation and documentation for various methods are not explored for lack of space, but Refs. [12, 22, 24, 29, 30, 34, 36, 39, 40, 41, 51, 59, 64, 65] should be consulted regarding these topics. Moreover, the integer code method for symbolic coding of the elements of the networks should also be consulted [30, 36, 40].

Recently, formula manipulation languages such as REDUCE, MACSYMA, and muMATH have shown remarkable progress and it is also hoped to apply these language programs to symbolic network analysis [66]. However, it is obvious that continued basic research on the usual symbolic network analysis as well as its applications, including nonnetwork ones, should be made, because the ability of formula manipulation languages is not enough to achieve our objectives.

REFERENCES

Many papers and books on symbolic network analysis published before 1973 are not covered in this list of references, but will be found in Refs. 9 and 18.

1. S. Seshu and M. B. Reed, *Linear Graphs and Electrical Networks*, Addison-Wesley, Reading, Mass., 1961.
2. D. K. Faddeev and V. N. Faddeeva, *Computational Methods of Linear Algebra*, Freeman, San Francisco, 1963.
3. J. H. Wilkinson, *The Algebraic Eigenvalue Problem*, Clarendon Oxford, England, 1965.
4. C. F. Kurth, A simple calculation of the determinant polynomial of general networks, *IEEE Trans. Circuit Theory*, vol. CT-14, pp. 234–236, 1967.
5. C. C. Someda, The bigenerator—an active pathological network, *IEEE Trans. Circuit Theory*, vol. CT-16, no. 1, pp. 125–126, 1969.

6. W. J. Troop and E. Peskin, The transfer function and sensitivity of a network with n variable elements, *IEEE Trans. Circuit Theory*, vol. CT-16, no. 2, pp. 242–244, 1969.
7. T. Downs, Inversion of the nodal admittance matrix for active networks in symbolic form, *Electron. Lett.*, vol. 6, pp. 690–691, Oct. 1970.
8. W. K. Chen, *Applied Graph Theory*, North-Holland, Amsterdam, 1971.
9. J. Katzenelson, Symbolic analysis of linear networks—a survey, NATO Advanced Study Institute on Network and Signal Theory, Bournemouth, U.K., Sept. 1972.
10. W. Mayeda, *Graph Theory*, Wiley-Interscience, New York, 1972.
11. K. Singhal and J. Vlach, Interpolation using the fast Fourier transform, *Proc. IEEE*, vol. 60, no. 12, p. 1558, 1972.
12. G. E. Anderson and P. M. Lin, Computer generation of symbolic network functions—a new theory and implementation, *IEEE Trans. Circuit Theory*, vol. CT-20, no. 1, pp. 48–56, 1973.
13. I. Kaufman, On poles and zeros of linear systems, *IEEE Trans. Circuit Theory*, vol. CT-20, no. 2, pp. 93–101, 1973.
14. C. B. Moler and G. Stewart, An algorithm for generalized matrix eigenvalue problems, *SIAM J. Numer. Anal.*, vol. 10, pp. 241–256, April 1973.
15. J. Numata and M. Iri, Mixed-type topological formulas for general linear networks, *IEEE Trans. Circuit Theory*, vol. CT-20, no. 5, pp. 488–494, 1973.
16. J. Katzenelson and S. Tsur, On the symbolic analysis of linear networks, *IEEE Trans. Circuit Theory*, vol. CT-20, no. 5, pp. 572–574, 1973.
17. L. Farber and N. R. Malik, A new technique for symbolic active network analysis by computer, *IEEE Trans. Circuit Theory*, vol. CT-20, pp. 426–429, July 1973.
18. P. M. Lin, A survey of applications of symbolic network functions, *IEEE Trans. Circuit Theory*, vol. CT-20, no. 6, pp. 723–737, Nov. 1973.
19. J. K. Fidler and J. I. Sewell, Symbolic analysis for computer-aided circuit design—the interpolative approach, *IEEE Trans. Circuit Theory*, vol. CT-20, no. 6, pp. 738–741, 1973.
20. E. Emre, O. Huseyin, and K. Abdullah, On the inversion of rational matrices, *IEEE Trans. Circuits Syst.*, vol. CAS-21, no. 1, pp. 8–10, 1974.
21. S. D. Shieu and S. P. Chan, Topological formulation of symbolic network functions sensitivity analysis of active networks, *IEEE Trans. Circuits Syst.*, vol. CAS-21, no. 1, pp. 39–45, 1974.
22. K. Singhal and J. Vlach, Generation of immittance functions in symbolic form for lumped distributed active networks, *IEEE Trans. Circuits Syst.*, vol. CAS-21, no. 1, pp. 57–67, 1974.

23. C. Fridas and J. I. Sewell, Symbolic analysis of networks by partitioned polynomial interpolation, *IEEE Trans. Circuits Syst.*, vol. CAS-21, no. 3, pp. 345–347, 1974.
24. C. F. Yokomoto, A simple bookkeeping scheme for computing sensitivities of symbolic transfer functions, *IEEE Trans. Circuits Syst.*, vol. CAS-21, no. 5, pp. 606–608, 1974.
25. E. Emre, O. Huseyin, and K. Abdullah, A new algorithm for the inversion of rational matrices, *Arch. Electron. Uebertragungstech.*, vol. 28, pp. 461–464, Nov. 1974.
26. E. O. Brigham, *The Fast Fourier Transform*, Prentice-Hall, Englewood Cliffs, N.J., 1974.
27. E. Emre and O. Huseyin, Generalization of Leverrier's algorithm to polynomial matrices of arbitrary degree, *IEEE Trans. Autom. Control*, vol. AC-22, p. 136, Feb. 1975.
28. S. E. Belter and S. C. Bass, Optimization of digital filters based on symbolic analysis, *IEEE Proc. 1975 ISCAS*, pp. 48–51.
29. S. E. Belter and S. C. Bass, Computer-aided analysis and design of digital filters with arbitrary topology, *IEEE Trans. Circuits Syst.*, vol. CAS-22, pp. 810–819, Oct. 1975.
30. L. O. Chua and P. M. Lin, *Computer-Aided Analysis of Electronic Circuits*, chapter 14, Prentice-Hall, Englewood Cliffs, N.J., 1975.
31. T. Lee, A simple method to determine the characteristic function $f(\lambda) = |\lambda I - A|$ by discrete Fourier series and fast Fourier transform, *IEEE Trans. Circuits Syst.*, vol. CAS-23, no. 6, p. 242, 1976.
32. L. E. Paccagnella and G. L. Pierobon, FFT calculation of a determinational polynomial, *IEEE Trans. Autom. Control*, vol. AC-21, pp. 401–402, June 1976.
33. R. Hashemian, Symbolic representation of network transfer functions using norator–nullator pairs, *Proc. Inst. Electr. Eng. Part G*, vol. 1, no. 6, pp. 193–197, 1977.
34. K. Singhal and J. Vlach, Symbolic analysis of analog and digital circuits, *IEEE Trans. Circuits Syst.*, vol. CAS-24, no. 11, pp. 598–609, 1977.
35. T. Matsumoto and K. Kanemaki, New topological necessary and sufficient conditions for N-port parameters to be nonzero, *Electron. Commun. Jpn.*, vol. 60-A, no. 12, pp. 1–9, 1977.
36. N. N. Puri, Symbolic fault diagnosis techniques, in *Rational Fault Analysis*, R. Saek and S. Liberty, eds., Marcel Dekker, New York, 1977.
37. Q. T. Nam and T. Matsumoto, A new calculating method for coefficients of Taylor's expansion of an N-variables function by using N-dimensional FFT algorithm, *Trans. IECE Jpn.*, vol. 61–A, no. 5, pp. 502–503, 1978.
38. R. R. Mielke, A new signal flowgraph formulation of symbolic network

functions, *IEEE Trans. Circuits Syst.*, vol. CAS-25, no. 6, pp. 334–340, 1978.

39. Q. T. Nam, Y. Ohta, and T. Matsumoto, Inversion of rational matrices by using FFT algorithm, *Trans. IECE Jpn.*, vol. 61-A, no. 9, pp. 813–819, 1978.
40. T. Hashimoto, Program for the generation of symbolic network functions for linear electric circuits, *Trans. IECE Jpn.*, vol. J62-A, no. 6, pp. 387–394, 1979.
41. R. Wehrhahn, New approach in the computation of poles and zeros in large networks, *IEEE Trans. Circuits Syst.*, vol. CAS-26, pp. 700–707, Sept. 1979.
42. J. A. Starzyk, Signal-flow-graph analysis by decomposition method, *Proc. Inst. Electr. Eng. Part G*, vol. 127, no. 2, pp. 81–86, 1980.
43. J. A. Starzyk and E. Sliwa, Hierarchic decomposition method for the topological analysis of electronic networks, *Int. J. Circuit Theory Appl.*, vol. 8, pp. 407–417, 1980.
44. B. G. Lee, The product matrices and new gain formulas, *IEEE Trans. Circuits Syst.*, vol. CAS-27, no. 4, pp. 284–292, 1980.
45. M. Sagawa, Symbolic analysis of linear networks, *Proc. IECE Jpn.*, vol. 63, no. 5, pp. 468–474, 1980.
46. P. Sannuti and N. N. Puri, Symbolic networks analysis—an algebraic formulation, *IEEE Trans. Circuits Syst.*, vol. CAS-27, no. 8, pp. 679–687, 1980.
47. E. Kabaya and M. Onoda, Computer generation of symbolic transfer functions for switched capacitor circuits, *J. IECE Jpn.*, Paper CAS80-112, pp. 21–28, 1981.
48. T. F. Gatts, Jr., Computer aided design using symbolic analysis, *IEEE Proc. 1981 ISCAS*, pp. 613–615.
49. K. Singhal and J. Vlach, Symbolic circuit analysis, *Proc. Inst. Electr. Eng. Part G*, vol. 128, no. 2, pp. 81–86, 1981.
50. H. Honma, N. Kanbayashi, and M. Sagawa, Symbolic analysis of switched capacitor networks using indefinite admittance matrix, *J. IECE Jpn.*, Paper CAS81-45, pp. 61–68, 1981.
51. H. Takamura, Y. Ohta, and T. Matsumoto, Symbolic analysis of linear networks using matrix partition method and FFT algorithm, *Trans. IECE Jpn.*, vol. J65-A, no. 11, pp. 1152–1159, 1982.
52. A. Ohshimo and M. Onoda, Symbolic analysis of SC network including some symbolic capacitors, *J. IECE Jpn.*, Paper CAS82-56, pp. 17–24, 1982.
53. H. Honma and M. Sagawa, Some developments of symbolic network analysis using interpolation, *J. IECE Jpn.*, Paper CAS82-75, pp. 37–44, 1982.

54. M. Tanaka, K. Murakami, and M. Yamagishi, Computer for symbolic analysis of active circuits by 2-graph method—tree generator, *Trans. IECE Jpn.*, vol. J65-D, no. 12, pp. 1467–1474, 1982.
55. K. Murakami, M. Tanaka, and K. Nakamura, Computer for symbolic analysis of active circuits by 2-graph method—tree and sign discriminators, *Trans. IECE Jpn.*, vol. J65-D, no. 12, pp. 1475–1482, 1982.
56. T. Matsumoto, S. Tanaka, and Y. Ohta, Topological formulas and generalized Feussner's principle for general linear networks, *J. IECE Jpn.*, Paper CAS83-22, pp. 41–48, June 1983.
57. T. Matsumoto, M. Kitai, and Y. Ohta, Systematic generations of symbolic network functions for general linear networks, *J. IECE Jpn.*, Paper CAS83-23, pp. 49–56, June 1983.
58. M. Kitai and T. Matsumoto, Symbolic network analysis of general linear networks by signal flowgraph approach, *Trans. IECE Jpn.*, vol. J66-A, no. 12, pp. 1259–1260, 1983.
59. J. Vlach and K. Singhal, *Computer Methods for Circuit Analysis and Design*, Van Nostrand-Reinhold, Princeton, N.J., 1983.
60. K. S. Yeung, Symbolic network function generation via discrete Fourier transform, *IEEE Trans. Circuits Syst.*, vol. CAS-31, no. 2, pp. 229–231, 1984.
61. J. A. Starzyk and E. Sliwa, Upward topological analysis of large circuits using directed graph representation, *IEEE Trans. Circuits Syst.*, vol. CAS-31, no. 4, pp. 410–414, 1984.
62. T. Matsumoto, M. Kitai, and Y. Ohta, Topological generation of symbolic network functions for general linear networks by signal flowgraph approach, *IEEE Proc. 1984 ISCAS*, pp. 1403–1406.
63. T. Matsumoto, M. Kitai, and Y. Kajitani, On distance between the common trees in two graphs, *IEEE Proc.* of *1985 ISCAS*, pp. 799–802.
64. H. Honma, K. Itoh, and M. Sagawa, A computing method for obtaining derivatives of denominator and numerator of network functions with respect to elements and sensitivity analysis, *Trans. IECE Jpn.*, vol. J68-A, no. 8, pp. 725–732, 1985.
65. J. A. Starzyk and A. Konczykowska, Flowgraph analysis of large electronic networks, *IEEE Trans. Circuits Syst.*, vol. CAS-33, no. 3, pp. 302–315, 1986.
66. K. Sugahara and K. Oohigashi, Symbolic analysis of digital networks by using symbolic and algebraic manipulation program, *Trans. IECE Jpn.*, vol. J70-A, no. 3, pp. 567–569, 1987.
67. T. Matsumoto, K. Hirabayashi, and S. Nakano, On generalized Feussner's principle in a two-graph, *IEEE Proc.* of *1987 ISCAS*, pp. 507–510.

68. T. Matsumoto, S. Nakano, and Y. Ohta, On the finest classification of all the common trees in a two-graph: Approach by a matroid with parity structure, *IEEE Proc.* of *1987 ISCAS*, WAM7.7, pp. 491–494.

69. Y. Cheng and P. M. Lin, Symbolic analysis of general switched-capacitor networks—new method and implementation, *IEEE Proc.* of *1987 ISCAS*, TAM3.1, pp. 55–59.

9
Diagnosability of Analog Circuits

Takao Ozawa

Department of Electrical Engineering, Kyoto University
Kyoto, Japan

1 INTRODUCTION

In recent years great research effort has been directed toward fault diagnosis of analog circuits. Many papers have been published on this subject [1, 2], and even if we restrict ourselves to the theoretical treatment of faults, there is a variety of problem formulations depending on fault models, measurement conditions, the final object of the fault diagnosis, and so forth. Key factors in the classification of diagnostic problems are the following.

1. Circuits under test
   a. Elements contained in the circuit: (1) *RLC* or *RC*, (2) controlled sources,* (3) operational amplifiers, (4) nullators and norators,† (5) nonlinear elements, (6) switches
   b. Excitation of the circuit: (1) DC excitation, (2) sinusoidal excitation—single-frequency or multifrequency
   c. Number of exciting sources (independent sources or inputs): (1) single exciting source, (2) multiple exciting sources

---

*A controlled source is a two-port element which consists of a sensor and a dependent source whose current or voltage is controlled by the voltage or current of the sensor.

†A nullator is an element whose voltage and current are both zero. A norator is an element whose voltage and current are arbitrary.

2. Fault models: (1) short circuits or open circuits (hard faults), (2) element- or parameter-value deviations outside the tolerance bounds (soft faults)
3. Measurements: (1) voltage measurements, (2) current measurements, (3) short-circuit transfer admittance measurements
4. Final object of fault diagnosis: (1) calculation of voltages and currents, (2) identification of faulty elements, (3) localization of faults within a subcircuit

In addition to problem formulations directly related to electrical and electronic circuits, attempts have been made to apply techniques of system diagnosis to analog circuit diagnosis.

In diagnosis of large-scale circuits, use of computers is inevitable. One special feature of circuit diagnosis which is quite different from those of circuit analysis is that the information for diagnosis or knowledge about the circuit under test is very restricted. Therefore diagnosability, or whether or not the diagnostic problem formulated is solvable under the specified conditions and the expected results are attainable, must be first investigated in order to distinguish instability intrinsic to the problem from that due to the computational method and errors. Since there are various problem formulations, diagnosability must be defined according to them.

In the following sections we consider the diagnosability of soft faults in a linear circuit which is in sinusoidal steady state. An advantage of assuming soft faults only is that the circuit topology or the graph of the circuit is known, and the equations derived from Kirchhoff's voltage and current laws (KVL and KCL equations) can be used. We assume that the circuit contains, as active elements, controlled sources, nullators, and norators only in addition to two-terminal passive elements such as resistors and capacitors. Most active elements can be represented by their controlled-source models or nullator-norator models. Therefore we do not suffer loss of generality. For simplicity of discussion we further assume that the circuit contains no voltage-controlled voltage sources or current-controlled current sources. Either of these controlled sources can be replaced by a cascade connection of a voltage-controlled current source and a current-controlled voltage source.

Computability of voltages and currents in the circuit from measured or known voltages, currents, and element values is investigated first, since it is the basis of fault diagnosis. Then the result is applied to fault location by the fault verification or assume-and-check method. It is shown that the diagnosability of an analog circuit, like the system diagnosability, depends on the connectivity of the circuit under test. Finally, a brief discussion is given on diagnosis by multiple circuit excitation.

2 PRELIMINARIES TO PROBLEM FORMULATION

2.1 Circuit Configuration

The circuit under consideration is denoted by N, and its graph by G. In order to overcome the difficulty arising from mutual coupling in controlled sources we use two circuits N_v and N_i and two graphs G_v and G_i. G_v and G_i are called the voltage and current graphs, respectively [3], and Kirchhoff's voltage and current laws are applied to G_v and G_i, respectively. These circuits and graphs are derived from N and G in the following way.

N_v is derived from N by contracting the current sensors and nullators and deleting dependent sources and norators. G_v is the graph of N_v. Next, N_i is the circuit which is derived from N by deleting voltage sensors and nullators and contracting dependent voltage sources and norators. G_i is the graph of N_i. Note that either the sensor or the dependent source of a controlled source remains in N_v or N_i, and a two-port element in N is represented by a two-terminal element in N_v and a two-terminal element in N_i, in the same way as a resistor. Thus there is no need to distinguish a controlled source from a resistor in N_v and N_i. The element in N_v and the element in N_i representing the same element in N are given the same label. Then N_v and N_i have a common element set, which is denoted by E. G_v and G_i also have a common edge set. Strictly speaking, circuits N, N_v, and N_i are constituted by "elements" which correspond to "edges" of graphs G, G_v, and G_i. For simplicity we will not distinguish edges from elements hereafter. Thus the common edge set of G_v and G_i is also denoted by E.

2.2 Formulation of Measurement Condition

Next let us formulate the measurements on N [4]. The element set E of N_v and N_i is partitioned into E_b, E_e, E_j, E_k, and E_u, which are defined as follows.

$E_b :=$ the set of elements whose voltages and currents can be both measured and known

$E_e :=$ the set of elements whose voltages only can be measured or known

$E_j :=$ the set of elements whose currents only can be measured or known

$E_k :=$ the set of elements whose voltages and currents are unknown but whose element values are known

$E_u :=$ the set of elements whose voltages and currents are unknown and whose element values are also unknown

More specifically, Table 9.1 applies to a resistor, inductor, capacitor, or controlled source. Table 9.2 applies to an independent voltage or current source.

Table 9.1 Classification of Elements I

Voltage	Current	Element value	Classification
Known	Known	Known	E_b
Known	Known	Unknown	E_b
Known	Unknown	Known	E_b
Unknown	Known	Known	E_b
Known	Unknown	Unknown	E_e
Unknown	Known	Unknown	E_j
Unknown	Unknown	Known	E_k
Unknown	Unknown	Unknown	E_u

Table 9.2 Classification of Elements II

Voltage	Current	Classification
Known	Known	E_b
Known	Unknown	E_e
Unknown	Known	E_j
Unknown	Unknown	E_u

The above classification of elements can be interpreted in terms of degrees of freedom as follows. Each element in the circuit originally has two degrees of freedom, because two variables, a voltage and a current, are associated with it. The degrees of freedom are decreased by the information obtained for the element or the restriction imposed on it. Thus an element in E_b has zero; one in E_e, E_j, or E_k has one; and one in E_u has two degrees of freedom. Note that in an ordinary circuit analysis each element in the circuit has one degree of freedom. The total number of KVL and KCL equations is equal to the number of elements, and thus the voltages and currents can be uniquely determined.

The measurement condition regarding a node can be expressed by an element which is connected to the node and the reference node, if such an element exists, or by an imaginary element which is added between the node and the reference node.

2.3 Graph Notation and Basic Propositions

For any graph G with edge set E and subset E_s of E, $G \cdot E_s$ (respectively $G \times E_s$) is the graph obtained from G by deleting (respectively contracting) the edges of $\bar{E}_s := E - E_s$. The rank and nullity of G are denoted by $r(G)$ and $n(G)$, respectively. $|E_s|$ is the cardinality of E_s and $+$ denotes the union of disjoint sets.

Regarding trees and cotrees of G we have the following propositions. For simplicity we use the same notation for a tree or cotree and its edge set.

Proposition 2.1 Let T_a and T_b be trees of $G \cdot E_s$ and $G \times E_s$, respectively. Then the union of T_a and T_b constitutes a tree of G, and

$$r(G) = r(G \cdot E_s) + r(G \times \bar{E}_s), \qquad n(G) = n(G \cdot E_s) + n(G \times \bar{E}_s) \tag{2.1}$$

holds.

Let T be a tree of G and K be the cotree of T.

Proposition 2.2 Given a subset E_s of E. Then

$$\max_{\text{all } T} |T \cap E_s| = r(G \cdot E_s), \qquad \max_{\text{all } K} |K \cap E_s| = n(G \times E_s) \tag{2.2}$$

where the maximums are taken over all the trees of G. The maximum in the first (second) equation is attained if and only if $T \cap E_s$ is a tree of $G \cdot E_s$ ($K \cap E_s$ is a cotree of $G \times E_s$).

3 DIAGNOSABILITY

3.1 Computability of Voltages and Currents

We first consider which voltages and currents in N can be computed from measurement data and known data [4]. This is because element or parameter values can be computed, in general, only from voltages and currents, and also it may be possible to diagnose N from voltages and currents.

Note that the voltage of an element in E_u and E_j can be obtained from a KVL equation only, since its element value is unknown. Suppose we use the fundamental tiesets determined by a cotree of G_v to derive KVL equations. Then the voltage of such an element can be computed if and only if the element is included in the cotree and all the voltages of the tree elements which belong to the fundamental tieset determined by this element are known. Therefore we want as many elements of E_u and E_j to be included in the cotree as possible, and as many elements of E_b and E_e to be included in the tree as possible.

Dually, the current of an element in E_e and E_u can be obtained from a KCL equation only. The current of such an element can be computed if and only if it is included in a tree of G_i and all the currents of the cotree elements which belong to the fundamental cutset determined by it are known. Thus we want as many elements of E_u and E_e to be included in the tree as possible, and as many elements of E_b and E_j to be included in the cotree as possible.

The above situation is the same as that of determining the voltages of current sources or the currents of voltages sources in conventional circuit analysis. These currents and voltages can be determined only after the currents and voltages of elements other than the sources are determined.

For the elements in E_k we can use their voltage versus current relations, that is,

$$i_k = Y_k v_k \tag{3.1}$$

where i_k and v_k are the current and voltage vectors of the elements in E_k, respectively, and Y_k is a diagonal matrix with admittances of the elements on the diagonal. We can get KVL and KCL equations for E_k using the cotree of G_v and the tree of G_i as stated above. They can be written as

$$B_k v_k = e_k \tag{3.2}$$

$$Q_k i_k = j_k \tag{3.3}$$

where e_k and j_k are vectors due to the known voltages and currents, respectively, and B_k and Q_k are the fundamental tieset and cutset matrices, respectively, which can be derived from graphs G_{vk} and G_{ik} defined as follows:

$$G_{vk} := G_v \times (E_u + E_j + E_k) \cdot E_k \tag{3.4}$$

$$G_{ik} := G_i \cdot (E_u + E_e + E_k) \times E_k \tag{3.5}$$

In order to get G_{vk} (G_{ik}) we contract the elements in E_b and E_e (E_u and E_e) which we want to be in the tree of G_v (G_i), and we delete those in E_u and E_j (E_b and E_j) which we want to be in the cotree.

Example 3.1 For the circuit shown in Figure 9.1a suppose that the voltages e_1 and v_6 (the subscripts correspond to the numbers on the edges in the figure) are measurable and that conductances g_3, g_4, g_5, and g_6 are known but g_2 is unknown. Then $E_b = \{6\}$, $E_e = \{1\}$, $E_j = \varnothing$, $E_k = \{3, 4, 5\}$, and $E_u = \{2\}$. Voltage graph G_v is shown in Figure 9.1b together with a tree T_v which is indicated by the dashed lines. T_v is chosen so that $T_v \ni 1, 6$ and its cotree K_v $(:= E - T_v) \ni 2$. Current graph G_i is shown in Figure 9.1c together with a tree T_i. T_i is chosen so that $T_i \ni 1, 2$ and its cotree K_i $(:= E - T_i) \ni 6$. G_{vk} and G_{ik} are given in Figures 9.1d and 9.1e, respectively. The KVL and KCL equations for E_k are

$$\begin{bmatrix} 1 & 0 & 1 \\ 0 & 1 & 0 \end{bmatrix} \begin{bmatrix} v_3 \\ v_4 \\ v_5 \end{bmatrix} = \begin{bmatrix} v_6 \\ e_1 - v_6 \end{bmatrix} \tag{3.6}$$

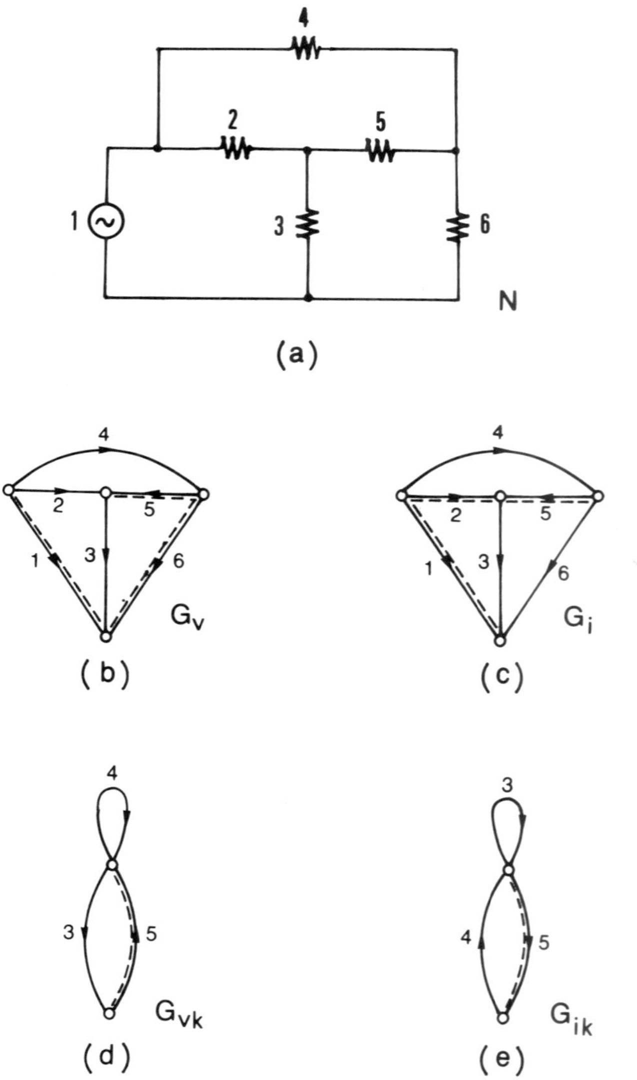

Figure 9.1 Example 3.1.

$$[0 \quad -1 \quad 1]\begin{bmatrix} i_3 \\ i_4 \\ i_5 \end{bmatrix} = -i_6 \tag{3.7}$$

respectively. We also have

$$i_3 = g_3 v_3, \qquad i_4 = g_4 v_k, \qquad i_5 = g_k v_k \tag{3.8}$$

Solving Eqs. (3.6)–(3.8) we can determine all the voltages and currents of the elements in E_k and then all the remaining voltages and currents in the circuit.

Equations (3.1)–(3.3) may or may not be solvable. We will consider topological conditions on the solvability of these equations, assuming that there exists no special relation among the element values, or all the element values are independent. This assumption is called the generality assumption on element values.

If we eliminate i_k using Eq. (3.1) we get a set of equations for v_k whose coefficient matrix is

$$\begin{bmatrix} B_k \\ Q_k Y_k \end{bmatrix} \tag{3.9}$$

It is known that this matrix can be, in general, transformed to a block diagonal matrix [5] as

$$\begin{bmatrix} M_{++} & 0 & 0 \\ M_{0+} & M_{00} & 0 \\ M_{-+} & M_{-0} & M_{--} \end{bmatrix} \tag{3.10}$$

and E_k is tripartitioned accordingly into E_{k+}, E_{k0}, and E_{k-}. In (3.10) M_{++} is a rectangular matrix with more rows that columns, M_{00} is a square matrix, and M_{--} is a rectangular matrix with fewer rows than columns; M_{++}, M_{00}, and M_{--} correspond to E_{k+}, E_{k0}, and E_{k-}, respectively; and 0 is a zero matrix.

Let v_{k+}, v_{k0}, and v_{k-} be the voltage vectors of the elements in E_{k+}, E_{k0}, and E_{k-}, respectively. Then M_{++} gives an overdetermined system of equations for v_{k+}; that is, there are more equations than unknown variables of v_{k+}. If e_k in Eq. (3.2) and j_k in Eq. (3.3) are obtained from measured voltages and currents, these equations for v_{k+} must be consistent, and we can determine v_{k+}. Then we can determine v_{k0}, since M_{00} is a square matrix and is nonsingular under the generality assumption on element values. We cannot, however, determine v_{k-}. In Example 3.1 we had a special case of $E_{k+} = E_{k-} = \varnothing$.

The partition of the matrix in (3.10) or the partition of E_k can be determined by Algorithm PART+ given below. This algorithm determines the "principal partition" of graphs G_{vk} and G_{ik} together with a special pair of trees, T_{vk} of G_{vk} and T_{ik} of G_{ik}, which have as many common edges as possible. Such a pair of trees is called a pair of maximally common trees (MCT). The cotrees of T_{vk} and T_{ik} are denoted by K_{vk} and K_{ik}, respectively, that is, $K_{vk} := E_k - T_{vk}$ and $K_{ik} := E_k - T_{ik}$.

We first give some definitions. Let e be a cotree edge in K_{vk}. We denote by $L_v(e/T_{vk})$ the fundamental tieset uniquely determined by e with respect to T_{vk}, and define

$$L_v(E_s/T_{vk}) := \bigcup_{e \in E_s} L_v(e/T_{vk}) \tag{3.11}$$

Similarly, if e is a tree edge in T_{ik}, $C_i(e/K_{ik})$ is the fundamental cutset uniquely determined by e with respect to K_{ik}, and

$$C_i(E_s/K_{ik}) := \bigcup_{e \in E_s} C_i(e/K_{ik}) \tag{3.12}$$

Likewise, for e in K_{ik}, $L_i(e/T_{ik})$ [respectively e in T_{vk} $C_v(e/K_{vk})$] denotes the fundamental tieset (cutset) uniquely determined by e with respect to T_{ik} (K_{vk}). $L_i(E_s/T_{ik})$ and $C_v(E_s/K_{vk})$ are defined similarly to Eqs. (3.11) and (3.12).

Algorithm PART+

Step 0. {Initialization}

Obtain an arbitrary pair of trees T_{vk} of G_{vk} and T_{ik} of G_{ik} (their cotrees are K_{vk} and K_{ik}, respectively).

Step 1.

(1.1) Set $X_1 := K_{vk} \cap T_{ik}$, and $m := 1$.

(1.2) If $X_1 = \varnothing$, go to step 7.

Step 2. {Beginning of the search for tree transformation}

(2.1) Set $m := 2$, and obtain $X_2 := C_i(X_1/K_{ik})$.

(2.2) If $X_2 \cap (T_{vk} \cap K_{ik}) \neq \varnothing$, go to step 5.

Step 3. {Search in G_{vk}}

(3.1) Set $m := m + 1$, and obtain

$$X_m := L_v(X_{m-1}/T_{vk}) - \bigcup_{n=1}^{m-1} X_n \tag{3.13}$$

(3.2) If $X_m = \varnothing$, go to step 7.

(3.3) If $X_m \cap (T_{vk} \cap K_{ik}) \neq \varnothing$, go to step 6.

Step 4. {Search in G_{ik}}

(4.1) Set $m := m + 1$, and obtain

$$X_m := C_i(X_{m-1}/K_{ik}) - \bigcup_{n=1}^{m-1} X_n \tag{3.14}$$

(4.2) If $X_m = \varnothing$, go to step 7.
(4.3) If $X_m \cap (T_{vk} \cap K_{ik}) = \varnothing$, go to step 3.

Step 5. {Tree transformation when search ends in G_{ik}}
There must be a sequence of edges $\{e_j, \ldots, e_{n-1}, e_n, \ldots, e_m\}$ such that $j = 1$ or 2, $e_j \in K_{vk} \cap T_{ik}$, $e_m \in T_{vk} \cap K_{ik}$, $e_n \in X_n$, and $e_n \in C_i(e_{n-1}/K_{ik})$ or $L_v(e_{n-1}/T_{vk})$. Perform either of the following tree transformations:

(5.1) If $j = 1$, $T_{vk} := T_{vk} \cup \{e_2, e_4, \ldots, e_{m-2}\} - \{e_3, e_5, \ldots, e_{m-1}\}$

$$T_{ik} := T_{ik} \cup \{e_2, e_4, \ldots, e_m\} - \{e_1, e_3, \ldots, e_{m-1}\}$$

(5.2) If $j = 2$, $T_{vk} := T_{vk} \cup \{e_2, e_4, \ldots, e_{m-2}\} - \{e_3, e_5, \ldots, e_{m-1}\}$

$$T_{ik} := T_{ik} \cup \{e_4, e_6, \ldots, e_m\} - \{e_3, e_5, \ldots, e_{m-1}\}$$

Go to step 1.

Step 6. {Tree transformation when search ends in G_{vk}}
There must be a sequence of edges $\{e_j, \ldots, e_{n-1}, e_n, \ldots, e_m\}$ such that $j = 1$ or 2, $e_j \in K_{vk} \cap T_{ik}$, $e_m \in T_{vk} \cap K_{ik}$, $e_n \in X_n$, and $e_n \in C_i(e_{n-1}/T_{ik})$ or $L_v(e_{n-1}/T_{vk})$. Perform either of the following tree transformations:

(6.1) If $j = 1$, $T_{vk} := T_{vk} \cup \{e_2, e_4, \ldots, e_{m-1}\} - \{e_3, e_5, \ldots, e_m\}$

$$T_{ik} := T_{ik} \cup \{e_2, e_4, \ldots, e_{m-1}\} - \{e_1, e_3, \ldots, e_{m-2}\}$$

(6.2) If $j = 2$, $T_{vk} := T_{vk} \cup \{e_2, e_4, \ldots, e_{m-1}\} - \{e_3, e_5, \ldots, e_m\}$

$$T_{vk} := T_{vk} \cup \{e_4, e_6, \ldots, e_{m-1}\} - \{e_3, e_5, \ldots, e_{m-2}\}$$

Go to step 1.

Step 7. {Search ends without breakthrough. T_{vk} and T_{ik} obtained are a pair of MCT.}

Set

$$E_{k+} := \bigcup_{n=1}^{m-1} X_n \tag{3.15}$$

Return T_{ik}, T_{vk}, and E_+.

Algorithm PART+ begins, at step 0, with an arbitrary pair of trees, T_{vk} of G_{vk} and T_{ik} of G_{ik}, and tries to increase $|T_{vk} \cap T_{ik}|$ by decreasing $|K_{vk} \cap T_{ik}|$ and $|T_{vk} \cap K_{ik}|$. To this end PART+ performs a breadth-first search for tree transformation of T_{vk} and T_{ik}. This search starts from the edges of $K_{vk} \cap T_{ik}$ (steps 1 and 2), aiming at a breakthrough to $T_{vk} \cap K_{ik}$, and is performed in G_{ik} and G_{vk} alternatingly (steps 3 and 4, respectively). If a breakthrough is obtained, tree transformation of T_{vk} and T_{ik} is performed in steps 5 and 6. In case of no breakthrough a pair of MCT and E_{k+} are obtained at step 7.

The search for tree transformation may be initiated in either G_{ik} or G_{vk}. We choose G_{ik} in Algorithm PART+, as given in step 2. Note that X_2 includes $K_{vk} \cap T_{ik}$, and if $X_2 \cap (T_{vk} \cap K_{iK}) = \varnothing$, the fundamental tiesets determined by the edges of $K_{vk} \cap T_{ik}$ are sought in G_{vk}. The sequence of edges obtained by the search initiated in this way begins with e_2, which corresponds to $j = 2$ in step 5 and step 6. $X_2, X_3, \ldots, X_{m-1}$ are mutually disjoint, and thus we only have to find new fundamental tiesets or cutsets.

Once a pair of MCT is obtained by Algorithm PART+, E_{k-} can be determined by the following algorithm PART−.

Algorithm PART−

Step 1.

(1.1) Using a pair of MCT T_{vk} and T_{ik}, set $X_1 =: T_{vk} \cap K_{ik}$, $m := 1$.

(1.2) If $X_1 = \varnothing$, go to step 5.

Step 2. Set $m := 2$, and obtain $X_2 := C_v(X_1/K_{vk})$.

Step 3.

(3.1) Set $m := m + 1$, and obtain

$$X_m := L_i(X_{m-1}/T_{ik}) - \bigcup_{n=1}^{m-1} X_n \tag{3.16}$$

(3.2) If $X_m = \varnothing$, go to step 5.

Step 4.

(4.1) Set $m := m + 1$, and obtain

$$X_m := C_v(X_{m-1}/K_{vk}) - \bigcup_{n=1}^{m-1} X_n \tag{3.17}$$

(4.2) If $X_m \neq \varnothing$, go to step 3.

Step 5.

Set

$$E_{k-} := \bigcup_{n=1}^{m-1} X_n \tag{3.18}$$

Return E_{k-}.

We have:

Theorem 3.1 T_{ik} and T_{vk} obtained at the termination of Algorithm PART+ is a pair of MCT.

Proof. For any tree pair T_{vk} and T_{ik} and an arbitrary edge subset E_{ks} of E_k, we have

$$\begin{aligned}|K_{vk} \cap T_{ik}| &\geqslant |K_{vk} \cap T_{ik} \cap E_{ks}| \\ &= |E_{ks}| - |T_{vk} \cap E_{ks}| - |K_{ik} \cap E_{ks}| + |T_{vk} \cap K_{ik} \cap E_{ks}| \\ &\geqslant |E_{ks}| - |T_{vk} \cap E_{ks}| - |K_{ik} \cap E_{ks}| \\ &\geqslant |E_{ks}| - r(G_{vk} \cdot E_{ks}) - n(G_{ik} \times E_{ks}) \\ &= r(G_{ik} \times E_s) - r(G_{vk} \cdot E_s) \end{aligned} \tag{3.19}$$

The last "$\geqslant$" in the above is due to Proposition 2.2. In (3.19) the equalities hold if and only if

$$K_{vk} \cap T_{ik} \subseteq E_{ks}, \qquad T_{vk} \cap K_{ik} \cap E_{ks} = \varnothing \tag{3.20}$$

$$|K_{vk} \cap E_{ks}| = r(G_v \cdot E_{ks}), \qquad |T_{ik} \cap E_{ks}| = n(G_{ik} \times E_{ks}) \tag{3.21}$$

It can be seen that T_{vk}, T_{ik}, and E_{k+} obtained at the termination of PART+ satisfy conditions (3.20) and (3.21) for the equalities. Thus $|K_{vk} \cap T_{ik}|$ and $|T_{vk} \cap K_{ik}|$ are the minimum, and $|T_{vk} \cap T_{ik}|$ is the maximum.

From the discussion in the above proof and its dual we can easily get the following minimax theorem.

Theorem 3.2

$$\min_{K_{vk}, T_{ik}} |K_{vk} \cap T_{ik}| = \max_{E_{ks} \subseteq E_k} \{r(G_{ik} \times E_{ks}) - r(G_{vk} \cdot E_{ks})\} := \delta_{k+} \tag{3.22}$$

$$\min_{T_{vk}, K_{ik}} |T_{vk} \cap K_{ik}| = \max_{E_{ks} \subseteq E_k} \{r(G_{vk} \times E_{ks}) - r(G_{ik} \cdot E_{ks})\} := \delta_{k-} \tag{3.23}$$

δ_{k+} and δ_{k-} defined in eqs. (3.22) and (3.23), respectively, are called the deficiencies. In fact, E_{k+} and E_{k-} are minimal subsets of E_k giving the deficiencies, that is, minimal subsets such that

$$r(G_{ik} \times E_{k+}) - r(G_{vk} \cdot E_{k+}) = \delta_{k+} \tag{3.24}$$

$$r(G_{vk} \times E_{k-}) - r(G_{ik} \cdot E_{k-}) = \delta_{k-} \tag{3.25}$$

E_{k+} and E_{k-} are uniquely determined irrespective of a pair of MCT obtained in PART+ and used in PART−. From Eqs. (3.24) and (3.25) we get

$$\delta_{k+} = r(G_{ik} \times E_{k+}) + n(G_{vk} \cdot E_{k+}) - |E_{k+}| \tag{3.26}$$

$$\delta_{k-} = |E_{k-}| - r(G_{ik} \cdot E_{k-}) - n(G_{vk} \times E_{k-}) \tag{3.27}$$

From Proposition 2.2 we see that $r(G_{ik} \times E_{k+})$ and $n(G_{vk} \cdot E_{k+})$ are the minimum numbers of KCL and KVL equations, respectively, which are obtained for E_{k+}, and $r(G_{ik} \cdot E_{k-})$ and $n(G_{vk} \times E_{k-})$ are the maximum numbers of KCL and KVL equations, respectively, which can be obtained for E_{k-}. Therefore Eq. (3.26) [respectively Eq. (3.27)] indicates that no matter how we choose trees of G_{vk} and G_{ik}, there are excess equations for v_{k+} (excess unknown variables in v_{k-}).

Suppose we have obtained a pair of MCT, T_{vk} of G_{vk} and T_{ik} of G_{ik}. Utilizing Proposition 2.1, we construct T_v of G_v and T_i of G_i as follows. Let

$$T_{vb} := \text{a tree of } G_v \cdot (E_b + E_e), \qquad T_{ib} := \text{a tree of } G_i \times (E_b + E_j)$$

$$T_{vu} := \text{a tree of } G_v \times (E_u + E_j), \qquad T_{iu} := \text{a tree of } G_i \cdot (E_u + E_e)$$

Then T_v and T_i and their cotrees are

$$T_v := T_{vk} + T_{vb} + T_{vu}, \qquad K_v := E - T_v \tag{3.28}$$

$$T_i := T_{ik} + T_{ib} + T_{iu}, \qquad K_i := E - T_i \tag{3.29}$$

Now the voltage of an element in K_{vu} can be computed if and only if the fundamental tieset determined by it consists of this element and elements from $E_b + E_e + E_{k+} + E_{k0}$ only. The set of all such voltage-computable elements in K_{vu} is denoted by E_{vd}. Likewise, the current of an element in T_{iu} can be computed if and only if the fundamental cutset determined by it consists of this element and elements from $E_b + E_j + E_{k+} + E_{k0}$ only. The set of all such current-computable elements in T_{iu} is denoted by E_{id}.

If the object of diagnosis is to know the voltages of elements in set F_v and the currents of elements in set F_i, we have the following theorem for diagnosability [4].

Theorem 3.3 The circuit is diagnosable if and only if $F_v \subseteq E_b + E_e + E_{k+} + E_{k0} + E_{vd}$ and $F_i \subseteq E_b + E_j + E_{k+} + E_{k0} + E_{id}$.

Example 3.2 Let us consider the circuit shown in Figure 9.2a. Element 13 is an imaginary one representing the voltage of node x with respect to the reference node. Suppose $E_b = \{11, 12, 13\}$, $E_e = \{1\}$, $E_j = \varnothing$, $E_u = \{2, 3, 4\}$ and $E_k = \{5, 6, 7, 8, 9, 10\}$. From $G_v = G_i$, which is shown in Figure 9.2b, we get G_{vk} and G_{ik}, shown in Figures 9.2c and 9.2d, respectively. We apply PART+ to these graphs.

Step 0. We choose $T_{vk} = \{5, 7\}$ and $T_{ik} = \{6, 8, 10\}$. Then $K_{vk} \cap T_{ik} = \{6, 8, 10\}$ and $T_{vk} \cap K_{ik} = \{5, 7\}$.
Step 1. $X_1 = \{6, 8, 10\}$. *Step 2.* $X_2 = \{6, 8, 7, 9\} \ni 7$.

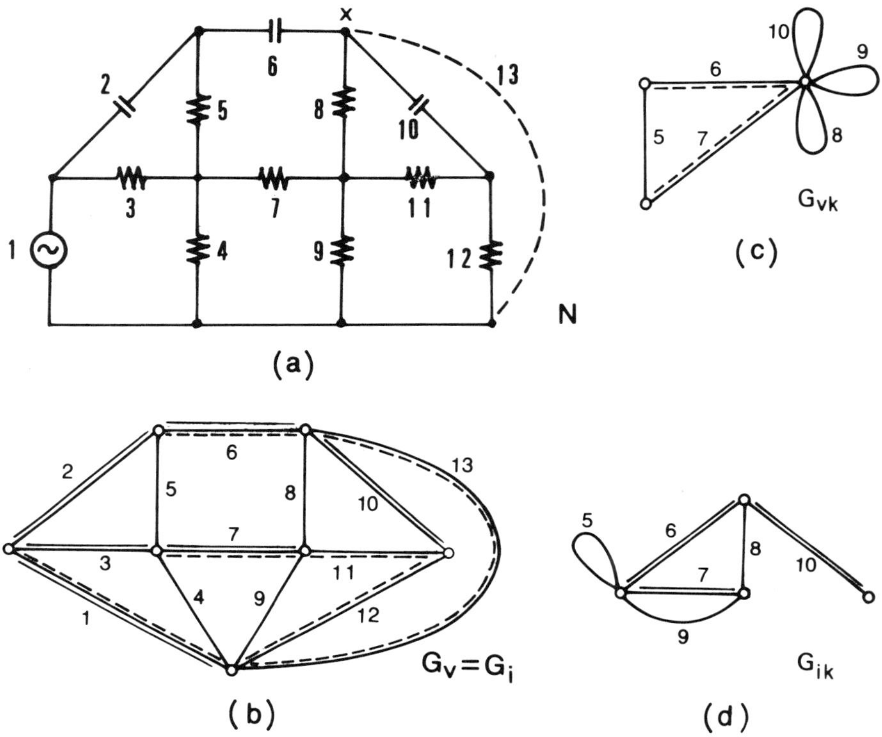

Figure 9.2 Example 3.2.

Step 5. $e_1 = 6$, $e_2 = 7$. We get new $T_{vk} = \{5, 7\}$ and $T_{ik} = \{7, 8, 10\}$. $K_{vk} \cap T_{ik} = \{8, 10\}$ and $T_{vk} \cap K_{ik} = \{5\}$.

Step 1. $X_1 = \{8, 10\}$. *Step 2.* $X_2 = \{8, 6\}$. $X_2 \cap \{5\} = \varnothing$.

Step 3. $X_3 = \{6, 5, 7\} - X_1 - X_2 = \{5, 7\} \ni 5$.

Step 6. $e_1 = 8$, $e_2 = 6$, $e_3 = 5$. We get new $T_{vk} = \{6, 7\}$ and $T_{ik} = \{6, 7, 10\}$. $K_{vk} \cap T_{ik} = \{10\}$, $T_{vk} \cap K_{ik} = \varnothing$.

Step 1. $X_1 = \{10\}$. *Step 2.* $X_2 = \{10\}$. *Step 3.* $X_3 = \{10\} - X_1 - X_2 = \varnothing$.

Step 7. $E_{k+} = \{10\}$.

Since $T_{vk} \cap K_{ik} = \varnothing$, we have $E_{k-} = \varnothing$. Then $E_{k0} = \{5, 6, 7, 8, 9\}$. Next we choose $T_{vb} = \{11, 12, 13\}$ and $T_{iu} = \{2, 3\}$. We have $T_{vu} = T_{ib} = \varnothing$. Finally, we get T_v of G_v and T_i of G_i as shown by the dashed lines and thin lines respectively in Figure 9.2b, and thus we get $E_{vd} = \{2, 3, 4\}$ and $E_{id} = \{2\}$.

3.2 Fault Localization

For an element in $E_{vd} \cap E_{id}$ we can calculate its element value, since its voltage and current are both known. Then we can determine whether or not it is faulty. Next, suppose we have only to localize the fault within a portion of the circuit. A classical but powerful way to do this is to assume the fault is localized in a certain subcircuit and then to check this assumption by some means or other. If the assumption is not verified, another part is assumed to be faulty, and the process is repeated. We say the fault within a portion is diagnosable if the assumption on it can be verified.

If the part assumed to be faulty is replaceable, the simplest way to check the assumption would be to replace it with a new good part and see if the circuit works well. In many cases this is not possible. The assumption must be checked by the measurement and equations we can get for the circuit. This assume-and-check method has been rigorously formulated and studied by several authors [6–11]. In the following we will apply the discussion of Section 3.1 to the assume-and-check method [10, 11].

Element sets E_b, E_e, and E_j are determined from the measurement condition. The remaining elements are partitioned into E_k and E_u, which are now redefined as follows.

$E_k :=$ the set of elements which are assumed to be fault-free
$E_u :=$ the element set which is assumed to contain faulty elements

We assume the effect of element value deviations is negligible and the nominal values can be used for the elements in E_k. The element values of those in E_u are unknown. Then we can derive exactly the same sets of equations as (3.1), (3.2), and (3.3) and get the principal partition of E_k into E_{k+}, E_{k0}, and E_{k-}.

We have more equations than unknown variables for E_{k+} and, under the generality assumption on element values, these equations are consistent if and only if E_{k+} contains no faulty element. Thus we have the following theorem.

Theorem 3.3 If $E_{k0} + E_{k-} = \varnothing$, then the assumption that the fault is localized in E_u can be checked (the assumption is correct if and only if the equations for E_{k+} are consistent), and the fault within E_u is diagnosable.

If $E_{k0} + E_{k-} \neq \varnothing$, we can redefine E_u, that is, replace it with $E_u + E_{k0} + E_{k-}$.

Corollary The fault in $E_u + E_{k-} + E_{k0}$ is diagnosable.

Suppose that another fault assumption is made, and $E - E_b - E_e - E_j$ is now partitioned into E_u^* and E_k^*. Suppose, for this partition, that E_k^* is further partitioned into E_{k+}^*, E_{k0}^*, and E_{k-}^*. It may be possible that $E_{k+}^* = E_{k+}$. Then faults in E_u and those in E_u^* cannot be distinguished by fault verification. In such a case E_u and E_u^* are said to belong to an ambiguity set.

Now a node is defined to be faulty if any element connected to it is faulty [9]. To find out whether or not a particular node is faulty, that is, whether or not the fault is localized within the set of elements which are incident on this node, we have only to set E_u equal to this element set and apply the above discussion. Node fault diagnosability can easily be obtained using Theorem 3.3. A disadvantage of considering node faults is that a single faulty branch not connected to the reference node will cause a two-node fault.

Next let us study how an ambiguity set arises. We consider the graphs obtained from G_v and G_i by contracting the elements of E_e and deleting those of E_j. For simplicity, the new pair of graphs is also denoted by G_v and G_i. It is known that the principal partition of G_{vk} and G_{ik} can be related to the partition with respect to electrical connectivities as follows [4].

The electrical connectivities are defined for E_b and E_u as [12]

$$\kappa_b := \min_{E_b \subseteq E_t \subseteq E - E_u} \{r(G_v \cdot E_t) - r(G_i \times E_t)\} \tag{3.30}$$

$$\kappa_u := \min_{E_u \subseteq E_t \subseteq E - E_b} \{r(G_i \cdot E_t) - r(G_v \times E_t)\} \tag{3.31}$$

where the minimums are taken as all possible subsets E_t such that $E_b \subseteq E_t \subseteq (E - E_u)$ and $E_u \subseteq E_t \subseteq (E - E_b)$, respectively. The minimal subsets which give κ_b and κ_u are denoted by E_c and E_w, respectively; that is, E_c and E_w are the minimal subsets such that

$$r(G_v \cdot E_c) - r(G_i \times E_c) = \kappa_b \tag{3.32}$$

$$r(G_i \cdot E_w) - r(G_v \times E_w) = \kappa_u \tag{3.33}$$

respectively.

If G_v and G_i have a common tree, that is, a tree which is a tree of G_v and a tree of G_i at the same time, it can be shown that $\kappa_b = \kappa_u$ and that $E - E_w$ $(E - E_c)$ is the maximal subset which gives κ_b (κ_u).

If $G_v = G_i := G$, it is rather easy to see the relation between the electrical connectivities and the conventional vertex connectivity. For easier understanding, suppose that E_b and E_u are the mutually disjoint sets of edges incident on certain vertices b and u, respectively. We note that $r(G \cdot E_t)$ and $r(G \times E_t)$ are equal to the numbers of edges belonging to trees of $G \cdot E_t$ and $G \times E_t$, respectively. The rank difference

$$\rho := r(G \cdot E_t) - r(G \times E_t); \qquad E_b \subseteq E_t \subseteq E - E_u \tag{3.34}$$

is equal to the difference between the numbers of these tree edges. By the contraction of the edges in $E - E_t$ to obtain $G \times E_t$ the connection vertices which connect $G \cdot E_t$ with the remaining part of G become a single vertex [for simplicity we assume that $G \cdot (E - E_t)$ is connected]. Thus ρ is equal to the number of the connection vertices minus one. The vertex connectivity between vertices b and u is defined as the minimum number of such connection vertices. For an electrical circuit a vertex connectivity of one is meaningless, hence the name electrical connectivity for κ_b or κ_u.

Example 3.3 In graph G shown in Figure 9.3a let E_t be the set constituted by the edges marked t. The connection vertices are marked c. $G \cdot E_t$ and $G \times E_t$ are shown in Figures 9.3b and 9.3c, respectively, and trees of these graphs are indicated by the dashed lines. We see that $r(G \cdot E_t) - r(G \times E_t) = 7 - 5 = 2 = 3 - 1$.

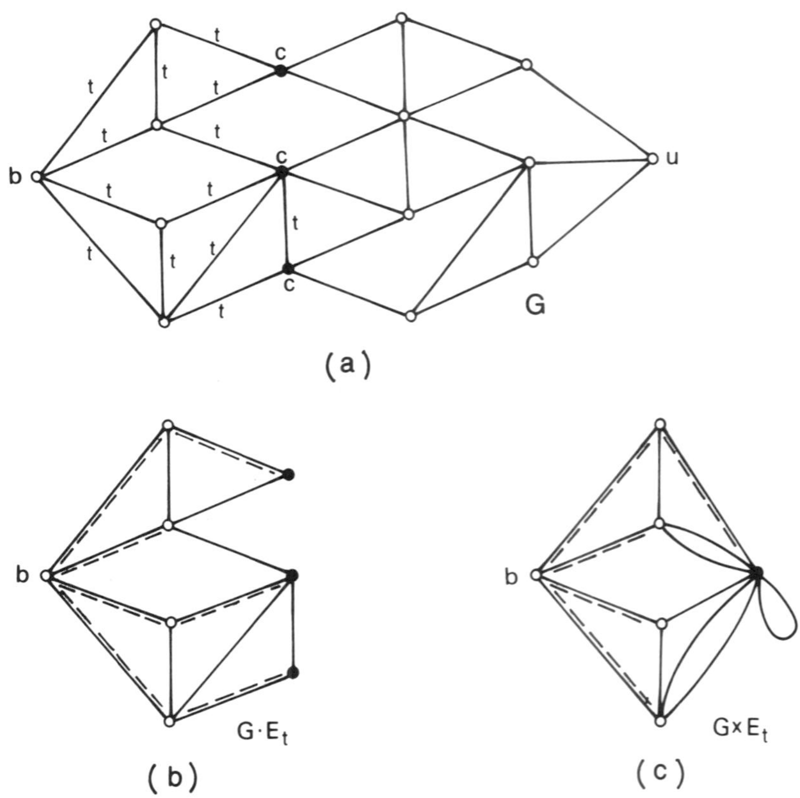

Figure 9.3 Example 3.3.

Let $E_{ks} := E_t - E_b$, $E_{ks} \subseteq E_k$. Using Proposition 2.1 we get

$$\kappa_b = \min_{E_b \subseteq E_t \subseteq E - E_u} \{r(G_v \cdot E_b) + r(G_v \cdot E_t \times E_{ks}) - r(G_i \times E_b) - r(G_i \times E_t \cdot E_{ks})\}$$

$$= r(G_v \cdot E_t) - r(G_i \times E_b) - \max_{E_{ks} \subseteq E_k} \{r(G_{ik} \times E_{ks}) - r(G_{vk} \cdot E_{ks})\} \tag{3.35}$$

Likewise, by setting $E_{ks} := E_t - E_u$, $E_{ks} \subseteq E_k$ we get

$$\kappa_u = r(G_i \cdot E_u) - r(G_v \times E_u) - \max_{E_{ks} \subseteq E_k} \{r(G_{vk} \times E_{ks}) - r(G_{ik} \cdot E_{ks})\} \tag{3.36}$$

Thus if we denote

$$\rho_b := r(G_v \cdot E_b) - r(G_i \times E_b) \tag{3.37}$$

$$\rho_u := r(G_i \cdot E_u) - r(G_i \times E_u) \tag{3.38}$$

we get

$$\delta_{k+} = \rho_b - \kappa_b \quad \text{and} \quad E_c = E_b + E_{k+} \tag{3.39}$$

$$\delta_{k-} = \rho_u - \kappa_u \quad \text{and} \quad E_w = E_u + E_{k-} \tag{3.40}$$

The above result is illustrated in Figure 9.4a and is interpreted as follows. Computability of voltages and currents in the circuit from measured and known data relies on the amount of "information" which can flow in the circuit. The amount of information flow is limited by the difference of ranks or the number of connection vertices which connect a part of the circuit with the remaining part. The rank difference ρ_b is the amount of information which can flow out from E_b where information is in excess (note that each edge in E_b has zero degree of freedom). The information flow to E_u through E_k is limited by the bottleneck which gives κ_b. This bottleneck for E_u can be that for another set $E_u^* \subseteq E_u + E_{k-} + E_{k0}$, as illustrated in Figure 9.4a. Then faults in E_u and E_u^* cannot be distinguished by our assume-and-check method, and E_u and E_u^* belong to an ambiguity set.

The above conclusion does not necessarily mean that the fault in $E_u + E_{k-} + E_{k0}$ cannot be further localized. It is possible that there exists a set $E_u^\circ \subsetneq E_u + E_{k-} + E_{k0}$ for which $\kappa_b^\circ = \kappa_u^\circ < \kappa_b = \kappa_u$ and $E_{k+}^\circ \supsetneq E_{k+}$. If the equations for E_{k+}° are consistent, the assumption that the fault is localized within E_u° is verified. This situation is illustrated in Figure 9.4b.

Example 3.4 Let us consider the circuit shown in Figure 9.5a. Elements 4 and 10 are voltage-controlled current sources. We assume the following measurement conditions. (1) The voltages of nodes a, d, and h with respect to the reference node g are measurable. (2) The current of the exciting voltage

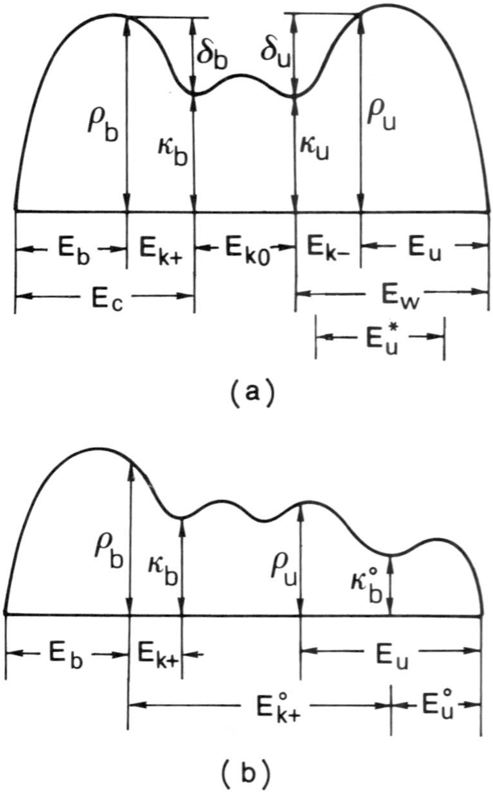

Figure 9.4 Illustration of Eqs. (3.39) and (3.40).

source 1 is measurable. (3) Resistor 14 is fault-free, and thus its resistance is known.

In order to represent the measurement condition for node h we add an imaginary element 15 between nodes h and g. Voltage graph G_v and current graph G_i for this circuit are shown in Figure 9.5b. From the measurement conditions we have $E_b = \{1, 14, 15\}$.

Let us first assume that the voltage-controlled current sources 4 and 10 are faulty but all the other elements are good. Then $E_u = \{4, 10\}$ and $E_k = \{2, 3, 5, 6, 7, 8, 9, 11, 12, 13\}$. We get G_{vk} and G_{ik} as shown in Figure 9.5c. We apply Algorithm PART+ to these graphs and get a pair of MCT, which are indicated by the dashed lines in Figure 9.5c. $K_{vk} \cap T_{ik} = \{6\}$ and from this we get $C_i(6/K_{ik}) = \{6, 12\}$, $L_v(6/T_{vk}) = \{6, 3\}$, $L_v(12/T_{vk}) = \{12\}$, $C_i(3/K_{ik}) = \{3, 2\}$, $L_v(2/T_{vk}) = \{2\}$. Thus $E_{k+} = \{2, 3, 6, 12\}$. $T_{vk} \cap K_{ik} = \varnothing$ and thus

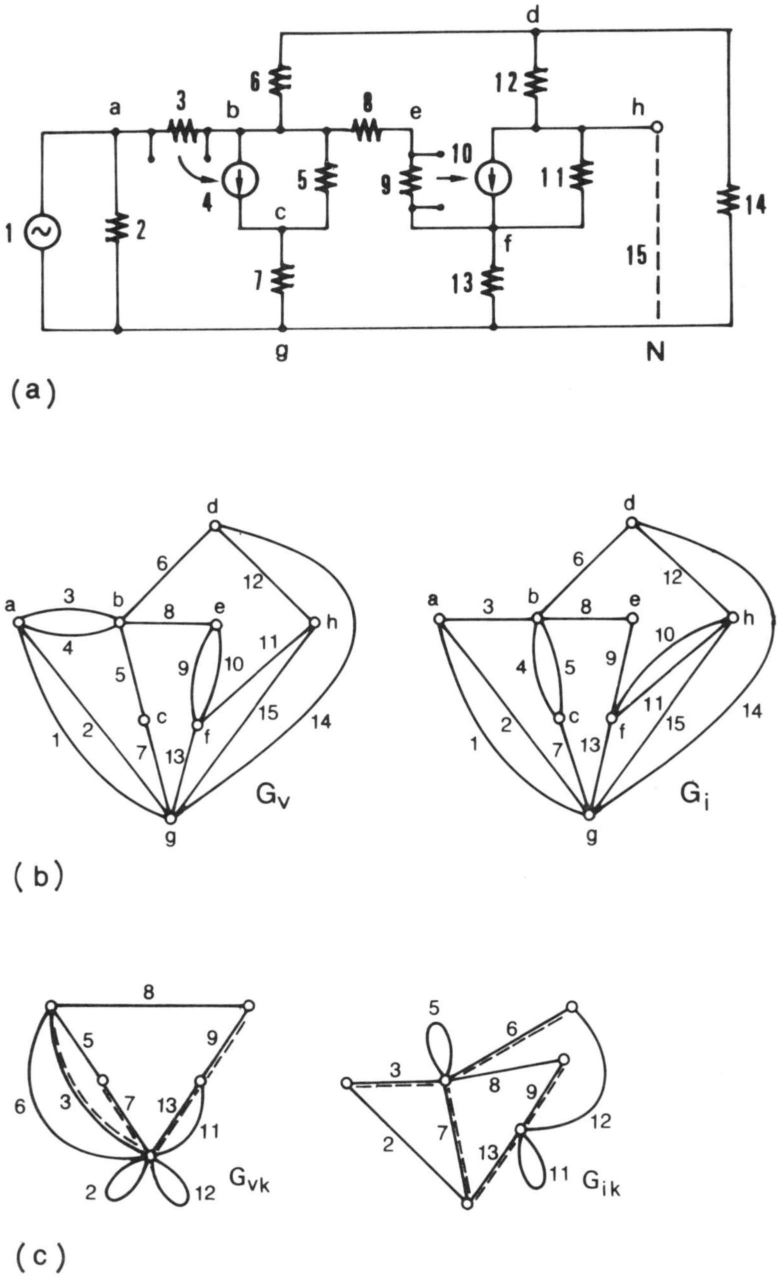
d
a
3
b
6
8
e
12
h
10
4
5
9
11
1
2
c
14
f
15
7
13
g
N
(a)
d
6
12
a
3
b
8
e
h
4
11
5
9
10
c
f
15
14
1
2
7
13
Gv
g
d
6
12
a
3
b
8
e
h
10
4
5
9
11
c
f
15
14
1
2
7
13
Gi
g
(b)
8
5
9
6
3
7
13
11
2
12
Gvk
5
6
3
8
9
7
12
2
13
11
Gik
(c)

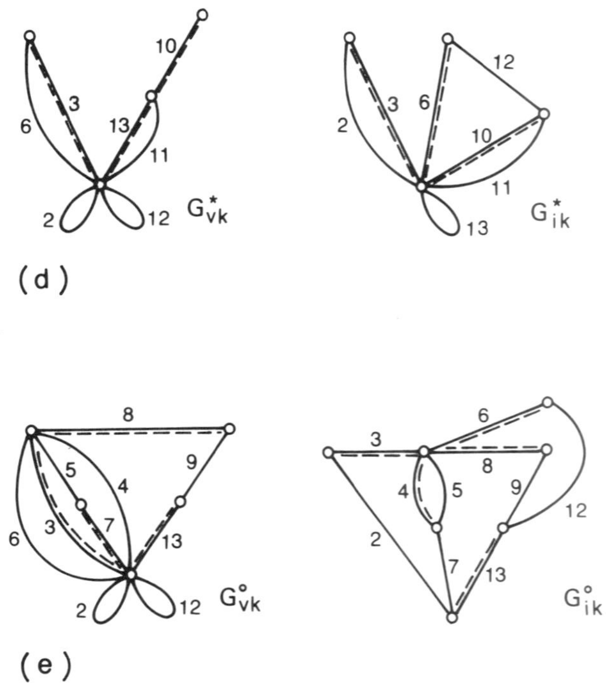

Figure 9.5 Example 3.4.

$E_{k-} = \varnothing$. Then $E_{k0} = \{5, 7, 8, 9, 11, 13\}$. We get $\delta_{k+} = 1$, $\rho_b = 3$, $\delta_{k-} = 0$, $\rho_u = 2$, $\kappa_b = \kappa_u = 2$.

Next let us assume that $E_u^* = \{4, 5, 7, 8, 9\} \subseteq E_u + E_{k0}$ is faulty. Then $E_k^* = \{2, 3, 6, 10, 11, 12, 13\}$ and we get G_{vk}^* and G_{ik}^* as shown in Figure 9.5d. A pair of MCT, T_{vk}^* and T_{ik}^*, are indicated by the dashed lines in the graphs. $K_{vk}^* \cap T_{ik}^* = \{6\}$ and $T_{vk}^* \cap K_{ik}^* = \{13\}$. From these sets we get $E_{k+}^* = \{2, 3, 6, 12\} = E_{k+}$, $E_{k-}^* = \{10, 11, 13\}$, and $E_{k0}^* = \varnothing$. Note that $E_u + E_{k0} + E_{k-} = E_{ku}^* + E_{k0}^* + E_{k-}^*$, and $\kappa_b = \kappa_b^*$. Therefore E_u and E_u^* belong to an ambiguity set.

Finally, let us assume that $E_u^\circ = \{10, 11\}$ is faulty. G_{vk}° and G_{ik}° for this assumption are shown in Figure 9.5e. Again a pair of MCT is indicated by the dashed lines in the graphs. $K_{vk}^\circ \cap T_{ik}^\circ = \{4, 6\}$, and from this set we get $E_{k+}^\circ = E_k^\circ = \{2, 3, 4, 5, 6, 7, 8, 9, 12, 13\}$. It is possible to check the fault assumption by the consistency of equations for E_{k+}°.

4 DIAGNOSIS BY MULTIPLE EXCITATIONS

The discussions in the previous sections concern a circuit with a particular excitation, that is, particular source voltages and currents with a fixed frequency. If the circuit has multiple exciting sources or the frequency of the excitation can be varied, we can get more measurement data. Even so, computable voltages and currents are the same if the measurable voltages and currents, or E_b, E_e, and E_j, are the same. Thus the following discussion is also based on the partition of the elements obtained in the previous sections.

Suppose all the elements in $E_b + E_{k+}$ are found to be fault-free. We assume the elements in E_{k0} are fault-free and the fault is localized in $E_w = E_u + E_{k-}$. We want to check this assumption by calculating element or parameter values which are independent of excitation or, equivalently, by checking the consistency of equations for such element or parameter values. Let $E_x := E - E_w$.

The voltages and currents of the elements in $E_{k+} + E_{k0}$ are computed using their nominal element values. Thus E_b in the previous sections is now replaced with E_x. For each excitation we get a set of equations for E_w which can be written in the same form as Eqs. (3.1), (3.2), and (3.3) except that the subscript k is now replaced with w. The coefficient matrix B_w and Q_w can be obtained from graphs

$$G_{vw} := G_v \times E_w \tag{4.1}$$

$$G_{iw} := G_i \cdot E_w \tag{4.2}$$

respectively. The equations for E_w contains the voltages, currents, and element values of the elements in E_w as unknowns. Thus they are nonlinear equations for unknown variables.

Suppose the frequency of the excitation can be varied. One way to check the fault assumption is use the method of Rapisarda and DeCarlo [13] (see also Chapter 11 in this book) and compute directly, if possible, the values of elements in E_w in more than one way and check their consistency.

Another way is to check the consistency of parameter values in the equations which relate the terminal voltages and currents of the subcircuit constituted by E_w [11]. To get such equations, the internal voltages and currents of the subcircuit must be eliminated. This can be done if the principal partition of G_{vw} and G_{iw} (the partition can be obtained by Algorithms PART+ and PART−) gives $E_{w+} = E_w$ and $E_{w0} = E_{w-} = \varnothing$. There is no need to express the parameters in terms of element values. They are rational functions of the frequency, and the coefficients of the functions are the constants which are independent of the excitation and whose consistency is to be checked.

5 CONCLUDING REMARKS

Diagnosability of analog circuits is investigated based on the computability of voltages and currents in the circuits. The results presented are graph theoretical and therefore give a necessary condition for diagnosability of practical circuits, for which measurement errors and element value deviations within tolerance bounds must be taken into consideration.

The results are applicable to circuit tuning or design where the graph of the circuit and some voltages and currents in the circuit are specified and element values are to be determined (thus unknown). For example, Nishikawa et al. [14] used the results in water distribution network expansion planning. The branches of the existing network and those of the network to be added constitute E_k and E_u, respectively. Waterheads (voltages) and waterflows (currents) are specified at certain points in the network, which determines E_b, E_e, and E_j. Thus, whether or not this planning is possible can be checked by using the diagnosability theorem given in Section 3.

Diagnosis by calculating element values is not discussed in detail. Multiple circuit excitations are inevitable in this case. Diagnosability or computability of element values has been investigated by many authors [15–22].

REFERENCES

1. Special Issue on Automatic Analog Fault Diagnosis, *IEEE Trans. Circuits Syst.*, vol. CAS-26, 1979.
2. J. W. Bandler and A. E. Salama, Fault diagnosis of analog circuits, *Proc. IEEE*, vol. 73, pp. 1279–1325, 1985.
3. W. Mayeda, *Graph Theory*, Wiley-Interscience, New York, 1972.
4. T. Ozawa and Y. Kajitani, Diagnosability of linear active networks, *IEEE Trans. Circuits Syst.*, vol. CAS-26, pp. 485–489, 1979.
5. T. Ozawa, Topological conditions for the solvability of linear active networks, *Int. J. Circuit Theory Appl.*, vol. 4, pp. 125–135, 1976.
6. R. M. Biernacki, and J. W. Bandler, Fault location of analog circuits, *1980 IEEE Int. Symp. Circuits Syst. Proc.*, pp. 1078–1081, 1980.
7. A. A. Sakla, E. I. El-Masry, and T. N. Trick, A sensitivity algorithm for fault detection in analog circuit, *1980 IEEE Int. Symp. Circuits Syst. Proc.*, pp. 1075–1080, 1980.
8. R. M. Biernacki and J. W. Bandler, Multiple-fault location of analog circuits, *IEEE Trans. Circuits Syst.*, vol. CAS-28, pp. 361–367, 1981.
9. Z. F. Huang, C.-S. Lin, and R.-W. Liu, Node-fault diagnosis and a design of testability, *IEEE Trans. Circuits Syst.*, vol. CAS-30, pp. 257–265, 1983.

10. T. Ozawa, Topological considerations on the diagnosability of analog circuits, *1984 IEEE Int. Symp. Circuits Syst. Proc.*, pp. 664–667, 1094.
11. T. Ozawa, Active circuit diagnosis and tuning based on the principal partition of two-graphs, *Proc. China 1985 Int. Conf. Circuits Syst.*, pp. 154–157, 1985.
12. N. Tomizawa, A practical criterion for the existence of a linkage pair of bases in a muoid and an algorithm for determining the maximally distant linkage pair of bases, *Trans. Inst. Electron. Commun. Eng. Jpn.*, vol. J59-A, pp. 280–286, 1976 (in Japanese).
13. L. Rapisarda and R. A. DeCarlo, Analog multifrequency fault diagnosis, *IEEE Trans. Circuits Syst.*, vol. CAS-30, pp. 223–234, 1983.
14. Y. Nishikawa, A. Udo, and H. Ozaki, Generalization of steady-state flow analysis for design and control of water distribution networks, *J. Jpn. Water Works Assoc.*, vol. 53, no. 2, pp. 1–20, 1984 (in Japanese).
15. R. S. Berkowitz, Condition for network-element-value solvability, *IRE Trans. Circuit Theory*, vol. CT-9, pp. 24–24, 1962.
16. S. D. Bedrosian and R. S. Berkowitz, Solution procedure for single element-kind networks, *IRE Int. Convention Rec.*, part 2, pp. 16–24, 1962.
17. S. Hayashi and Y. Hattori, and T. Sasaki, Considerations on network-element-value evaluation, *Proc. Inst. Electron. Commun. Eng. Jpn.*, vol. 50, pp. 2361–2368, 1967 (in Japanese, translated in *Electron. Commun. Jpn.*, vol. 50, pp. 118–127, 1967).
18. N. Navid and A. N. Willson, Jr., A theory and an algorithm for analog fault diagnosis, *IEEE Trans. Circuits Syst.*, vol. CAS-26, pp. 441–457, 1979.
19. T. Ozawa, S. Sinoda, and M. Yamada, An equivalent-circuit transformation and its application to network-element-value calculation, *IEEE Trans. Circuits Syst.*, vol. CAS-30, pp. 432–441, 1983.
20. T. Ozawa and M. Yamada, Conditions for determining parameter values in a linear active network from node voltage measurements, *1981 IEEE Int. Symp. Circuits Syst. Proc.*, pp. 274–277, 1981.
21. T. Ozawa and M. Yamada, Conditions for network-element-value determination by multifrequency measurements, *1982 IEEE Int. Symp. Circuits Syst. Proc.*, pp. 1156–1159, 1982.
22. J. A. Starzyk, R. M. Biernacki, and J. W. Bandler, Evaluation of faulty elements within linear subnetworks, *Int. J. Circuit Theory Appl.*, vol. 12, pp. 23–37, 1984.

10
Fault Location by Nodal Equations

Janusz A. Starzyk and Mohamed A. El-Gamal

Ohio University
Athens, Ohio

1 INTRODUCTION

Fault analysis of analog circuits has gained considerable interest during the past 10 years. This is due to the progress in the area of electronic design, which has not been accompanied by equal progress in the area of maintenance. Increasing diagnosability requirements of large systems caused intensification of efforts to develop effective fault location techniques.

In this chapter we present fault diagnosis techniques utilizing nodal equations. Node voltage measurements are used [1, 2] instead of port voltages [3] or branch voltages [4]. The main objective of the node fault diagnosis discussed is to search for faulty nodes.

The chapter consists of four parts. In the first part necessary and sufficient algebraic conditions for isolating the faulty nodes are formulated [1, 2]. We then present different topological interpretations of these algebraic conditions [1, 2, 5, 6]. These topological conditions are helpful in the design stage, especially in choosing measurement points to increase the testability of the network.

In the second part the problem of locating faulty regions in a faulty network is discussed. With the increase in the size and complexity of analog circuits it becomes apparent that location of faulty regions within a large network is as important as locating faulty elements (branches). A method for localizing the effect of faults in subnetworks is discussed [7]. Next a topological algorithm is presented, which can be used to detect the fault regions taking into account the topology of the network.

In the third part two different methods for location of faulty branches are presented. In the first method, which uses multiple excitations, the faulty branches can be identified after isolating the faulty nodes [2]. In the second method, under the assumption that all network nodes are accessible, we identify all network elements [8–10]. The minimum number of necessary and sufficient excitations for identifying network elements from node voltage measurements is discussed.

Finally, the fault diagnosis technique utilizing multifrequency tests is addressed [11–13]. A quantitative measure of solvability is presented based on algebraic properties of the Jacobian matrix.

2 MULTIPLE FAULT LOCATION BY NODAL EQUATIONS

Nodal equations are a convenient tool for approaching multiple fault location in analog circuits. While slightly restrictive in the range of networks one may consider, they are very handy in developing topological conditions for testability. For some applications modified nodal or tableau approaches may be preferred [14].

One of the practical constraints in fault location is that the number of measurements performed is usually less than the number of elements in the circuit. That is why the identification of all network elements is impossible and fault location is performed by identifying the faulty elements only, under the assumption that good elements are at their nominal values.

In what follows we present techniques that address the problem of fault location using the nodal equations and a limited number of independent measurements. Techniques in which we first assume that the fault has occurred in a part of the network and then check whether the assumption is correct are emphasized. This can be done by examining the consistency of certain linear equations invariant on faulty elements [1, 2].

First an algebraic formulation of such equations is presented. Their topological equivalence is then discussed in detail. For passive networks a simple topological condition for fault diagnosis is given. The Coates flow graph representation of the network is used to derive a necessary topological condition for both passive and active networks. Finally, a necessary and almost sufficient condition based on the representation of the network through a pair of graphs and their common trees is discussed. It is shown that this condition is valid for passive as well as active networks.

2.1 Nodal Equations of the Faulty Network [1]

Assume that a network S has $(n + 1)$ nodes, m of them accessible for excitation and measurement, with f faulty nodes and $f < m$.

The nodal equations of the network S are used to formulate an overdetermined system of equations. Consistency of this system of equations is a necessary condition to identify the faulty nodes. For the nominal values of the elements the nodal equations which describe the network S have the form

$$\mathbf{Y}_n\mathbf{V}_n = \mathbf{I}_n \tag{1}$$

where $\mathbf{Y}_n$ is the nodal admittance matrix, $\mathbf{V}_n$ is the vector of nodal voltages with respect to a selected reference node g, and $\mathbf{I}_n$ is the vector of nodal currents.

If S is perturbed to $(S + \Delta S)$ with the same excitation, we obtain

$$(\mathbf{Y}_n + \Delta\mathbf{Y}_n)(\mathbf{V}_n + \Delta\mathbf{V}_n) = \mathbf{I}_n \tag{2}$$

Subtracting (1) from (2) yields

$$\mathbf{Y}_n\Delta\mathbf{V}_n = -\Delta\mathbf{Y}_n\mathbf{V}'_n = \Delta\mathbf{I}_n \tag{3}$$

where $\mathbf{V}'_n = \mathbf{V}_n + \Delta\mathbf{V}_n$ is the vector of nodal voltages in the perturbed (faulty) network and $\Delta\mathbf{I}_n$ represents changes in nodal currents caused by faulty elements.

Assuming that $\mathbf{Y}_n$ is nonsingular, we can rewrite (3) as

$$\mathbf{Z}_n\Delta\mathbf{I}_n = \Delta\mathbf{V}_n \tag{4}$$

where $\mathbf{Z}_n = \mathbf{Y}_n{}^{-1}$. Equation (4) is used to develop fault diagnosis conditions.

2.2 Algebraic Conditions of Node Fault Diagnosis [1, 2]

The purpose of node fault diagnosis is to determine faulty nodes. By a fault we mean any change in the element value which can cause failure of the whole circuit. Accordingly, a node is faulty if any branch incident on it is faulty.

In the next section we present necessary and almost sufficient algebraic conditions to detect the faulty nodes.

Node diagnosis equations

Recalling equation (4), we may rewrite it in the following way:

$$\begin{bmatrix} \mathbf{Z}_{MN} \\ \mathbf{Z}_{N-M,N} \end{bmatrix} \Delta\mathbf{I}_n = \begin{bmatrix} \Delta\mathbf{V}_n{}^M \\ \Delta\mathbf{V}_n{}^{N-M} \end{bmatrix} \tag{5}$$

where M is the set of measurement nodes and N is the set of all nodes excluding the reference node. As a result, we have

$$\Delta \mathbf{V}_n{}^M = \mathbf{Z}_{MN}\Delta \mathbf{I}_n \tag{6}$$

Equations (3) and (6) are called the node diagnosis equations [2]. $\mathbf{Z}_{MN}$ and $\Delta \mathbf{V}_n{}^M$ are known; therefore we can solve for $\Delta \mathbf{I}_n$ first and then estimate $\Delta \mathbf{Y}_n$ from (3). However, since not all the nodes are accessible, $\Delta \mathbf{I}_n$ is not unique. This difficulty can be alleviated by the assumption that the number of faulty nodes is less than the number of measurement nodes. It is required to determine the nonzero components of $\Delta \mathbf{I}_n$ since they represent the faulty nodes.

Assuming that a few elements are faulty, $\Delta \mathbf{I}_n$ takes the form

$$\Delta \mathbf{I}_n = \begin{bmatrix} \Delta \mathbf{I}_n{}^F \\ \mathbf{0} \end{bmatrix} \tag{7}$$

where F is the set of faulty nodes. We can rewrite (6) as follows:

$$[\mathbf{Z}_{MF} \quad \mathbf{Z}_{M,N-F}] \begin{bmatrix} \Delta \mathbf{I}_n{}^F \\ \mathbf{0} \end{bmatrix} = \Delta \mathbf{V}_n{}^M \tag{8}$$

hence,

$$\mathbf{Z}_{MF}\Delta \mathbf{I}_n{}^F = \Delta \mathbf{V}_n{}^M \tag{9}$$

where $\Delta \mathbf{I}_n{}^F$ is the nonzero part of $\Delta \mathbf{I}_n$ and consists of f components. Equation (9) is an overdetermined system of equations since $m > f$. The least-squares solution of (9) is given by

$$\Delta \mathbf{I}_n{}^F = [\mathbf{Z}_{MF}{}^T \quad \mathbf{Z}_{MF}]^{-1} \quad \mathbf{Z}_{MF}{}^T \quad \Delta \mathbf{V}_n{}^M \tag{10}$$

Eliminating $\Delta \mathbf{I}_n{}^F$ from (9) we get

$$[\mathbf{Z}_{MF} \quad (\mathbf{Z}_{MF}{}^T\mathbf{Z}_{MF})^{-1} \quad \mathbf{Z}_{MF}{}^T - \mathbf{1}] \quad \Delta \mathbf{V}_n{}^M = \mathbf{0} \tag{11}$$

The above equation designates a necessary condition for isolating the faulty nodes. This equation is satisfied regardless of the values of the fault currents $\Delta \mathbf{I}_n{}^F$ and depends on their location only [13].

Rank test

To address the uniqueness of the solution obtained, i.e., whether the faulty nodes are uniquely located or not, we refer to the concept of testability [2].

Definition 2.1 A network is said to be f-node fault testable if one will be able to determine from the measurements at the accessible nodes

1. Whether the network has no more than f faulty nodes
2. If affirmative, whether the faulty nodes can be uniquely located

Any f faulty nodes can be uniquely located if the following rank test, known as the *f-node fault testability condition*, is satisfied:

$$\text{Rank } \mathbf{Z}_{MQ} = f + 1 \tag{12}$$

for all possible Q, where Q refers to $(f + 1)$ columns of $\mathbf{Z}_{MN}$. It can be shown that a network S is f-node fault testable if the f-node fault testability condition (12) is satisfied. The concept of f-node fault testability is very useful at the design stage, when a designer intends to build a network such that any set of f-node faults will be testable. On the other hand, this condition is too strong if we are interested in detecting a certain set of faults. Considering a specific candidate for the set of faulty nodes F, the following condition must be satisfied:

$$\text{Rank } \mathbf{Z}_{MX} = f + 1 \tag{13a}$$

where X refers to the set of columns of the matrix $\mathbf{Z}_{MN}$ such that

$$X = F \cup \{y\}, \qquad y \in N - F \tag{13b}$$

The testing process based on (13) is facilitated when information is available about the most likely faulty elements. The above condition is also equivalent to the existence of a square nonsingular submatrix of $\mathbf{Z}_{MX}$ of order $(f + 1)$. An equivalent testability condition can be stated in terms of the nodal admittance matrix using the following equivalence relation [15]:

$$\det \mathbf{Z}_{EX} \neq 0 \Leftrightarrow \det \mathbf{Y}(X|E) \neq 0 \tag{14}$$

where $\mathbf{Y}(X|E)$ is the matrix obtained from $\mathbf{Y}_n$ by removing X rows and E columns and E is a subset of M with cardinality $f + 1$.

Example 1 Consider the ladder network given in Figure 10.1, which has 4 nodes and 5 conductances with nominal values $G_i = 1$ S, $i = 1, 2, \ldots, 5$.

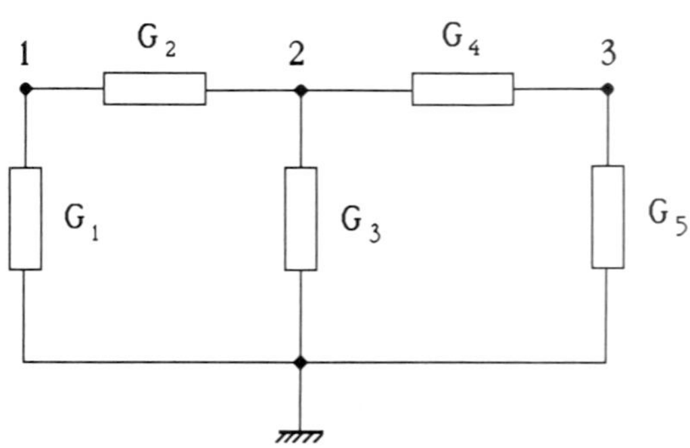

Figure 10.1 Resistive network.

Nodes 1 and 3 are chosen as measurement nodes. The nominal responses are $V_1 = \frac{5}{8}\,\mathrm{V}$, $V_3 = \frac{1}{8}\,\mathrm{V}$.

These measurements are simulated for the faulty network, where we decrease the value of the conductance G_3 by 0.5 S. Accordingly, we have $V_1' = \frac{2}{3}\,\mathrm{V}$ and $V_3' = \frac{1}{6}\,\mathrm{V}$. Constructing equation (6), we get

$$\begin{bmatrix} \Delta V_1{}^M \\ \Delta V_3{}^M \end{bmatrix} = \frac{1}{8}\begin{bmatrix} 5 & 2 & 1 \\ 1 & 2 & 5 \end{bmatrix} \Delta \mathbf{I}_n$$

Since every two columns of $\mathbf{Z}_{MN}$ are linearly independent, this network is 1-node fault testable. In order to determine which node is faulty we examine relation (9) for the three possible nodes and check which one gives a consistent system. For node 1 we have

$$\begin{bmatrix} \dfrac{1}{24} \\ \dfrac{1}{24} \end{bmatrix} = \frac{1}{8}\begin{bmatrix} 5 \\ 1 \end{bmatrix} \Delta I_1{}^F$$

which is inconsistent. For node 2 we have

$$\begin{bmatrix} \dfrac{1}{24} \\ \dfrac{1}{24} \end{bmatrix} = \frac{1}{8}\begin{bmatrix} 2 \\ 2 \end{bmatrix} \Delta I_2{}^F$$

which has the solution $\Delta I_2{}^F = \frac{1}{6}$. Finally, for node 3 we have

$$\begin{bmatrix} \dfrac{1}{24} \\ \dfrac{1}{24} \end{bmatrix} = \frac{1}{8}\begin{bmatrix} 1 \\ 5 \end{bmatrix} \Delta I_3{}^F$$

and this is inconsistent too. Accordingly, node 2 is faulty since the corresponding $\Delta \mathbf{I}_n{}^F$ is nonzero and the 1-node fault testability condition given in (12) is satisfied. The main difficulty with this algebraic approach is that checking the rank of a matrix is usually a computationally demanding procedure, especially for large networks. Besides, it is subject to numerical instability when the values of the network elements are scattered over a wide range. The main purpose of the topological conditions discussed next is to establish nonsingularity of the matrix $\mathbf{Y}(X\,|\,E)$ on the basis of the network topology.

2.3 Topological Conditions of Node Fault Diagnosis [1, 2, 5]

In this section we present topological conditions to examine network testability. One common advantage of these topological conditions is that they depend only on the network topology and not on the element values. Therefore the problem of tolerance (elements deviating from their nominal values) does not appear. However, for large-scale networks, a direct approach using these topological conditions could be inefficient, as in the case of symbolic network analysis. In such cases the decomposition technique [16] may be used and then the topological conditions could be applied to the decomposed network.

Linear graph representation

Let G be the linear graph of the network. Another graph G_t can be constructed from G in the following way. First we delete all branches which are incident between any two accessible nodes, and then connect all accessible nodes except the reference node to a new node t. A simple topological interpretation of the f-node fault testability condition in the case of linear passive networks is given in the following theorem [2].

Theorem 2.1 The network is *f-fault testable* if there exist at least $f + 1$ independent paths from any inaccessible node to the node t in G_t (the reference node is deleted from the network).

It should be noted that two paths are independent if they do not have any common node except the terminal nodes. An interesting result here is that branches between accessible nodes have no effect on the testability of the network. Considering the ladder network of Figure 10.1, we have node 2 as the only inaccessible node. Since there are two independent paths to the accessible (measurement) nodes 1 and 3, respectively, we conclude that the network is 1-node fault testable. The same result was obtained before using algebraic analysis.

Coates flow graph representation

Another topological condition of fault diagnosis, which capitalizes on (14) is derived on the basis of the Coates flow graph representation of a network. In this analysis a topological criterion is developed to check nonsingularity of the matrix $\mathbf{Y}(X|E)$ with X containing specific candidates for the set F of faulty nodes.

Let G_c denote a directed Coates graph [17] of the network S and let P denote a set of node pairs of G_c, namely $P = \{(v_{s1}, v_{e1}), \ldots, (v_{sk}, v_{ek})\}$, where $v_{pl} \neq v_{nm}$ for $l \neq m$ $(p, n = s, e)$. We start by defining a k-connection of G_c [18].

Definition 2.2 A k-connection of a graph G_c is a subgraph c_P of the graph such that elements of c_P form a set of k node-disjoint directed paths and node-disjoint directed circuits incident with all graph nodes. The start and end points of the paths are indicated by the pairs of P.

We also define $G_c(X \mid E)$ as the graph obtained from G_c after deleting all the edges incoming to nodes X and all the edges outgoing from nodes E. Let P contain pairs (v_{si}, v_{ei}) such that $v_{si} \in X$ and $v_{ei} \in E$. The following topological condition can be formulated [1].

Theorem 2.2 A necessary condition for $\det \mathbf{Y}(X \mid E) \neq 0$ is the existence of at least one $(f + 1)$-connection c_P in the graph $G_c(X \mid E)$.

The above theorem simply states that the existence of $(f + 1)$ connection is a necessary condition for the assumed set F to include all faulty nodes. The above theorem is applicable to passive as well as active networks. It should be noted that the condition is also sufficient under the assumption that there is no special relation between weights of the graph edges. However, for specific values of these weights it could fail.

Example 2 Consider the active network shown in Figure 10.2. Let the measurement nodes be 1 and 2; thus we have the set $E = \{1, 2\}$. The nodal admittance matrix is given by

$$\mathbf{Y}_n = \begin{bmatrix} Y_1 + Y_2 & 0 & -Y_2 & 0 \\ 0 & Y_4 + Y_6 & -Y_4 & g_2 \\ -Y_2 - g_1 & -Y_4 & Y_4 + Y_2 + g_1 & 0 \\ g_1 & 0 & -g_1 & Y_5 \end{bmatrix}.$$

The associated Coates graph G_c of the network is shown in Figure 10.3. Assume that node 3 is faulty, i.e., $F = \{3\}$, thus $y \in N - F = \{1, 2, 4\}$. For each X, where $X = F \cup \{y\}$, we draw the corresponding $G_c(X \mid E)$ and check to see if there exists at least one 2-connection c_P in each case. Consider $X = \{3, 4\}$. Figure 10.4 shows the corresponding $G_c(X|E)$ and one of the 2-connections required by Theorem 2.2. The other two possibilities of the set X, namely $X = \{2, 3\}$ and $X = \{1, 3\}$, are shown in Figures 10.5 and 10.6 with the associated Coates graph and the corresponding 2-connection for each case. Accordingly, the necessary topological condition stated in Theorem 2.2 is satisfied for the specified selection of the measurement and faulty nodes.

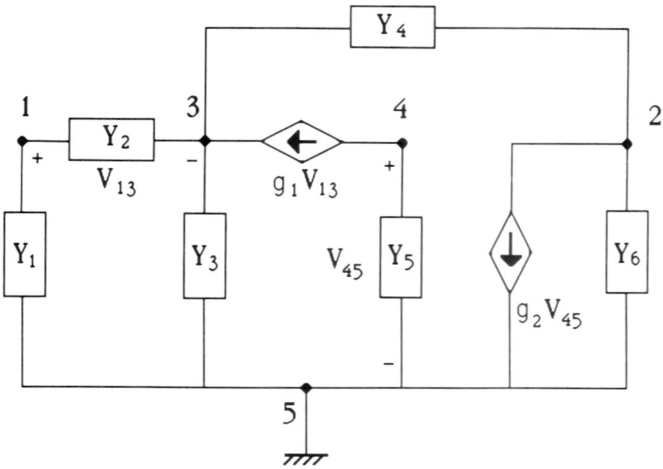

Figure 10.2 Active network.

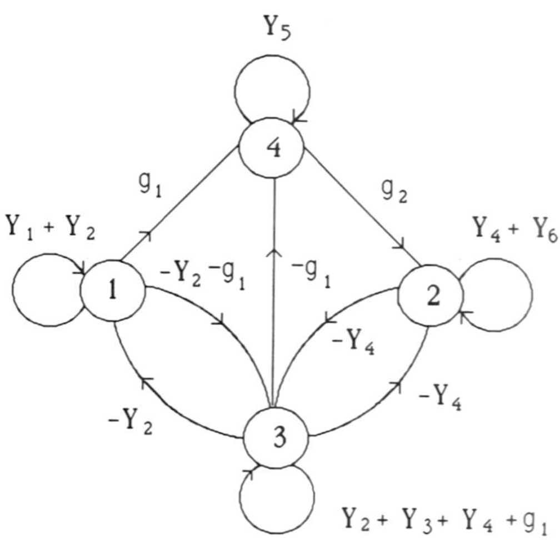

Figure 10.3 Associated Coates graph of the active network.

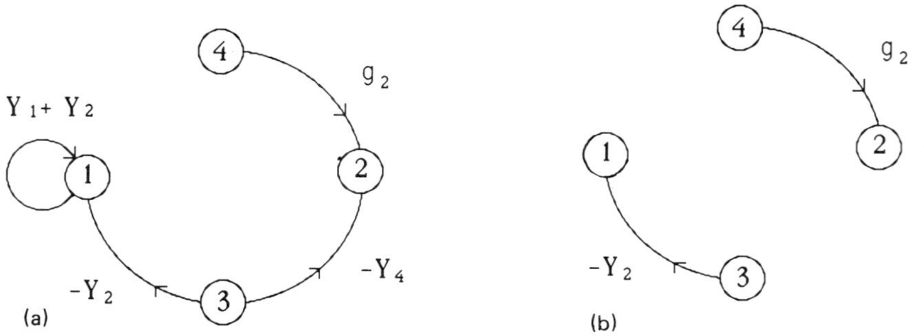

Figure 10.4 (a) Coates graph $G_c(\{3, 4\}|\{1, 2\})$. (b) A 2-connection c_p with $P = \{(3, 1), (4, 2)\}$.

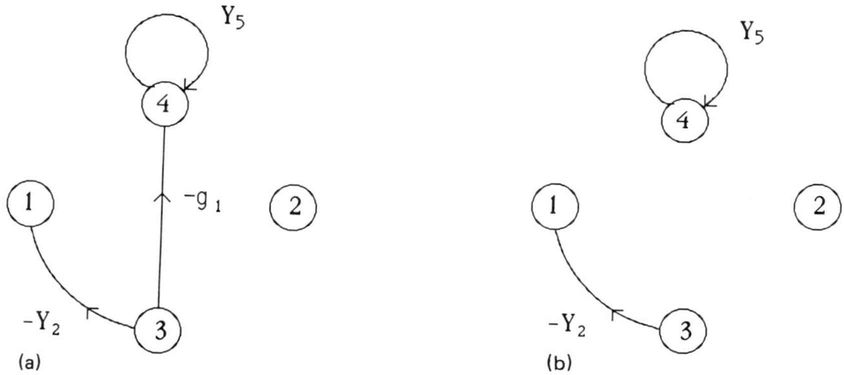

Figure 10.5 (a) Coates graph $G_c(\{2, 3\}|\{1, 2\})$. (b) A 2-connection c_p with $P = \{(3, 1), (2, 2)\}$.

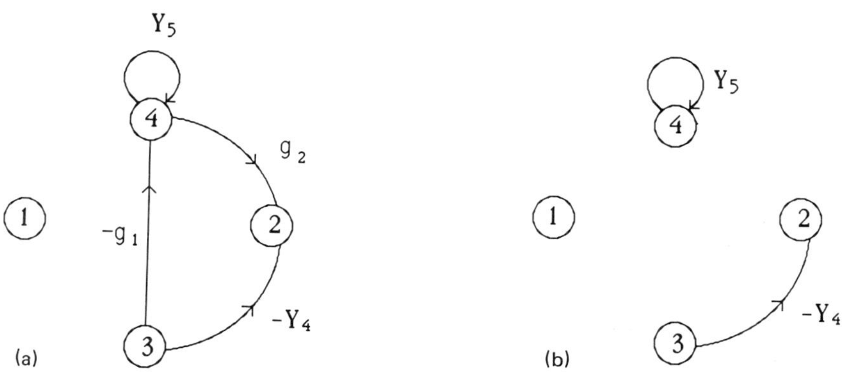

Figure 10.6 (a) Coates graph $G_c(\{1, 3\}|\{1, 2\})$. (b) A 2-connection c_p with $P = \{(3, 2), (1, 1)\}$.

Two-graph representation

In this method a topological condition is derived [5] on the basis of the two-graph representation of the active network, namely the current graph and the voltage graph [19]. This two-graph representation together with the concept of a common tree is used to give a topological equivalence for det $\mathbf{Y}(X|E)$ to be nonzero. Let G be the current or voltage graph of the network and an $(f+1)$ element subset of the set of its vertices be $D = \{v_1, v_2, \ldots, v_f, g\}$. Let $G(D)$ denote the graph obtained from G by identification of all the vertices of D (i.e., by shorting vertices of D to the reference node g). G_i and G_v are the current and voltage graphs of the network, respectively. A common tree is a set of edges, which is a tree of both voltage and current graphs.

Theorem 2.3 The existence of a common tree of both $G_i(X \cup \{g\})$ and $G_v(E \cup \{g\})$ is a necessary and almost sufficient condition for det $\mathbf{Y}(X|E)$ to be nonzero.

The set E is a subset of the set of measurement nodes M, i.e., E is known. Assuming that we are able to guess the set of faulty nodes F we can form the set X. Therefore $G_i(X \cup \{g\})$and $G_v(E \cup \{g\})$ are directly formulated and the existence of a common tree of these two graphs guarantees the testability of the network for the assumed set of faulty nodes F. An equivalent condition can be formulated and checked directly from G_i and G_v. As shown in [5], this condition requires the existence of a common $(f+2)$-tree of both G_i (with each node of the set X and reference node in different components) and G_v (with each node of the set E and the reference node in different components). These two equivalent topological conditions are both necessary and almost sufficient for passive and active networks described by nodal equations. The sufficiency follows from the fact that the edges of the two-graph representation of the network have unique weights. Therefore there is no symbolic cancelation of terms, which can occur in the case of the Coates flow graph representation. For passive networks G_i is the same as G_v and the topological condition for testability can be reduced to the existence of an $(f+2)$-tree in the linear graph G of the network.

Example 3 Consider once again the active network discussed in Example 2 with the same set of measurement and faulty nodes. We will show how the topological condition given in Theorem 2.3 can be used to identify the faulty nodes. The current and voltage graphs of the network are shown in Figure 10.7. Since $E = \{1, 2\}$ the graph $G_v(E \cup \{5\})$ is obtained from G_v by shorting nodes 1 and 2 to the reference node 5. For $F = \{3\}$ we have $y \in N - F = \{1, 2, 4\}$. If there exists a common tree of both $G_v(E \cup \{5\})$ and

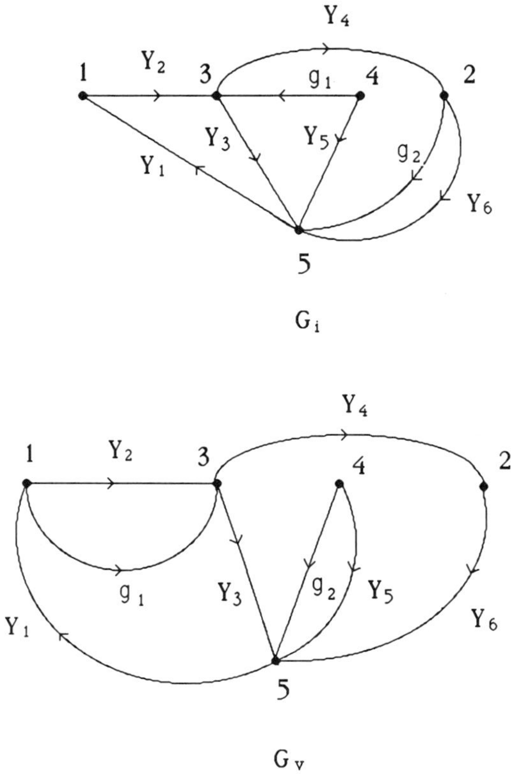

Figure 10.7 Current and voltage graphs of the network.

$G_i(X \cup \{5\})$ where $X = F \cup \{y\}$, then $\mathbf{Y}(X|E)$ is nonsingular and we can uniquely identify node 3 as faulty.

First, consider $X = \{3, 4\}$. We can see from Figure 10.8 that $Y_2 g_2$ is a common tree of both $G_i(X \cup \{5\})$ and $G_v(E \cup \{5\})$. This can be verified by examining the determinant of the matrix $\mathbf{Y}(X|E)$, which in this case has the form

$$\mathbf{Y}(X|E) = \begin{bmatrix} -Y_2 & 0 \\ -Y_4 & g_2 \end{bmatrix}$$

Similarly, current graphs which correspond to the other two choices of the set X are shown in Figures 10.9 and 10.10. $Y_2 Y_5$ is a common tree of both $G_i(X \cup \{5\})$ shown in Figure 10.9 and $G_v(E \cup \{5\})$ (Figure 10.8b). Finally, we find that $Y_4 Y_5$ and $g_1 g_2$ are common trees of both $G_i(X \cup \{5\})$ shown in

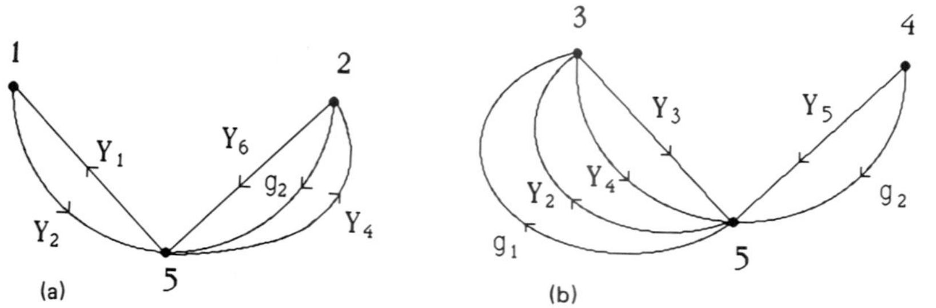

Figure 10.8 (a) Current graph $G_i(\{3, 4, 5\})$. (b) Voltage graph $G_v(\{1, 2, 5\})$.

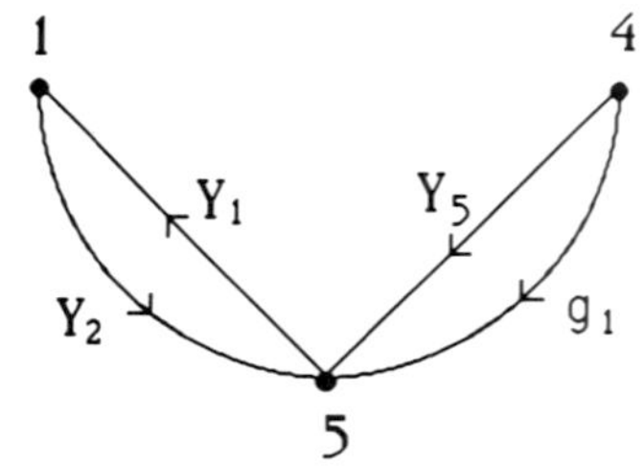

Figure 10.9 Current graph $G_i(\{2, 3, 5\})$.

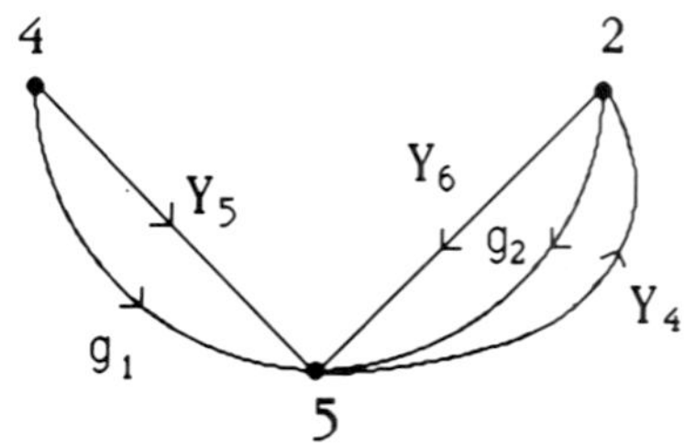

Figure 10.10 Current graph $G_i(\{1, 3, 5\})$.

Figure 10.10 and $G_v(E \cup \{5\})$. Hence, the topological condition stated in Theorem 2.3 is satisfied and we conclude that if node 3 is faulty it can be uniquely located from measurement nodes 1 and 2.

3 LOCATION OF FAULTY REGIONS

Most of the proposed techniques do not seem to be practical when dealing with large networks. Considering the rapid increase in the size and complexity of analog circuits, it becomes apparent that the ability to locate faulty subnetworks or regions has become as important as locating faulty elements. Location of faulty regions reduces the effort needed to isolate faulty elements since it works with a subnetwork that is usually much smaller than the network.

Any number of faults in one subnetwork can be represented by faults at common nodes with the other subnetwork. This representation makes it possible to solve the fault evaluation problem locally at the subnetwork level. The theoretical basis of the decomposition technique given in Ref. [7] can be summarized briefly as follows.

Let us decompose the graph G of the network into subgraphs $G_1, \ldots, G_k$. Let c_j denote the cardinality of the set C_j of these nodes of G_j, which are incident to the other subgraphs. Consequently, we have

$$C_j \triangleq \bigcup_{\substack{l=1 \\ l \neq j}}^{k} N_l \cap N_j \tag{15}$$

where N_l, N_j represent sets of nodes of subgraphs G_l and G_j, respectively. Let M_j denote the set of measurement nodes which belongs to G_j and $m_j = \operatorname{card} M_j$. The faulty nodes in the subgraph G_j can be detected if the conditions stated in the following theorem are satisfied.

Theorem 3.1 If subgraph G_j contains f_j faults with

$$m_j > c_j + f_j \tag{16}$$

and the conditions stated in (13) are satisfied for $M = M_j$, $F = C_j \cup F_j$, $N = N_j$, and $f = \operatorname{card} F$, then F_j contains all faulty nodes in G_j.

The significance of this theorem is clear. It allows us to apply the testability conditions given in the previous section to the subnetwork level. Moreover, if any subnetwork was found to be fault-free, we can remove the corresponding set of nodes from (15). Also, if a set of faulty nodes F_l in any subnetwork was previously established, we can use the set directly rather than its effect at common nodes. Accordingly, as the search for faulty subnetworks progresses, C_j in (15) can be replaced by C'_j,

$$C'_j = \bigcup_{\substack{l=1 \\ l \neq j}}^{k_1} N_l \cap N_j \cup \bigcup_{l=k_1+1}^{k} F_l \tag{17}$$

where k_1 denotes the number of subgraphs where faulty nodes have not been evaluated. It should be noted that if F_l has been uniquely evaluated, then we have $m_l > f_l$ and measurements m_l can be used together with m_j to evaluate faulty nodes F_j. To this end, let us assume that

$$M'_j = M_j \cup \bigcup_{i=k_1}^{k} M_i \tag{18}$$

Theorem 3.1 can be modified to use previously tested subnetworks.

Theorem 3.2 If the conditions stated in (13) are satisfied for $M = M'_j$, $F = C'_j \cup F_j$, $N = N_j$, and $f = \text{card}\, F$, then F_j contains all faulty nodes in G_j.

The above theorem together with Theorem 3.1 is the basis for partitioning the network into subnetworks, which will then be tested for the presence of faults. The ability to evaluate faults within a subnetwork depends on the actual number of faults, the number of measurements within the subnetwork, and the information obtained through the nodes common with the rest of the network.

3.1 Network Partitioning into Fault Regions [7]

As should be clear from our previous discussion, an important problem is to guess the set that contains all faulty nodes. However, if we do not have initial information about the network the probability of guessing the proper set F is low, because we have $\binom{n}{f}$ different combinations to choose from. A topological algorithm given in Ref. [7] can be used to detect the faulty region, taking into account the network topology and utilizing Theorems 3.1 and 3.2. The main steps of this topological algorithm are as follows.

Topological algorithm

Step 1. Decompose the Coates signal flow graph G_c of the network into subgraphs $G_1, \ldots, G_k$ separated by a small number of nodes.

Step 2. Choose the subgraph G_j (or combination of subgraphs) containing m_j measurement nodes such that $m_j > c_j$. If there is no such subgraph, stop.

Step 3. If the chosen subgraph G_j contains f_j faults such that $m_j > c_j + f_j$, evaluate them using Theorem 3.1.

Step 4. If no subgraph chosen in step 2 satisfies the condition stated in step 3, then try different combinations of two or more subgraphs and check if step 3 may be realized for the combination considered. If not, stop.

Step 5. For the remaining subgraphs use Theorem 3.2. If there is no success, stop.

One of the main advantages of this algorithm is that it allows us to decompose the network and detect faults in a subnetwork level even if the number of measurements is less than the number of faults.

Example 4 Consider the resistive network shown in Figure 10.11, which has 20 nodes and 39 resistors with nominal values $R_i = 1\,\Omega$ for $i \neq 12$ and $R_{12} = 2\,\Omega$. Nodes 9, 11, 13, and 19 are the measurement nodes. The value of the resistors R_k ($k = 5, 6, \ldots, 12$) and R_{37} increased by $1\,\Omega$ and $I_{in} = 1$ A. The measurements are simulated for the faulty network. They are equal to $V_9 = 0.1316$ V, $V_{11} = 0.06177$ V, $V_{13} = 0.03797$ V, $V_{19} = 0.0535$ V. We start by decomposing the graph of the network into three subgraphs as shown in Figure 10.12. All the measurements are placed in subgraph G_2. If we apply the topological algorithm it is clear that subgraph G_2 has a number of measurements m_2 larger than c_2. Next we will check the inequality $m_2 > C_2 + f_2$. Since it is valid only for $f_2 = 0$, we can only check whether subgraph G_2 is nonfaulty. We take X as in Theorem 3.1 having $F_2 = \varnothing$. In this case $F = N_1 \cap N_2 \cup N_3 \cap N_2 = \{9, 13, 18\}$. Now we can check the conditions stated in (13). In other words, we verify that the rank of Z_{MX} is 4

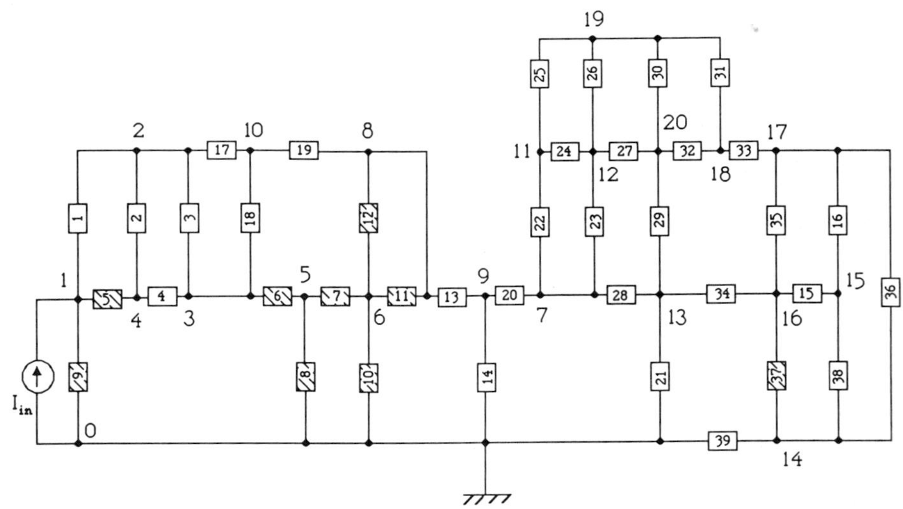

Figure 10.11 Restive network. (From Ref. 7.)

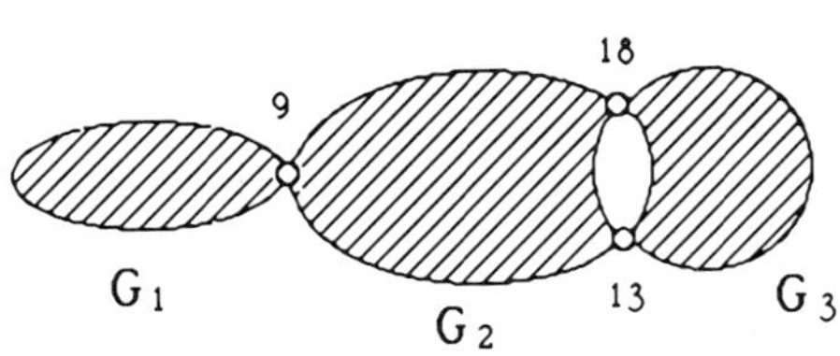

Figure 10.12 Decomposition of the graph of the resistive network into subgraphs. (From Ref. 7.)

for all $y \in N_2 - F = \{7, 11, 12, 19, 20\}$. Next we use equation (9) to determine $\Delta\mathbf{I}_n{}^F$, which in this case will represent all faulty elements. Equation (9) is of the form

$$\begin{bmatrix} \Delta V_9{}^M \\ \Delta V_{11}{}^M \\ \Delta V_{13}{}^M \\ \Delta V_{19}{}^M \end{bmatrix} = \begin{bmatrix} 0.0676 \\ 0.0319 \\ 0.0197 \\ 0.0277 \end{bmatrix} = \begin{bmatrix} 0.506 & 0.144 & 0.170 \\ 0.237 & 0.384 & 0.572 \\ 0.144 & 0.536 & 0.381 \\ 0.205 & 0.396 & 0.698 \end{bmatrix} \begin{bmatrix} \Delta I_9{}^F \\ \Delta I_{13}{}^F \\ \Delta I_{18}{}^F \end{bmatrix}$$

Solving for $\Delta\mathbf{I}_n{}^F$, we obtain

$$\Delta I_9{}^F = 0.133\ \text{A}, \qquad \Delta I_{13}{}^F = 0.00094\ \text{A}, \qquad \Delta I_{18}{}^F = -3.1 \times 10^{-15}\ \text{A}$$

From the solution obtained, the requirements of Theorem 3.1 for $F_2 = \varnothing$ are satisfied, so we can be sure that subgraph G_2 is nonfaulty. If G_3 contains only one faulty element as in this example, we can locate it exactly using the reduction technique described in Ref. [7]. What we need to do is check the combination of every two nodes in G_3 which are connected by a resistor. After subtracting column 16 from column 14 in $\mathbf{Z}_{MN}$, (9) can be written as

$$\begin{bmatrix} 0.506 & -0.0289 \\ 0.237 & -0.0769 \\ 0.144 & -0.0107 \\ 0.205 & -0.0792 \end{bmatrix} \begin{bmatrix} \Delta I_9{}^F \\ \Delta I_{14-16}{}^F \end{bmatrix} = \begin{bmatrix} 0.0676 \\ 0.0319 \\ 0.0197 \\ 0.0277 \end{bmatrix}$$

which gives us the solution $\Delta I_{14-16}{}^F = 0.0475$ A. This proves that the faulty element is between nodes 14 and 16. Moreover, the value of the faulty element can be determined as shown in Ref. [7].

4 EVALUATION OF FAULTY ELEMENTS

Fault diagnosis and automatic testing for analog circuits often require parameter identification. Several techniques have been presented for the calculation of element values of the network using a linear system of equations [13].

One can distinguish two main approaches. In the first approach a single excitation is used and the basic assumption is that the branch currents and voltages can be measured. Therefore this approach is not very practical. In the second approach multiple excitations are used to calculate the elements based on voltage measurements only [8–10]. Since we are mainly concerned with methods that utilize nodal equations, our emphasis is on the second approach. Two different methods are discussed.

In the first method, a graph-theoretical condition for determination of all parameter values from node voltage measurements is given [8]. In the second method the faulty branches are identified after isolating the faulty nodes, using the concept of f-node fault testability [2]. A minimum sufficient number of independent excitations that would enable us to identify all elements within a faulty subnetwork is also discussed [9–10].

4.1 Multiple Excitation Element Evaluation Technique [8–10]

In this technique the main assumption is that all the nodes of the network are accessible. Starting from the nodal equations of the network

$$\mathbf{Y}_n\mathbf{V}_n = \mathbf{I}_n \tag{19}$$

with n independent excitations, we have

$$\mathbf{Y}_n\hat{\mathbf{V}}_n = \hat{\mathbf{I}}_n \tag{20}$$

where

$$\hat{\mathbf{V}}_n = [\mathbf{V}_n{}^1 \quad \mathbf{V}_n{}^2 \quad \cdots \quad \mathbf{V}_n{}^n] \tag{21}$$

and

$$\hat{\mathbf{I}}_n = [\mathbf{I}_n{}^1 \quad \mathbf{I}_n{}^2 \quad \cdots \quad \mathbf{I}_n{}^n] \tag{22}$$

If $\hat{\mathbf{V}}_n$ is nonsingular, then the unknown matrix $\mathbf{Y}_n$ is given by

$$\mathbf{Y}_n = \hat{\mathbf{I}}_n\hat{\mathbf{V}}_n{}^{-1} \tag{23}$$

As a consequence of equations (19) and (23), the following theorem provides sufficient conditions for the evaluation of $\mathbf{Y}_n$.

Theorem 4.1 If a given linear network can be described by nodal equations and the current excitations are chosen in such a way that $\hat{\mathbf{I}}_n$ is a nonsingular matrix, then $\hat{\mathbf{V}}_n$ is also nonsingular and the solution (23) exists.

If we choose to apply a unit current consecutively to all nodes, then $\hat{\mathbf{I}}_n = \mathbf{1}$. This together with (23) gives us an important relation,

$$\mathbf{Y}_n = \hat{\mathbf{V}}_n{}^{-1} \tag{24}$$

which can be used to find $\mathbf{Y}_n$ and hence to identify element values.

Example 5 Consider the passive network shown in Figure 10.13. We excite the network at nodes 1, 2, 3, and 4 successively. The corresponding matrix of

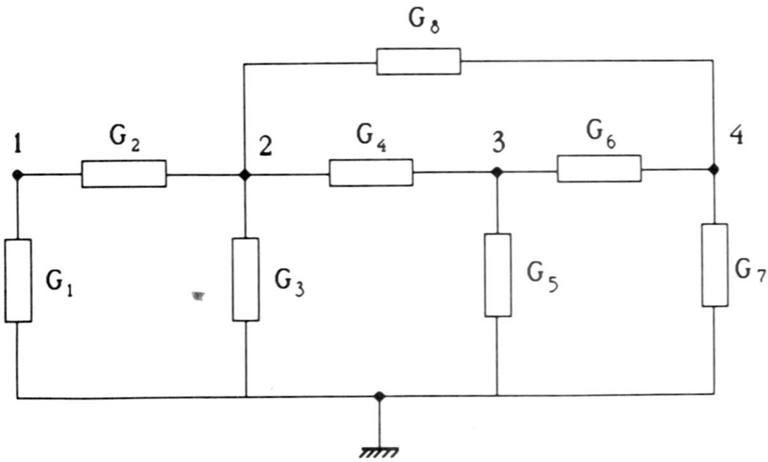

Figure 10.13 Resistive network.

voltage responses is given by

$$\hat{\mathbf{V}}_n = \begin{bmatrix} \frac{35}{59} & \frac{11}{59} & \frac{5}{59} & \frac{4}{59} \\ \frac{11}{59} & \frac{22}{59} & \frac{10}{59} & \frac{8}{59} \\ \frac{5}{59} & \frac{10}{59} & \frac{26}{59} & \frac{9}{59} \\ \frac{4}{59} & \frac{8}{59} & \frac{9}{59} & \frac{19}{59} \end{bmatrix}$$

Therefore

$$\mathbf{Y}_n = \hat{\mathbf{V}}_n^{-1} = \begin{bmatrix} 2 & -1 & 0 & 0 \\ -1 & 4 & -1 & -1 \\ 0 & -1 & 3 & -1 \\ 0 & -1 & -1 & 4 \end{bmatrix}$$

Consequently, we can identify the elements of the network as $G_i = 1$ S, $i = 1, 2, \ldots, 6, 8$ and $G_7 = 2$ S.

An important question arises: Is it necessary to excite all the nodes of the network to identify its element values? The answer is no. The number of necessary and sufficient excitations to identify all network elements is usually much smaller than the number of network nodes. A practical problem is to determine a reasonably small number of excitation nodes for the identification of all faulty element values within a network.

4.2 Node Fault Diagnosis Approach [2]

In this approach, branches which are incident on faulty nodes can be isolated and identified through the use of multiple excitations to a network which is f-node fault testable.

Assume for simplicity that a passive network N is f-node fault testable (the analysis can be generalized to an active network case). Recalling (3), we have

$$-\Delta\mathbf{I}_n = \Delta\mathbf{Y}_n(\mathbf{V}_n + \Delta\mathbf{V}_n) \tag{3}$$

with $\Delta\mathbf{I}_n^F$ the nonzero part of $\Delta\mathbf{I}_n$ given by

$$\Delta\mathbf{I}_n^F = [\mathbf{Z}_{MF}^T \quad \mathbf{Z}_{MF}]^{-1} \quad \mathbf{Z}_{MF}^T \quad \Delta\mathbf{V}_n^M \tag{10}$$

On the other hand, $\mathbf{V}_n + \Delta\mathbf{V}_n$ can be calculated in the following way. We have

$$\Delta\mathbf{V}_n = \mathbf{Z}_n\Delta\mathbf{I}_n \tag{4}$$

and

$$\mathbf{V}_n = \mathbf{Z}_n\mathbf{I}_n = \mathbf{Z}_n\begin{bmatrix}\mathbf{I}_m \\ \mathbf{0}\end{bmatrix} \tag{25}$$

where $\mathbf{I}_m$ is the current excitation vector at the measurement nodes.

Combining (4) and (25), we get

$$\mathbf{V}_n + \Delta\mathbf{V}_n = \mathbf{Z}_n\left(\begin{bmatrix}\mathbf{I}_m \\ \mathbf{0}\end{bmatrix} + \Delta\mathbf{I}_n\right) \tag{26}$$

and (3) can be used to identify $\Delta\mathbf{Y}_n$. If $\mathbf{H}$ is a column selector matrix such that $\Delta\mathbf{Y}_n\mathbf{H}$ is an $n \times f'$ matrix with $f' \leqslant f$ and $\Delta\mathbf{Y}_n\mathbf{H}$ retains all nonzeros of $\Delta\mathbf{Y}_n$, then (3) can be rewritten as

$$-\Delta\mathbf{I}_n = \Delta\mathbf{Y}_n\mathbf{H}\mathbf{H}^T(\mathbf{V}_n + \Delta\mathbf{V}_n) \tag{27}$$

Applying m independent excitations we have the matrix equation

$$-\Delta\hat{\mathbf{I}}_n = \Delta\mathbf{Y}_n\mathbf{H}\mathbf{H}^T(\hat{\mathbf{V}}_n + \Delta\hat{\mathbf{V}}_n) \tag{28}$$

where $\Delta\hat{\mathbf{I}}_n = [\Delta\mathbf{I}_n^1, \ldots, \Delta\mathbf{I}_n^m]$. Finally, the nonzero columns of $\Delta\mathbf{Y}_n$ are evaluated by

$$\Delta\mathbf{Y}_n\mathbf{H} = -\Delta\hat{\mathbf{I}}_n\mathbf{L}^T(\mathbf{L}\mathbf{L}^T)^{-1} \tag{29}$$

where $L = \mathbf{H}^T(\hat{\mathbf{V}}_n + \Delta\hat{\mathbf{V}}_n)$ and has a full row rank. Using (29), we can directly locate and evaluate the faulty branches, as can be seen from the following example.

Example 6 Consider the ladder network of Figure 10.1 with the same fault as before (i.e., $G_3 = 0.5$ S, $M = \{1, 3\}$, $F = \{2\}$). We excite the network twice, first at node 1 and then at node 3. The nominal responses at the measurement nodes are

$$\mathbf{V}_n{}^M = \begin{bmatrix} \frac{5}{8} & \frac{1}{8} \\ \frac{1}{8} & \frac{5}{8} \end{bmatrix}$$

These responses simulated for the faulty network are

$$\mathbf{V}_n{}^M + \Delta\mathbf{V}_n{}^M = \begin{bmatrix} \frac{2}{3} & \frac{1}{6} \\ \frac{1}{6} & \frac{2}{3} \end{bmatrix}$$

Therefore $\Delta\mathbf{V}_n{}^M$ is given by

$$\Delta\mathbf{V}_n{}^M = \begin{bmatrix} \frac{1}{24} & \frac{1}{24} \\ \frac{1}{24} & \frac{1}{24} \end{bmatrix}$$

Since the network is 1-node fault testable with node 2 as the faulty node, $\Delta I_2{}^F$ is calculated using (10) as follows. For the unit excitation at node 1 we have

$$\Delta I_2{}^F = \left(\begin{bmatrix} \frac{2}{8} & \frac{2}{8} \end{bmatrix} \begin{bmatrix} \frac{2}{8} \\ \frac{2}{8} \end{bmatrix} \right)^{-1} \begin{bmatrix} \frac{2}{8} & \frac{2}{8} \end{bmatrix} \begin{bmatrix} \frac{1}{24} \\ \frac{1}{24} \end{bmatrix} = \frac{1}{6}$$

Similarly, for the unit excitation at node 3 we get $\Delta I_2{}^F = \frac{1}{6}$. Therefore $\Delta\hat{\mathbf{I}}_n$ is

$$\Delta\hat{\mathbf{I}}_n = \begin{bmatrix} 0 & 0 \\ \frac{1}{6} & \frac{1}{6} \\ 0 & 0 \end{bmatrix}$$

However, the fact that the first and the third row of $\Delta\hat{\mathbf{I}}_n$ are zero implies that the first and third row of $\Delta\mathbf{Y}_n$ are zero [see (3)]. But $\Delta\mathbf{Y}_n$ is symmetrical, because we are dealing with a passive network, therefore the first and the third columns of $\Delta \mathbf{Y}_n$ are also zero. Using (20) for both current excitations, we can calculate $(\hat{\mathbf{V}}_n + \Delta\hat{\mathbf{V}}_n)$ and for $\mathbf{H}^T = [0 \quad 1 \quad 0]$ we find

$$\mathbf{L} = \mathbf{H}^T(\hat{\mathbf{V}}_n + \Delta\hat{\mathbf{V}}_n) = \begin{bmatrix} \frac{1}{3} & \frac{1}{3} \end{bmatrix}$$

Therefore $\Delta \mathbf{Y}_n \mathbf{H}$ can be obtained from (29) as

$$\Delta \mathbf{Y}_n \mathbf{H} = \begin{bmatrix} 0 \\ \frac{-1}{2} \\ 0 \end{bmatrix}$$

Since $\Delta \mathbf{Y}_n \mathbf{H}$ retains all nonzero columns of $\Delta \mathbf{Y}_n$ we conclude that

$$\Delta \mathbf{Y}_n = \begin{bmatrix} 0 & 0 & 0 \\ 0 & \frac{-1}{2} & 0 \\ 0 & 0 & 0 \end{bmatrix}$$

and we have G_3 as the faulty element with $\Delta G_3 = -0.5$ S.

4.3 Conditions for Sufficient Excitations [10]

A topologically based condition for the determination of the minimum number of excitations has been discussed in Refs. [8–10]. The basic concept is to identify a good sequence of cutsets T_i, $i = 1, 2, \ldots, n$, in such a way that the element values of the branches associated with these cutsets can be determined from the node voltage measurements [13]. Rewrite (20) in the form

$$\hat{\mathbf{V}}_n{}^T \mathbf{Y}_n{}^T = \hat{\mathbf{I}}_n{}^T \tag{30}$$

and consider the product of $\hat{\mathbf{V}}_n{}^T$ and the jth column of $\mathbf{Y}_n{}^T$. We have

$$\hat{\mathbf{V}}_n{}^T \mathbf{y}_j = \begin{bmatrix} (\mathbf{V}_n{}^1)^T \\ (\mathbf{V}_n{}^2)^T \\ \vdots \\ (\mathbf{V}_n{}^n)^T \end{bmatrix} \begin{bmatrix} y_{j1} \\ y_{j2} \\ \vdots \\ y_{jn} \end{bmatrix} = \mathbf{I}_j \tag{31}$$

Let the k unknown elements be identified by the set of indices $C = \{j_1, \ldots, j_k\}$. The set of elements y_{ji}, $i \in C$, is called a reduced cutset. Transferring the known terms from the left-hand side to the right-hand side of (31) and adjusting $\mathbf{I}_j$ properly, we get

$$\hat{\mathbf{V}}_n{}^T \begin{bmatrix} \mathbf{0} \\ y_{jj_1} \\ \vdots \\ y_{jj_k} \\ \mathbf{0} \end{bmatrix} = \hat{\mathbf{V}}_{NC}{}^T \mathbf{y}_j{}^C = \mathbf{I}_j^* \tag{32}$$

where $\mathbf{I}_j^*$ is the modified right-hand side, $\mathbf{y}_j{}^C$ is the reduced cutset admittance vector, and $\hat{\mathbf{V}}_{NC}{}^T$ consists of columns C from $\hat{\mathbf{V}}_n{}^T$.

To determine $\mathbf{y}_j{}^C$ we have to find k rows of (32) such that the resulting square submatrix of $\hat{\mathbf{V}}_{NC}{}^T$ is nonsingular. Let the set $B = \{i_1, \ldots, i_k\}$ determine such rows. Accordingly, we may write (32) as

$$\hat{\mathbf{V}}_{BC}{}^T \mathbf{y}_j{}^C = \mathbf{I}_{jB}^* \tag{33}$$

where $\hat{\mathbf{V}}_{BC}{}^T$ consists of rows B from $\hat{\mathbf{V}}_{NC}{}^T$ and $\mathbf{I}_{jB}^*$ consists of rows B from $\mathbf{I}_j^*$.

According to (30), $\hat{\mathbf{V}}_{BC}{}^T$ can be defined as

$$\hat{\mathbf{V}}_{BC}{}^T = \hat{\mathbf{I}}_{BN}{}^T (\mathbf{Y}^T)_{NC}{}^{-1} \tag{34}$$

where $\hat{\mathbf{I}}_{BN}{}^T$ consists of rows B from $\hat{\mathbf{I}}_n{}^T$ and $(\mathbf{Y}^T)_{NC}{}^{-1}$ consists of columns C from $(\mathbf{Y}_n{}^T)^{-1}$.

Consequently, if the matrix $\hat{\mathbf{V}}_{BC}{}^T$ is nonsingular, there exists D such that $\hat{\mathbf{I}}_{BD}{}^T$ and $(\mathbf{Y}^T)_{DC}{}^{-1}$ are nonsingular. From matrix theory if $(\mathbf{Y}^T)_{DC}{}^{-1}$ is nonsingular then $\mathbf{Y}_n(D|C)$ is nonsingular, where $\mathbf{Y}_n(D|C)$ is the matrix obtained from $\mathbf{Y}_n$ after deleting D rows and C columns. Consider a sequence of sets $T_j, j = j_1, \ldots, j_m$, which correspond to a sequence of reduced cutsets of the network. The following theorem can be formulated.

Theorem 4.2 If independent excitations applied at a subset of network nodes A are sufficient for the identification of all elements of $\mathbf{Y}_n$ then

$$\forall C_j \exists \mathrm{B}_j \subset A \text{ and } \exists D_j\text{: } \det \hat{\mathbf{I}}_{B_j D_j}{}^T \neq 0 \text{ and } \det \mathbf{Y}_n(C_j | D_j) \neq 0 \tag{35}$$

where

$$\operatorname{card} B_j = \operatorname{card} C_j = \operatorname{card} D_j \tag{36}$$

Nodes A in the above theorem are called the injection nodes. It was shown in Ref. [10] that all the corner nodes must be injection nodes. A node is said to be a corner if there exists a complete subgraph containing (1) all edges incoming to this node and (2) all edges having the same weight as any of the incoming ones.

An efficient heuristic algorithm which can be adopted to find injection nodes is presented in Ref. [9]. The algorithm searches for a nearly minimal set of injection nodes in a time that depends linearly on the network size.

Other topological conditions for determining parameter values from node voltage measurements are presented in Refs. [20, 21].

Example 7 Consider the network of Figure 10.13 whose parameters we want to design. The Coates graph of the network is shown in Figure 10.14. Let us assume for simplicity that the independent current excitation $\hat{\mathbf{I}} = \mathbf{1}$. This can easily be achieved when elements are identified through direct voltage measurements. There are three corners in this network, namely nodes 1, 3, and 4. They constitute a sufficient set of injection nodes for this network. Table 10.1 illustrates the reduced cutsets considered and elements associated with them. For identification of network elements, we apply excitations at

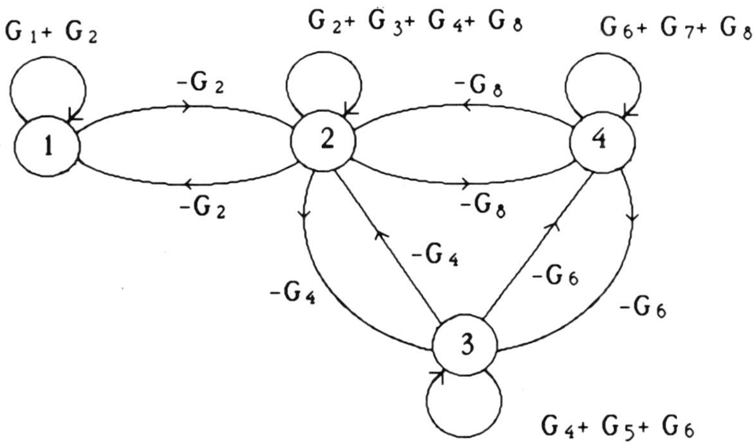

Figure 10.14 Coates signal flow graph.

Table 10.1 Reduced Cutsets

Step i	Nodes in reduced cutset	Elements in reduced cutset to be found
1	1, 2	G_1, G_2
2	2, 3, 4	G_3, G_4, G_8
3	3, 4	G_5, G_6
4	4	G_7

Table 10.2 Nodal Voltages at Excitation Nodes

Excitation at node number	Voltage at node number 1	2	3	4
1	$\frac{35}{59}$	$\frac{11}{59}$	$\frac{5}{59}$	$\frac{4}{59}$
3	$\frac{5}{59}$	$\frac{10}{59}$	$\frac{26}{59}$	$\frac{9}{59}$
4	$\frac{4}{59}$	$\frac{8}{59}$	$\frac{9}{59}$	$\frac{19}{59}$

nodes 1, 3, and 4. The nodal voltages measured with unit excitations at different nodes are shown in Table 10.2.

We formulate equations (33) for successive reduced cutsets and compute element values. The first equation with $B = \{1, 3\}$, $C = \{1, 2\}$, and $j = 1$ is

$$\begin{bmatrix} V_{11} & V_{12} \\ V_{31} & V_{32} \end{bmatrix} \begin{bmatrix} G_1 + G_2 \\ -G_2 \end{bmatrix} = \begin{bmatrix} 1 \\ 0 \end{bmatrix}$$

Therefore we have

$$\begin{bmatrix} \frac{35}{59} & \frac{11}{59} \\ \frac{5}{59} & \frac{10}{59} \end{bmatrix} \begin{bmatrix} G_1 + G_2 \\ -G_2 \end{bmatrix} = \begin{bmatrix} 1 \\ 0 \end{bmatrix}$$

and we obtain $G_1 = 1$, $G_2 = 1$.

The second equation with $B = \{1, 3, 4\}$, $C = \{2, 3, 4\}$, and $j = 2$ can be obtained from

$$\begin{bmatrix} V_{11} & V_{12} & V_{13} & V_{14} \\ V_{31} & V_{32} & V_{33} & V_{34} \\ V_{41} & V_{42} & V_{43} & V_{44} \end{bmatrix} \begin{bmatrix} -G_2 \\ G_2 + G_3 + G_4 + G_8 \\ -G_4 \\ -G_8 \end{bmatrix} = \begin{bmatrix} 0 \\ 0 \\ 0 \end{bmatrix}$$

Since G_2 is known it can be transformed as follows:

$$\begin{bmatrix} V_{12} & V_{13} & V_{14} \\ V_{32} & V_{33} & V_{34} \\ V_{42} & V_{43} & V_{44} \end{bmatrix} \begin{bmatrix} G_3 + G_4 + G_8 \\ -G_4 \\ -G_8 \end{bmatrix} = \begin{bmatrix} (V_{11} - V_{12})G_2 \\ (V_{31} - V_{32})G_2 \\ (V_{41} - V_{42})G_2 \end{bmatrix}$$

$$\begin{bmatrix} \frac{11}{59} & \frac{5}{59} & \frac{4}{59} \\ \frac{10}{59} & \frac{26}{59} & \frac{9}{59} \\ \frac{8}{59} & \frac{9}{59} & \frac{19}{59} \end{bmatrix} \begin{bmatrix} G_3 + G_4 + G_8 \\ -G_4 \\ -G_8 \end{bmatrix} = \begin{bmatrix} \frac{24}{59} \\ \frac{-5}{59} \\ \frac{-4}{59} \end{bmatrix}$$

and we obtain

$$G_3 = 1, \qquad G_4 = 1, \qquad G_8 = 1$$

The third equation with $B = \{1, 4\}$, $C = \{3, 4\}, j = 3$ is given by

$$\begin{bmatrix} V_{13} & V_{14} \\ V_{43} & V_{44} \end{bmatrix} \begin{bmatrix} G_5 + G_6 \\ -G_6 \end{bmatrix} = \begin{bmatrix} (V_{12} - V_{13})G_4 \\ (V_{42} - V_{43})G_4 \end{bmatrix}$$

or

$$\begin{bmatrix} \frac{5}{59} & \frac{4}{59} \\ \frac{9}{59} & \frac{19}{59} \end{bmatrix} \begin{bmatrix} G_5 + G_6 \\ -G_6 \end{bmatrix} = \begin{bmatrix} \frac{6}{59} \\ -\frac{1}{59} \end{bmatrix}$$

and we obtain $G_5 = 1$, $G_6 = 1$. Continuing this procedure, we obtain $G_7 = 2$. Hence, we identify all element values exciting nodes $A = \{1, 3, 4\}$ only instead of exciting all the nodes, as required by (29).

5 MULTIFREQUENCY FAULT DIAGNOSIS

In all the fault diagnosis techniques presented in previous sections it was assumed that the measurements are performed at a single frequency. In general, performing measurements at different frequencies would provide more information about the network we are testing.

A question is how to establish a measure of solvability of test equations. Moreover, what are the test frequencies that should be employed to both optimize solvability and minimize the prediction variances for element values?

These topics are discussed in Refs. [11, 12, 22]. In Ref. [11] the component connection model (CCM) was utilized to derive the fault diagnosis equations in the form of a transfer function matrix. In Ref. [12] the modified nodal analysis was used.

Because the theoretical results appear to be independent of the form of the equations used to represent the network, the classical nodal approach is used here to obtain the fault diagnosis equations [13]. The measure of solvability of these equations is then discussed.

5.1 Multifrequency Fault Diagnosis Equations [11—13]

With M being the set of measurement nodes and N the set of all nodes excluding the reference node, the nodal equations in (1) can be partitioned as

$$\begin{bmatrix} \mathbf{Y}_{MM} & \mathbf{Y}_{M,N-M} \\ \mathbf{Y}_{N-M,M} & \mathbf{Y}_{N-M,N-M} \end{bmatrix} \begin{bmatrix} \mathbf{V}^{M} \\ \mathbf{V}^{N-M} \end{bmatrix} = \begin{bmatrix} \mathbf{I}^{M} \\ \mathbf{I}^{N-M} \end{bmatrix} \tag{37}$$

Assuming $\mathbf{I}^{N-M} = \mathbf{0}$ we can represent the relation between the measurement voltage vector $\mathbf{V}^M$ and the current excitation vector $\mathbf{I}^M$ in the form

$$(\mathbf{Y}_{MM} - \mathbf{Y}_{M,N-M}\mathbf{Y}_{N-M,N-M}{}^{-1}\mathbf{Y}_{N-M,M})\mathbf{V}^M = \mathbf{I}^M \tag{38}$$

From (38) we may define the transfer function matrix

$$\mathbf{Y}(s, r) = \mathbf{Y}_{MM} - \mathbf{Y}_{M,N-M}\mathbf{Y}_{N-M,N-M}{}^{-1}\mathbf{Y}_{N-M,M} \tag{39}$$

where $\mathbf{r} = [r_i]$, $i = 1, 2, \ldots, k$, is the vector of the potentially faulty parameters (elements) and s is the complex frequency. The coefficient matrix $\mathbf{Y}(s, \mathbf{r})$ can be determined by voltage measurements taken under different current excitations and (39) can be used as fault diagnosis equations.

5.2 Measure of Solvability of Fault Diagnosis Equations [11–13]

The fault diagnosis equations (39) are nonlinear with respect to the unknown parameters $\mathbf{r}$. Several such equations can be written for different frequencies while the number of unknowns remains invariant.

Without loss of generality, assume that $\text{vec}(\mathbf{Y}(s, \mathbf{r}))$ transforms $\mathbf{Y}(s, \mathbf{r})$ to a column vector. The fault diagnosis equations take the form

$$\mathbf{E}(\mathbf{r}) = \begin{bmatrix} \text{vec}(\mathbf{Y}(s_1, \mathbf{r})) \\ \text{vec}(\mathbf{Y}(s_2, \mathbf{r})) \\ \vdots \\ \text{vec}(\mathbf{Y}(s_l, \mathbf{r})) \end{bmatrix} \tag{40}$$

where l is the number of test frequencies.

From the implicit function theorem [23] the measure of solvability $\delta(\mathbf{r}_0)$ of the fault diagnosis equations is established by the rank of the Jacobian matrix $\mathbf{J}(\mathbf{r})$ of (40) calculated at some prefixed point $\mathbf{r}_0$ as follows:

$$\delta(\mathbf{r}_0) = k - \rho \tag{41}$$

where $\rho = \text{rank}\,\mathbf{J}(\mathbf{r}_0)$. If $\delta(\mathbf{r}_0) = 0$ this implies that the diagnosis equation has a local unique solution. If $\delta = 1$ the solution is determined up to one arbitrary parameter, and so on, with increasing values of δ representing decreasing measures of solvability.

Since the Jacobian matrix $\mathbf{J}(\mathbf{r})$ is rational in $\mathbf{r}$, then ρ is constant almost everywhere [11]. This in turn permits us to consider the rank of $\mathbf{J}(\mathbf{r})$ which is conditioned by the set of selected test frequencies almost independent of $\mathbf{r}$. As a result, global solvability is determined by the maximum of the rank of the Jacobian matrix $\mathbf{J}(\mathbf{r})$, as formulated in the following theorem [11].

Theorem 5.1 If $\bar{\rho}$ is the maximum number of linearly independent columns of the Jacobian matrix $\mathbf{J}(\mathbf{r})$ evaluated at a prefixed vector $\mathbf{r}$ of arbitrary values over the field of complex numbers, then the minimum value of the measure of solvability $\delta_{\min}$ is given by

$$\delta_{\min} = k - \bar{\rho} \tag{42}$$

and it is achieved by almost any choice of $k - \delta_{\min}$ distinct complex frequencies.

Although the theorem implies that we can randomly choose almost any $k - \delta_{\min}$ test frequencies to maximize the solvability of the fault diagnosis equations, it was observed [11, 22] that the solution is quite sensitive to the choice of test frequencies.

In Ref. [12] another measure of solvability was developed which requires evaluation of the rank of a suitable numerical matrix obtained from knowledge of the Jacobian matrix at a number of fixed frequencies. The basic procedure for obtaining this matrix is outlined below.

Referring to (39), consider as before

$$\text{vec}(\mathbf{Y}(s, \mathbf{r})) = \frac{\mathbf{h}(s, \mathbf{r})}{q(s, \mathbf{r})} \tag{43}$$

The Jacobian matrix evaluated at an arbitrary $\mathbf{r}_0$ is given by

$$\mathbf{J}(s) = \left.\frac{d\,\text{vec}(\mathbf{Y}(s, \mathbf{r}))}{d\mathbf{r}}\right|_{\mathbf{r}=\mathbf{r}_0} = \left[\frac{\mathbf{p}_1(s)}{\Delta(s)}, \ldots, \frac{\mathbf{p}_k(s)}{\Delta(s)}\right] \tag{44}$$

where $\Delta(s) = q^2(s, \mathbf{r}_0)$, and

$$\mathbf{p}_i(s) = q(s, \mathbf{r}_0)\,\frac{\partial \mathbf{h}(s, \mathbf{r})}{\partial r_i} - \mathbf{h}(s, \mathbf{r}_0)\left.\frac{\partial q(s, \mathbf{r})}{\partial r_i}\right|_{\mathbf{r}=\mathbf{r}_0} \tag{46}$$

with $i = 1, 2, \ldots, k$.

Let the matrix $\mathbf{P}(s)$ be defined as

$$\mathbf{P}(s) = [\mathbf{p}_1(s), \ldots, \mathbf{p}_k(s)] \tag{47}$$

An upper limit to the degrees of the polynomials $\mathbf{h}(s, \mathbf{r})$ and $q(s, \mathbf{r})$ is determined by the number of frequency-dependent elements, say x_0. Therefore with the aid of (45), we conclude that $d = 2x_0$ represents an upper limit to the degrees of the polynomials $\mathbf{p}_i(s)$, $i = 1, \ldots, k$.

In general, for n_i inputs and n_o outputs each $\mathbf{p}_i(s)$ column of the $\mathbf{P}(s)$ matrix can be expressed in terms of the following Stirling expansion [12]:

$$\mathbf{p}_i(s) = \sum_{h=0}^{d} S_h(s)\mathbf{b}_{hi} \tag{48}$$

where the Stirling polynomials $S_h(s)$ are defined as

$$S_h(s) = \begin{cases} 1, & h = 0 \\ \prod_{j=1}^{h} (s - s_j), & h > 0 \end{cases} \tag{49}$$

and $\mathbf{b}_{hi}$ are suitable real vectors of order $(n_i \cdot n_o)$ and $s_1, \ldots, s_{d+1}$ are *a priori* fixed frequencies.

Let $\mathbf{B} = [\mathbf{b}_{hi}]$ be the matrix whose ith column ($i = 1, 2, \ldots, k$) is composed of all the elements of vectors $\mathbf{b}_{0i}, \ldots, \mathbf{b}_{di}$, respectively, which are the Stirling coefficients of all the polynomials (46).

Accordingly, $\mathbf{B}$ is composed of $(d + 1)n_i \cdot n_o$ rows and k columns. This numerical matrix $\mathbf{B}$ is useful in establishing the column rank of $\mathbf{J}(s)$, as shown in the following theorem.

Theorem 5.2 The maximum number of linearly independent columns of the Jacobian matrix $\mathbf{J}(s)$ is equal to the rank of the matrix $\mathbf{B}$.

Using this theorem, the global solvability can be determined from

$$\delta_{\min} = k - \operatorname{rank} \mathbf{B} \tag{50}$$

where $\delta_{\min}$ determines the degree of solvability of the diagnosis equations given an optimal choice of test frequencies.

Example 8 Consider the passive network of Figure 10.15. The transfer function V_2/I_{in} is given by

$$\frac{V_2}{I_{\text{in}}} = \frac{G_2}{sC(G_1 + G_2) + G_1G_2 + G_1G_3 + G_2G_3}$$

and $\mathbf{r} = [G_1, G_2, C, G_3]^T$.

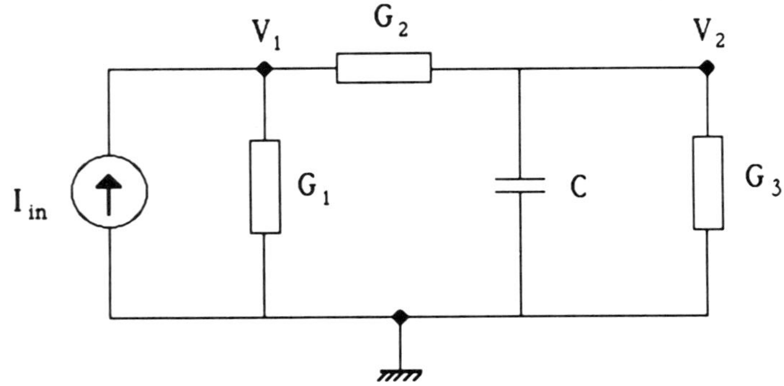

Figure 10.15 Passive network.

The Jacobian matrix $d(V_2/I_{in})/d\mathbf{r}$ is

$$\mathbf{J}(r) = \left[\frac{\partial(V_2/I_{in})}{\partial G_1} \quad \frac{\partial(V_2/I_{in})}{\partial G_2} \quad \frac{\partial(V_2/I_{in})}{\partial C} \quad \frac{\partial(V_2/I_{in})}{\partial G_3} \right]$$

$$= \left[\frac{p_1}{\Delta^2} \quad \frac{p_2}{\Delta^2} \quad \frac{p_3}{\Delta^2} \quad \frac{p_4}{\Delta^2} \right]$$

where

$$\Delta = sC(G_1 + G_2) + G_1G_2 + G_1G_3 + G_2G_3$$

and

$$p_1 = -G_2(sC + G_2 + G_3)$$

$$p_2 = \Delta - G_2(sC + G_1 + G_3)$$

$$p_3 = -sG_2(G_1 + G_2)$$

$$p_4 = -G_2(G_1 + G_2)$$

For a unity nominal value (i.e., $\mathbf{r}_0 = [1 \quad 1 \quad 1 \quad 1]^T$) we have

$$\mathbf{J}(s) = \left[\frac{-(s+2)}{2s+3} \quad \frac{s+1}{2s+3} \quad \frac{-2s}{2s+3} \quad \frac{-2}{2s+3} \right]$$

which has two independent columns over the field of complex numbers, Consequently we obtain $\delta_{min} = 2$ and hence only a single fault can be diagnosed using multifrequency measurements of this transfer function.

Alternatively, we can find the measure of solvability by determining the rank of **B** as follows. Since we have only one frequency-dependent element C, the maximum degree of the polynomials p_i, $i = 1, 2, 3, 4$, is two. Moreover, the Stirling coefficients of these polynomials are obtained using (48) and (49) as follows:

$$p_1(s) = b_{01} + b_{11}(s - s_1)$$

If we choose the test frequencies $s_1 = 1$ and $s_2 = 2$ then

$$b_{01} = p_1(1) = -G_2(C + G_2 + G_3) = -3$$

and

$$\begin{aligned} b_{11} &= p_1(2) - b_{01} = -G_2(2C + G_2 + G_3) + G_2(C + G_2 + G_3) \\ &= -G_2C = -1 \end{aligned}$$

Similarly, the Stirling coefficients of the other three polynomials can be obtained. Consequently the matrix **B** is given by

$$\mathbf{B} = \begin{bmatrix} -3 & 2 & -2 & -2 \\ -1 & 1 & -2 & 0 \end{bmatrix}$$

which is of rank 2. The measure of solvability given by (50) is $\delta_{\min} = 2$, which is the same result as obtained before using (42).

6 CONCLUSIONS

The techniques of fault diagnosis presented in this chapter are based on nodal equations. Using these equations we can formulate the fault diagnosis problem and establish testability conditions, presented in both algebraic and topological forms. We can study the problem of locating faulty regions whenever full testability cannot be attained or solution of fault diagnosis equations is too cumbersome. We can also evaluate faulty branches using relationships between nodal and branch equations expressed through the network topology. Finally, by differentiating the nodal equations, we can find multifrequency conditions for the solvability of the fault diagnosis problem.

REFERENCES

1. J. A. Starzyk and J. W. Bandler, Nodal approach to multiple fault location in analog circuits, *Proc. IEEE Int. Symp. Circuits Syst.*, Rome, pp. 1136–1139, 1982.
2. Z. F. Huang, L. S. Lin, and R. W. Liu, Node fault diagnosis and a design of testability, *IEEE Trans. Circuits Syst.*, vol. CAS-30, pp. 257–265, 1983.
3. J. A. Starzyk and J. W. Bandler, Multiport approach to multiple fault location in analog circuits, *IEEE Trans. Circuits Syst.*, vol. CAS-30, pp. 762–765, 1983.

4. A. A. Sakla, E. I. El-Masry, and T. N. Trick, A sensitivity algorithm for fault location in large analog circuits, *Proc. IEEE Int. Symp. Circuits Syst.*, Houston, pp. 1075–1077, 1980.
5. J. A. Starzyk and M. A. El-Gamal Topological conditions for element evaluation, presented at the 28th Midwest Symp. on Circuits and Systems, Louisville, Kentucky, 1985.
6. M. A. El-Gamal Fault analysis in analog circuits, Ph.D. Dissertation, Ohio Univ., Athens, Ohio, in preparation.
7. J. A. Starzyk and J. W. Bandler, Location of fault regions in analog circuits, Rep. SOS-81-17-R, Simulation Optimization Systems Research Laboratory, McMaster University, Hamilton, Canada, 1981.
8. R. M. Biernacki and J. A. Starzyk, Sufficient test conditions for parameter identification of analog circuits based on voltage measurements, *Proc. Eur. Conf. Circuit Theory and Design*, Warsaw, vol. 2, pp. 233–244, 1980.
9. R. M. Biernacki and J. A. Starzyk, A test generation algorithm for parameter identification of analog circuits, *Proc. Eur. Conf. Circuit Theory and Design*; The Hague, pp. 993–997, 1981.
10. J. A. Starzyk, R. M. Biernacki, and J. W. Bandler, Evaluation of faulty elements within linear subnetworks, *Int. J. Circuit Theory Appl.*, vol. 12, pp. 23–37, 1984.
11. N. Sen and R. Saeks, Fault diagnosis for linear systems via multifrequency measurements, *IEEE Trans. Circuits Syst.*, vol. CAS-26, pp. 457–465, 1979.
12. G. Iuculano, A. Liberatore, S. Manetti, and M. Marini, Multifrequency measurement of testability with application to large linear analog systems, *IEEE Trans. Circuits Syst.*, vol. CAS-33, pp. 644–648, 1986.
13. J. W. Bandler and A. E. Salma, Fault diagnosis in analog circuits, *Proc. IEEE*, vol. 73, pp. 1279–1325, 1985.
14. J. Vlach and K. Singhal, *Computer Methods for Circuit Analysis and Design*, Van Nostrand-Reinhold, New York, 1983.
15. E. T. Browne, *Introduction to the Theory of Determinants and Matrices*, Univ. of North Carolina Press, Chapel Hill, 1958.
16. A. E. Salama, J. A. Starzyk, and J. W. Bandler, A unified decomposition approach for fault location in large analog circuits, *IEEE Trans. Circuits Syst.*, vol. CAS-31, pp. 602–622, 1984.
17. W. K. Chen, *Applied Graph Theory—Graphs and Electrical Networks*, North-Holland, London, 1976.
18. J. A. Starzyk, Signal flow graph analysis by decomposition method, *IEE Proc.*, vol. 127, pt. G, pp. 81–86, 1980.
19. W. Mayeda, *Graph Theory*, Wiley-Interscience, New York, 1972.

20. T. Ozawa and M. Yamada, Conditions for network element value determination by multifrequency measurements, *Proc. IEEE Int. Symp. Circuits Syst.*, Rome, pp. 1156–1159, 1982.
21. T. Ozawa and M. Yamada, Conditions for determining parameter values from node voltage measurements, *Proc. IEEE Int. Symp. Circuits Syst.*, Chicago, pp. 274–277, 1981.
22. G. N. Stenbakken and T. M. Souders, Test point selection and testability measures via QR factorization of linear models, *Proc. 29th Midwest Symp. on Circuits and Systems*, Lincoln, Nebraska, 1986.
23. W. Fleming, *Functions of Several Variables*, Addison-Wesley, Reading, Mass., 1965.

11
Tableau Approach to Fault Diagnosis

Lawrence A. Rapisarda

U.S. Military Academy
West Point, New York

Raymond A. DeCarlo

Purdue University
West Lafayette, Indiana

1 INTRODUCTION

The proliferation of large circuits and systems of ever-increasing complexity has stirred great interest in automated methods for troubleshooting or fault diagnosis. One philosophical approach to fault diagnosis uses a two-stage procedure: (1) DC testing to determine hard faults (shorts, opens, catastrophic changes in bias points, etc.) and (2) multifrequency testing of the system/circuit linearized about its operating points to identify soft faults (parameter variations inimical to system performance). This chapter addresses stage 2 of such a perspective and presents the so-called tableau approach to multifrequency testing of linearized circuits. A scheme for stage 1 follows in Chapter 12.

The philosophy underlying the tableau approach merits some discussion, which is best undertaken by drawing an analogy between two types of circuit models. Suppose one wished to determine the frequency response of a linearized circuit. The direct approach would be to combine the circuit element information with the Kirchhoff voltage and current laws (KVL and KCL) to produce a transfer function model of the circuit. Evaluation of the transfer function over the proper frequency range would produce the desired frequency response. Alternatively, one could arrange the device equations and the KVL and KCL equations into a large structured table (or tableau) without combining them together. On specification of a frequency or range of frequencies, the tableau becomes a matrix equation whose solution determines all voltages and/or currents, from which the circuit response is found. Although the latter approach includes a large number of superfluous variables, it avoids the difficulty of computing a transfer function of a large circuit, is well suited to implementation on a digital computer, and turns out to be a numerically well-conditioned representation solvable by numerically well-conditioned methods such as the LU decomposition and Gauss elimination.

The tableau approach to fault diagnosis also computes superfluous variables but again avoids the need to compute a circuit transfer function model. In addition, it is well suited to the digital computer, has reasonable numerical conditioning, and permits the selection of an optimum step size for each interaction of a Newton-Raphson solution technique normally used to solve large sets of nonlinear equations.

The next section describes the component connection model (CCM), which is the circuit model underlying the tableau approach.

2 COMPONENT CONNECTION MODEL

2.1 Introduction

Underlying the forthcoming fault diagnosis approach is an interconnected system model called the component connection model, abbreviated CCM [1–3]. The purpose of this section is to introduce the CCM notation needed to develop the fault diagnosis tableau.

Two sets of equations constitute the CCM: (1) component characteristic equations and (2) interconnection or topological equations. Basically, all system models are equivalent. The differences lie in the way the system information is displayed. The CCM maintains separate descriptions of the component dynamics and system topology. Such descriptions result in large numbers of equations and unknowns. In matrix form the equations are very sparse and hence admit the use of sparse matrix storage and manipulation techniques [4]. For large systems, storage requirements are often lower than those for smaller nonsparse composite system representations. In some applications, use of the CCM has produced dramatic improvements in the use of computing resources. The most notable example is the MARYSAS program, which used the CCM in a simulation of a Space Shuttle engine model. The program performed the simulation 26 times faster than previous simulations used by NASA [5].

2.2 CCM Preliminaries

Figure 11.1 shows a linear system consisting of N components. The components are shown explicitly as numbered blocks. The horseshoe labeled "interconnections" represents only the information describing how the components are connected to each other and to the outside world.

The system input is the vector u and the system output is the vector y. Each component of the system has input and output vectors a_i and b_i, respectively ($i = 1, 2, \ldots, N$). The component inputs and outputs will often be handed collectively, so for convenience define the column vectors

$$a = \text{col}(a_1, a_2, \ldots, a_N)$$

$$b = \text{col}(b_1, b_2, \ldots, b_N) \tag{1}$$

The vectors a and b denote the composite component input and composite component output vectors. The composite component output b is related to the composite component input a via the component characteristics. The composite component input a is related to both b and u (the external system input) through the interconnection or topological equations. Finally, the system output y depends on the composite component output b and the system input u.

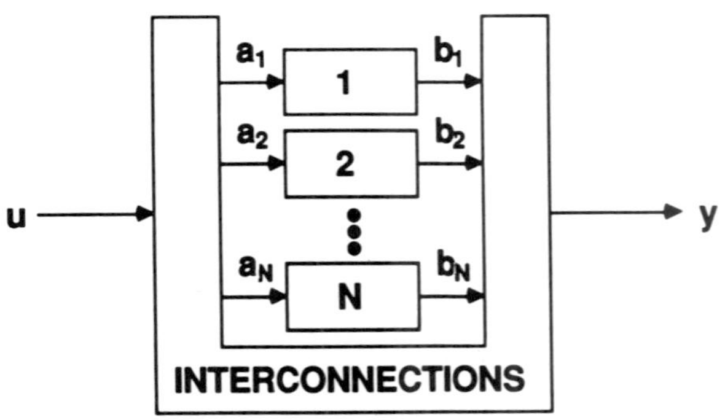

Figure 11.1 Linear system with N components.

2.3 Component Equations

Since the focus here is linear systems, the components can be characterized by a transfer function in the frequency domain. Let $Z_i(s_i \to s, r_i)$ denote the transfer function matrix for component i, where s is the Laplace transform variable and r_i is a vector parameter which characterizes component i. The object of the fault diagnosis procedure developed in this chapter is to identify (diagnose) the value of r_i ($i = 1, 2, \ldots, N$).

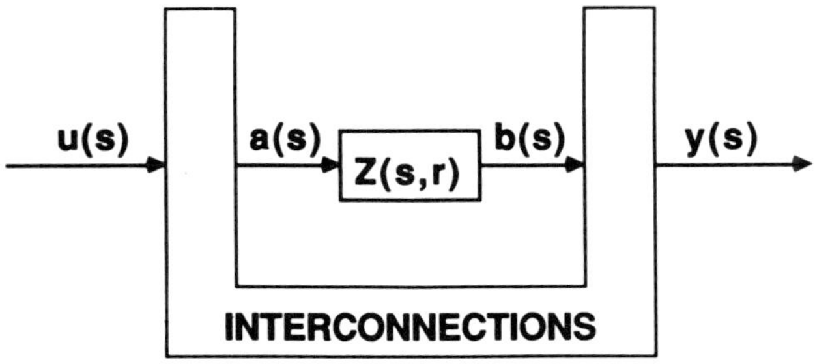

Figure 11.2 Illustration of the relationship of the composite transfer function to the entire system.

Let $a_i(s)$ and $b_i(s)$ be the Laplace transforms of the component input and output vectors. Then the component characteristic equation for component i is

$$b_i(s) = Z_i(s, r_i)a_i(s) \tag{2}$$

Define

$$r = \text{col}(r_1, r_2, \ldots, r_N) \tag{3}$$

and

$$Z(s, r) = \text{block-diag}[Z_1(s, r_1), Z_2(s, r_2), \ldots, Z_n(s, r_n)] \tag{4}$$

The characteristic relation for all the components can now be written compactly as

$$b(s) = Z(s, r)a(s) \tag{5}$$

where $a(s)$ and $b(s)$ are the Laplace transforms of the composite component input and composite component output vectors. The matrix $Z(s, r)$ is called the composite component transfer function matrix. It is sparse due to its block diagonal structure.

Figure 11.2 illustrates the relationship of the composite component transfer function to the entire system.

2.4 Connection Equations

The connection equations model the component interconnection constraints. These constraints are linear and algebraic, representing conservation laws such as Kirchhoff's current and voltage laws. Let $u(s)$ be the Laplace transform of the system input vector and $y(s)$ the Laplace transform of the system output vector. From Figure 11.2, note that the inputs to the interconnections are $u(s)$ and $b(s)$ and the outputs from the interconnections are $a(s)$ and $y(s)$. This leads, naturally, to the following form for the connection equations:

$$a(s) = L_{11}b(s) + L_{12}u(s) \tag{6}$$

$$y(s) = L_{21}b(s) + L_{22}u(s) \tag{7}$$

where the L_{ij} are called the connection matrices and are generally very sparse. This occurs because most circuit elements and/or subsystem blocks have physical connections to only a few "neighbors."

A small example described in the next section best summarizes the above development.

2.5 CCM Example

Figure 11.3 is a circuit consisting of three components, two resistors and a capacitor. The components are shown separated from their positions in the circuit to emphasize the difference between the connection equations and the component equations. The circuit input is u and the output is $y = [y_1, y_2]^t$. Using the usual resistor and capacitor equations as component models produces the following composite component transfer function matrix equation:

$$\begin{bmatrix} b_1(s) \\ b_2(s) \\ b_3(s) \end{bmatrix} = \begin{bmatrix} r_1 & 0 & 0 \\ 0 & r_2/s & 0 \\ 0 & 0 & r_3 \end{bmatrix} \begin{bmatrix} a_1(s) \\ a_2(s) \\ a_3(s) \end{bmatrix} \tag{8}$$

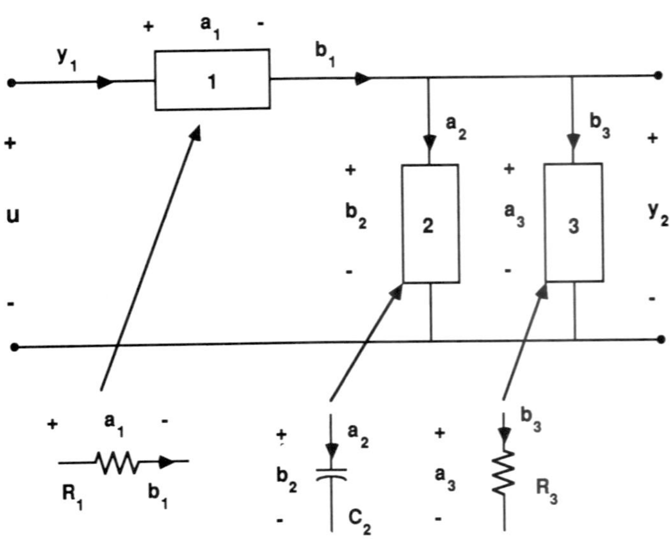

Figure 11.3 CCM example circuit.

where $r_1 = 1/R_1$, $r_2 = 1/C_2$, and $r_3 = 1/R_3$. Note that this equation is independent of the connections. It was derived by relating the component outputs and inputs through the component dynamics.

Next, consider the connections. By using KVL and KCL on the circuit, the following equations result:

$$\begin{bmatrix} a_1(s) \\ a_2(s) \\ a_3(s) \end{bmatrix} = \begin{bmatrix} 0 & -1 & 0 \\ 1 & 0 & -1 \\ 0 & 1 & 0 \end{bmatrix} \begin{bmatrix} b_1(s) \\ b_2(s) \\ b_3(s) \end{bmatrix} + \begin{bmatrix} 1 \\ 0 \\ 0 \end{bmatrix} u(s) \tag{9}$$

$$\begin{bmatrix} y_1(s) \\ y_2(s) \end{bmatrix} = \begin{bmatrix} 1 & 0 & 0 \\ 0 & 1 & 0 \end{bmatrix} \begin{bmatrix} b_1(s) \\ b_2(s) \\ b_3(s) \end{bmatrix} + \begin{bmatrix} 0 \\ 0 \end{bmatrix} u(s) \tag{10}$$

Note also that the interconnection equations did not require any knowledge of the actual component dynamics.

Most notable in the example is the large number of zero entries in the $Z(s, r)$ and L_{ij} matrices. In fact, the number of nonzero entries in the system matrices usually increases as the order of the number of components (i.e., linearly), resulting in extremely sparse matrices for large systems.

2.6 Simulation

The tableau approach to simulation requires solving the following matrix equation, which amounts to a simultaneous statement of (5) and (6).

$$\begin{bmatrix} Z(s, r) & -I \\ -I & L_{11} \end{bmatrix} \begin{bmatrix} a(s) \\ b(s) \end{bmatrix} = \begin{bmatrix} 0 \\ -L_{12}u(s) \end{bmatrix} \tag{11}$$

For any value of complex frequency s and input $u(s)$, the solution of the sparse system (11) becomes the input to (7) to establish the system response. For example, Figure 11.3 yields the following tableau:

$$\begin{bmatrix} r_1 & 0 & 0 & -1 & 0 & 0 \\ 0 & r_2/s & 0 & 0 & -1 & 0 \\ 0 & 0 & r_3 & 0 & 0 & -1 \\ -1 & 0 & 0 & 0 & -1 & 0 \\ 0 & -1 & 0 & 1 & 0 & -1 \\ 0 & 0 & -1 & 0 & 1 & 0 \end{bmatrix} \begin{bmatrix} a_1(s) \\ a_2(s) \\ a_3(s) \\ b_1(s) \\ b_2(s) \\ b_3(s) \end{bmatrix} = \begin{bmatrix} 0 \\ 0 \\ 0 \\ -u(s) \\ 0 \\ 0 \end{bmatrix} \tag{12}$$

Conceptually, the problem of fault diagnosis is the inverse of simulation. The development of a set of fault diagnosis equations then requires a special rearrangement of the system simulation equations to permit a viable solution for the component parameter values.

3 DEVELOPMENT OF THE TABLEAU EQUATIONS

3.1 PROBLEM STATEMENT

The general fault diagnosis problem can be formulated as follows. Given the following information:

1. An appropriately modeled linear network containing N components, each component characterized by a parameter r_i, $i = 1, 2, \ldots, N$
2. A set of test input measurements
3. A set of test output measurements

determine the parameters r_i, $i = 1, 2, \ldots, N$. Measurements at a single test frequency may be insufficient to determine all the parameters. Thus it is necessary to make a series of measurements at enough different test frequencies to provide sufficient data to uniquely specify all parameters.

There are two major approaches to multifrequency fault diagnosis for linear systems based on the use of the CCM:

1. The composite transfer function approach developed by Sen and Saeks [6]
2. The tableau approach developed in Refs. [7–9]

In conformance with the perspective presented in the Introduction, our concentration is on the tableau approach, the solution of the sparse system (11).

3.2 Derivations of the Fault Diagnosis Equations

The development of the fault diagnosis equations begins with the frequency domain tableau of equations (7) and (11):

$$\begin{bmatrix} Z(s, r) & -I \\ -I & L_{11} \end{bmatrix} \begin{bmatrix} a(s) \\ b(s) \end{bmatrix} = \begin{bmatrix} 0 \\ -L_{12}u(s) \end{bmatrix} \tag{11}$$

$$y(s) = L_{21}b(s) + L_{22}u(s) \tag{7}$$

Suppose that the output $y^M(s)$ is observed. The superscript M emphasizes the test measurement status of the system output $y(s)$. Apply the simulation procedure in reverse by putting $y^M(s)$ into the output equation (7) and gathering known quantities together to obtain

$$L_{21}b(s) = y^M(s) - L_{22}u(s) \tag{13}$$

The only unknown in (13) is the composite component output vector $b(s)$. A closer look at the properties of L_{21} is necessary in order to determine the nature of the solution.

In any practical situation the number of system outputs is less than the number of component outputs. (Measurement at essentially every point within a system makes the fault diagnosis problem trivial but it is unfortunately seldom practical.) To be consistent with this practical consideration, make the following assumption:

Assumption 1 For the $n_y \times n_b$ matrix L_{21}, where n_y = number of outputs and n_b = dimension of $b(\cdot)$, *assume* $n_b > n_y$.

Furthermore, it is reasonable to assume the observations are independent, that is, each row of L_{21} (each row determines an output) is independent of the other rows. Hence:

Assumption 2 The matrix L_{21} has full row rank.

To solve (13) note that assumption 2 ensures that L_{21} has a right inverse, say $L_{21}{}^{-R}$ [10], and therefore a solution to (13) must exist. Unfortunately, assumption 1 also implies that L_{21} must have a nontrivial null space and therefore there are infinitely many solutions to (13). The solution family may be characterized in the following way [7–9].

$$b(s) = b_0(s) + V\alpha(s) \tag{14}$$

where (1) $b_0(s) = L_{21}{}^{-R}[y^M(s) - L_{22}u(s)]$ is a particular solution to (13); (2) $V = [v_1, \ldots, v_p]$ has columns which are a basis for the p-dimensional null space of L_{21}; and (3) $\alpha(s) = \mathrm{col}[\alpha_1(s), \alpha_2(s), \ldots, \alpha_p(s)]$ is a vector of possibly complex scalar functions of s.

As $b_0(s)$ can be thought of as a particular solution to (13), $V\alpha(s)$ lives in the null space of L_{21} and characterizes the ambiguity in determining $b(s)$ given the input-output measurement $[u(s), y^M(s)]$. The use of multiple test frequencies arises from the need to resolve such ambiguity intrinsically present in any realistic formulation of the problem.

Since diagnosis typically requires more than one test frequency and/or input vector [remember $u(s)$ can be multidimensional], let q equal the required number of test frequencies with corresponding inputs denoted $s = s_i$ and $u(s) = u(s_i)$, $i = 1, 2, \ldots, q$. Then (14) becomes a family of equations:

$$b(s_i) = b_0(s_i) + V\alpha(s_i) \qquad i = 1, 2, \ldots, q \tag{15}$$

A little thought suggests that $a(s_i)$ also has a form similar to (15). In particular, one may write

$$a(s_i) = a_0(s_i) + L_{11}V\alpha(s_i) \qquad i = 1, 2, \ldots, q \tag{16}$$

where

$$a_0(s_i) = L_{11}b_0(s_i) + L_{21}u(s_i) \tag{17}$$

This relationship follows after substituting (15) into the connection equation, $a(s) = L_{11}b(s) + L_{12}u(s)$, and making the identification given in (17).

Combining (15) and (16) with the composite component equation, $b(s) = Z(s, r)a(s)$, yields the family of diagnosis equations:

$$b_0(s_i) + V\alpha(s_i) = Z(s_i)[a_0(s_i) + L_{11}V\alpha(s_i)] \qquad i = 1, 2, \ldots, q \tag{18}$$

which must be solved simultaneously for r and $\alpha(s_i)$, $i = 1, 2, \ldots, q$. Finally, these equations (18) can be succinctly rewritten in the following product form [7–9]:

$$[Z(s_i, r) | -V]\begin{bmatrix} L_{11}V\alpha(s_i) + a_0(s_i) \\ \alpha(s_i) \end{bmatrix} = b_0(s_i) \qquad i = 1, 2, \ldots, q \tag{19}$$

The family of equations thus defined constitute the tableau form of the fault diagnosis equations. Notice that this set of equations does not require the computation of the composite transfer function matrix. The nonlinear aspect of these equations resides in the terms $Z(s_i, r)L_{11}V\alpha(s_i)$, and the order of the nonlinearity does not increase as the size of the system increases. In fact, for systems where the components have the form $Z_i(s, r_i) = r_i Z_i(s)$ the equations are quadratic regardless of system size. Further discussion of these points follows.

4 SOLUTION OF THE FAULT DIAGNOSIS EQUATIONS

4.1 Product Formulation

The product form of (19) lends itself to the following compact characterization of the fault diagnosis equations [7–9]:

$$F(x) = \begin{bmatrix} f_1(r)g_1(\boldsymbol{\alpha}_1) - \beta_1 \\ \vdots \\ f_q(r)g_q(\boldsymbol{\alpha}_q) - \beta_q \end{bmatrix} = \theta \tag{20}$$

where

1. $\boldsymbol{\alpha}_i = \alpha(s_i)$
2. $x = \text{col}(\boldsymbol{\alpha}_1, \boldsymbol{\alpha}_2, \ldots, \boldsymbol{\alpha}_q, r)$

3. $f_i(r) = [Z(s_i, r)| - V]$
4. $g_i(\boldsymbol{\alpha}_i) = \begin{bmatrix} L_{11}V\boldsymbol{\alpha}_i + a_0(s_i) \\ \boldsymbol{\alpha}_i \end{bmatrix}$
5. $\beta_i = b_0(s_i)$
6. θ is the zero vector

The solution to (20) is readily determined by employing the Newton-Raphson iteration scheme:

$$J_F(x^k)(x^{k+1} - x^k) = -F(x^k) \tag{21}$$

where

1. x^k is the kth estimate of the root
2. J_F is the Jacobian of $F(\cdot)$

The dimension of r is N, the dimension of $\boldsymbol{\alpha}_i$ is p, and the dimension of x is $N + pq$.

There are two special characteristics of this formulation which may be exploited to improve the efficiency of the N-R iteration: (1) the sparseness of J_F in (21) and (2) the quadratic nature of $F(x)$, which arises in many situations of interest.

4.2 Sparse Jacobian

As a result of the product structure of (20) the Jacobian has a sparse elegant structure [7–9]:

$$J_F(x) = \begin{bmatrix} f_1(r)\dfrac{\partial g_1}{\partial \boldsymbol{\alpha}_1}(\boldsymbol{\alpha}_1) & 0 & \cdot & 0 & \dfrac{\partial f_1}{\partial r}(r)g_1(\boldsymbol{\alpha}_1) \\ 0 & f_2(r)\dfrac{\partial g_2}{\partial \boldsymbol{\alpha}_2}(\boldsymbol{\alpha}_2) \cdot & & \cdot & \cdot \\ \cdot & 0 & \cdot & 0 & \cdot \\ \cdot & \cdot & & \cdot\, f_q(r)\dfrac{\partial g_q}{\partial \boldsymbol{\alpha}_q}(\boldsymbol{\alpha}_q) & \dfrac{\partial f_q}{\partial r}(r)g_q(\boldsymbol{\alpha}_q) \end{bmatrix} \tag{22}$$

where

$$f_i(r)\frac{\partial g_i}{\partial \boldsymbol{\alpha}_i}(\boldsymbol{\alpha}_i) = Z(s_i, r)L_{11}V - V \tag{23}$$

and

$$\frac{\partial f_i}{\partial r}(r)g_i(\boldsymbol{\alpha}_i) = \left[\frac{\partial Z}{\partial r_1}(s_i, r)[L_{11}V\boldsymbol{\alpha}_i + a_0(s_i)]\right|\cdots\left|\frac{\partial Z}{\partial r_N}(s_i, r)[L_{11}V\boldsymbol{\alpha}_i + a_0(s_i)]\right] \tag{24}$$

Note that

$$f_i(r)\frac{\partial g_i}{\partial \alpha_i}(\boldsymbol{\alpha}_i)$$

is independent of $\boldsymbol{\alpha}_i$. Also notice that when the components have the form $Z_j(s, r_j) = r_j Z_j(s)$ (e.g., *RLC* circuit elements) then

$$\frac{\partial f_i}{\partial r}(r) g_i(\boldsymbol{\alpha}_i)$$

forms a diagonal block of $J_F(\cdot)$ which is independent of r. Thus the Jacobian associated with the tableau fault diagnosis equations has an elegant simple sparse structure which allows greater efficiency in programming a solution to (20) than is generally possible [4].

4.3 Exploitation of the Quadratic Form of the Tableau

An extremely important special case arises when all of the entries of the component transfer function matrix have the form

$$Z_i(s, r_i) = r_i Z_i(s) \tag{25}$$

In this case one readily notices that each of the product terms of (20) is affine [11] and the components of $F(x)$ are always quadratic polynomials in x, regardless of the number of components in the system! In the case of electrical networks this form of component transfer function suffices for modeling resistors, inductors, capacitors, and dependent sources. This means that (20) has this quadratic form for any circuit modeled by an interconnection of the above components. This is an extremely large category of possible circuits.

The significance of this special form is that it represents specific information about tableau fault diagnosis equations which, under appropriate circumstances, is useful in determining their solution. Specifically, the quadratic form permits an exact characterization of its behavior along an N-R search direction. This provides a simple means of precisely establishing the point along the search direction at which the norm of the nonlinear function $F(x)$ is a minimum. Use of this "minimum point" as the next estimate of the solution is designed to guarantee and streamline the convergence of the N-R iteration.

Consider the following modification of the N-R algorithm. Let the next estimate of the solution to $F(x) = \theta$ be $x^{k+1} = x^k + \lambda d$, where d satisfies $J_F(x^k)d = -F(x^k)$. One chooses λ by selecting the value which minimizes

$$\|F(x^{k+1})\|^2 = \|F(x^k + \lambda d^k)\|^2 \tag{26}$$

over λ.

For circumstances which ordinarily might cause the N-R algorithm to diverge, this modification results in a nondiverging algorithm [12]. The quadratic form of $F(x)$ means that (26) is a fourth-order polynomial in λ. This permits the following simple and exact method for determining λ:

Step 1. Evaluate $\|F(x^k + \lambda d^k)\|^2$ at five values of λ. Call these $G_i \triangleq G(\lambda_i)$, $i = 1, \ldots, 5$.

> *Remark:* Because of the form of the tableau fault diagnosis equations, this requires matrix additions and multiplications only. No matrix inverses are necessary.

Step 2. Generate a fourth-order interpolant $h(\lambda)$ for the data from step 1.

> *Remark:* Although it is possible to generate the coefficients of $\|F(x^k + \lambda d^k)\|^2$ by substituting $x^k + \lambda d^k$ into the expression for F and using algebra to reduce it to a polynomial in λ, it is far simpler in a computer implementation to use steps 1 and 2 for the following reasons. First, any computer implementation of the Newton-Raphson algorithm must already have a routine for computing the value of F. Second, since the $\|F\|^2$ is a fourth-degree polynomial in λ, then $h(\lambda)$ is equal to $\|F(x^k + \lambda d^k)\|^2$ for all λ (since the interpolant is the same order as F). Specifically, if we express $h(\lambda)$ as the polynomial $c_1\lambda^4 + \cdots + c_5$, then the coefficients c_i are found by solving

$$\begin{bmatrix} c_1 \\ c_2 \\ c_3 \\ c_4 \\ c_5 \end{bmatrix} = \begin{bmatrix} \lambda_1{}^4 & \lambda_1{}^3 & \lambda_1{}^2 & \lambda_1 & 1 \\ \lambda_2{}^4 & \lambda_2{}^3 & \lambda_2{}^2 & \lambda_2 & 1 \\ \lambda_3{}^4 & \lambda_3{}^3 & \lambda_3{}^2 & \lambda_3 & 1 \\ \lambda_4{}^4 & \lambda_4{}^3 & \lambda_4{}^2 & \lambda_4 & 1 \\ \lambda_5{}^4 & \lambda_5{}^3 & \lambda_5{}^2 & \lambda_5 & 1 \end{bmatrix}^{-1} \begin{bmatrix} G_1 \\ G_2 \\ G_3 \\ G_4 \\ G_5 \end{bmatrix} \tag{27}$$

Step 3. Find the roots of the equation $dh(\lambda)/d\lambda = 0$.

> *Remark:* This solution is easily computed since $dh(\lambda)/d\lambda$ is a third-degree polynomial.

Step 4. Let λ equal that root for which (26) is minimum.

The result of this procedure is a value for λ which minimizes $\|F(x^k - \lambda d^k)\|^2$ along the search direction, d^k. This is the optimum choice for λ made possible by the quadratic nature of the tableau fault diagnosis equations.

We next turn to a discussion of the conditions necessary for a solvable set of fault diagnosis equations.

5 DIAGNOSABILITY AND WELL POSEDNESS

5.1 Diagnosability and Its Consequences

Before attempting to determine a solution for (20), it is reasonable to ask whether such a venture is worthwhile. Specifically, if the test data are insufficient, it is impossible to determine uniquely the faulty parameter vector r. This leads naturally to the following definition.

Definition 1 A circuit/system modeled by (11) and (7) (the CCM) is said to be *diagnosable* if and only if there exist frequency, input pairs $[s_i, u(s_i)]$ $i = 1, 2, \ldots, q$, with q finite, for which a solution to (20) exists and is an isolated solution.

To determine whether a circuit with specified test frequencies and corresponding inputs and measured outputs is *diagnosable* use

Theorem 1 Suppose a circuit/system is characterized by a parameter vector r. Let x be a solution to (20) which includes the subvector r. Then the circuit/system is diagnosable for the parameter vector r if there are sufficient test frequencies s_i and corresponding inputs $u(s_i)$, $i = 1, 2, \ldots, q$, such that $J_F(x)$ has full column rank.

Proof. References [8] and [9] provide the details of the proof. The basis for the truth of Theorem 1 is the fact that a local inverse for $F(\cdot)$ must exist at x if $J_F(x)$ has full column rank and the inverse function theorem ensures that $F(x + e)$ is not equal to θ (e is a vector of very small entries). Hence the solution is isolated, satisfying the definition above.

To be of any practical use, the fact that $J_F(\cdot)$ has full column rank at some specific solution point must imply that it has full column rank elsewhere. This is important for two reasons. First, the N-R iteration scheme requires that $J_F(x)$ have full column rank to uniquely solve the N-R step for a sequence of estimates x^k. If at any point there is no unique solution, the iteration scheme could not proceed. Second, it would be reassuring to know that when a circuit/system is designed to be diagnosable for some nominal parameter vector r, it will still be diagnosable should the parameter vector change due to aging or other environmental disturbance.

In practice, the use of the N-R iteration scheme requires that $J_F(x)$ have full column rank almost everywhere. In this context almost everywhere means everywhere except in a lower-dimensional algebraic variety [13]. If this is true, then whenever the algorithm encounters a “bad” value for x an arbitrarily small perturbation of x will yield a value from which the iteration can continue.

Theorem 2 Suppose $x^* \in R^{N+pq}$ and $J_F(x^*)$ has full column rank. Then $J_F(x)$ has full column rank for almost all $x \in R^{N+pq}$.

Proof. Again, details are available in Ref. [8] or [9]. The set of points for which the Jacobian fails to have full rank is the zero set of a polynomial in x which is not identical to zero [since there is at least one point (x^*) for which the Jacobian has full rank]. Such a zero set must have a dimension less than $N + pq$ (the dimension of x).

The question still remains: Can the parameter vector change to make a diagnosable circuit nondiagnosable? Diagnosability is defined only for those points $x \in R^{N+pq}$ which are possible solutions to (20), and this is an N-dimensional subset of R^{N+pq}. Clearly, measure over R^{N+pq} is not appropriate to this situation. Since the solution space is isomorphic to R^N [8] the measure over R^N is used in the following:

Theorem 3 Suppose a circuit/system whose component characteristics are rational functions of r is known to be diagnosable via Theorem 1 for parameter vector r^*. Then it is diagnosable for almost all $r \in R^N$.

Proof. The proof is similar to (but more involved than) the proof of Theorem 2 and is found in Refs. [8, 9].

Theorems 2 and 3 are quite subtle but important. Theorem 2 ensures that the solution algorithm is robust. Theorem 3 means that diagnosability is a generic property of the circuit/system and is independent of the actual parameter values.

5.2 Test Frequency Requirements

The use of Theorem 1 requires the selection of appropriate test frequencies. Selection of the "best" test frequencies for the solution algorithm depends on the parameter values of the circuit under diagnosis. Although nominal values for the parameter vector are known, the faulted values are unpredictable. Hence it is not possible to make this selection in an optimal manner. Nevertheless, it is possible to place some simple bounds on the number of test input/frequency combinations necessary to satisfy the conditions of Theorem 1. We present the bounds for both real and complex test frequencies. The use of real test frequencies is more suitable for problem illustration, while complex frequencies (sinusoidal test signals) are more commonly used for actual testing.

Theorem 4 (lower bound) Suppose a circuit/system has N real parameters and $\mathrm{Dim}\{\mathrm{null}[L_{21}]\} = p$. The minimum number of test frequencies (with corresponding inputs), $q_{\min}$, required to make the circuit/system diagnosable is $\lceil N/(M - p) \rceil$ for real test frequencies and $\lceil N/[2(M - p)] \rceil$ for complex test frequencies, where the $\lceil \; \rceil$ indicates "least upper-bounding integer" and M is the row dimension of $Z(\cdot, \cdot)$.

Proof. A proof for complex frequencies appears in Refs. [8] and [9] and is similar to the following proof for real test frequencies. Each of the terms $f_i(r)g_i(\boldsymbol{\alpha}_i) - \beta_i = 0$ in (20) consists of M scalar equations in $N + p$ unknowns. (Recall that $f_i(r) = [Z(s_i\ r)| - V]$.) N unknowns correspond to the parameter subvector r and are common to each set. Thus for q test frequencies there will be qM equations with $N + qp$ unknowns. A necessary condition for this system of equations to have a solution is $qM \geqslant N + qp$; hence the bound given above.

Note: Implicit in the above proof is the fact that M must be greater than p in order for q to be positive and finite. Intuitively, if the dimension of ambiguity at any single test frequency is not strictly less than the number of scalar equations generated by each test frequency, no choice of test frequencies could possibly resolve it.

Theorem 5 (upper bound) Consider the same circuit/system as in Theorem 4. If it is diagnosable, the maximum number of test inputs/frequencies necessary is N.

Proof. Again for real test frequencies: Each test frequency yields M scalar equations in $N + p$ unknowns. Therefore the first test input/frequency produces $N + p$ unknowns and each subsequent measurement introduces p more. Clearly, if each such set of M equations contributes p (or fewer) independent equations to the entire set, there could be no locally unique solution. On the other hand, if each contributes $p + 1$, a locally unique solution is possible. Since the circuit/system is diagnosable by hypothesis, then the worst case (requiring the most test frequencies) is $p + 1$ independent equations per test frequency. In this case q must satisfy: $q(p + 1) \geqslant N + pq$ and therefore $q \geqslant N$. Since $q = N$ is the minimum integer which satisfies the worst case, this must be the most test frequencies necessary.

N is also the upper limit for complex test frequencies (the theorem statement made no distinction). This proof appears in Refs. [8] and [9].

For a given circuit it is now possible to choose test frequencies and determine whether the choice renders the circuit diagnosable for some nominal set of parameters. After a circuit is found to be diagnosable, the Newton-Raphson iteration scheme can be used to solve for the actual values for those parameters from measurements taken at the selected frequencies. An example is now in order.

6 EXAMPLES

6.1 Simple First Example

The example presented below is the same example used to illustrate the CCM at the beginning of the chapter (Figure 11.3). Recall that the following CCM equations form this example:

$$\begin{bmatrix} b_1(s) \\ b_2(s) \\ b_3(s) \end{bmatrix} = \begin{bmatrix} r_1 & 0 & 0 \\ 0 & r_2/s & 0 \\ 0 & 0 & r_3 \end{bmatrix} \begin{bmatrix} a_1(s) \\ a_2(s) \\ a_3(s) \end{bmatrix} \tag{8}$$

$$\begin{bmatrix} a_1(s) \\ a_2(s) \\ a_3(s) \end{bmatrix} = \begin{bmatrix} 0 & -1 & 0 \\ 1 & 0 & -1 \\ 0 & 1 & 0 \end{bmatrix} \begin{bmatrix} b_1(s) \\ b_2(s) \\ b_3(s) \end{bmatrix} + \begin{bmatrix} 1 \\ 0 \\ 0 \end{bmatrix} u(s) \tag{9}$$

$$\begin{bmatrix} y_1(s) \\ y_2(s) \end{bmatrix} = \begin{bmatrix} 1 & 0 & 0 \\ 0 & 1 & 0 \end{bmatrix} \begin{bmatrix} b_1(s) \\ b_2(s) \\ b_3(s) \end{bmatrix} + \begin{bmatrix} 0 \\ 0 \end{bmatrix} u(s) \tag{10}$$

In addition to the information provided in (8), (9), and (10), the tableau approach requires a right inverse for L_{21} and V, a basis for the null space of L_{21}. These can be computed very efficiently using singular value decomposition techniques [14] such as those found in IMSL [15] or LINPACK [16]. In this example L_{21} is small enough to note that $p = 1$ and to compute the following by inspection.

$$L_{21}{}^{-R} = \begin{bmatrix} 1 & 0 \\ 0 & 1 \\ 0 & 0 \end{bmatrix} \tag{28}$$

$$V = [v_1] = \begin{bmatrix} 0 \\ 0 \\ 1 \end{bmatrix} \tag{29}$$

Notice also that $N = 3$ (the number of parameters) and $M = 3$ (the row dimension of Z). According to Theorem 4, the minimum number of real test frequencies needed to diagnose this circuit is $[N/(M - p)] = [3/(3 - 1)] = 2$. Choose two real test frequencies: $s_1 = 1$ and $s_2 = 10$. Let $u(s_1) = 1$ and $u(s_2) = 1$. Suppose the measurements which result are

$$y^M(s_1) = \begin{bmatrix} 1.091 \\ 0.7273 \end{bmatrix} \quad \text{and} \quad y^M(s_2) = \begin{bmatrix} 2.4 \\ 0.4 \end{bmatrix} \tag{30}$$

If the above information is substituted into the fault diagnosis equations, (20), the following set of nonlinear simultaneous equations result:

$$\begin{bmatrix} r_1 & 0 & 0 & 0 \\ 0 & r_2 & 0 & 0 \\ 0 & 0 & r_3 & -1 \end{bmatrix} \begin{bmatrix} 0.2727 \\ 1.091 - \alpha_1(s_1) \\ 0.7273 \\ \alpha_1(s_1) \end{bmatrix} - \begin{bmatrix} 1.091 \\ 0.7273 \\ 0 \end{bmatrix} = 0 \tag{31}$$

$$\begin{bmatrix} r_1 & 0 & 0 & 0 \\ 0 & 0.1r_2 & 0 & 0 \\ 0 & 0 & r_3 & -1 \end{bmatrix} \begin{bmatrix} 0.6 \\ 2.4 - \alpha_1(s_2) \\ 0.4 \\ \alpha_1(s_2) \end{bmatrix} - \begin{bmatrix} 2.4 \\ 0.4 \\ 0 \end{bmatrix} = 0 \tag{32}$$

These two equations are the fault diagnosis equations for the example circuit. The first test frequency yields (31) and the second yields (32). Together they form six equations in five unknowns. The unknowns are

$$x = \text{col}(\alpha_1(s_1), \alpha_1(s_2), r_1, r_2, r_3) \tag{33}$$

To determine the solution to (31) and (32) use the Newton-Raphson scheme by repeatedly solving $J_F(x^k)d = -F(x^k)$. The vector d is used to update the estimate via $x^{k+1} = x^k + \lambda d$. If $\lambda = 1$ this is the standard N-R iteration. One might also choose λ as discussed in Section 4.3. In either case the Jacobian used is

$$J_F(x) = \begin{bmatrix} 0 & 0 & 0.2727 & 0 & 0 \\ -r_2 & 0 & 0 & 1.091 - \alpha_1(s_1) & 0 \\ -1 & 0 & 0 & 0 & 0.7273 \\ 0 & 0 & 0.6 & 0 & 0 \\ 0 & -0.1r_2 & 0 & 0.1[2.4 - \alpha_1(s_2)] & 0 \\ 0 & -1 & 0 & 0 & 0.4 \end{bmatrix} \tag{34}$$

The resulting solution is

$$x^* = \text{col}(0.7273, 0.4, 4, 2, 1) \tag{35}$$

See the Appendix for a rudimentary but illustrative computer program which implements a solution to this example.

6.2 Additional Example

This example is based on the AC equivalent circuit of the single-stage transistor amplifier in Figure 11.4 selected from Ref. [6]. The component connection equations are shown below. [Note: The control voltage for the dependent source is defined differently than it was in [6], making $Z(s, r)$ diagonal and changing one entry in L_{11}.] The input, output, component input, and component output vectors are defined as

$$u = V_1 \qquad y = \begin{bmatrix} V_0 \\ I_{C_1} \\ I_E \end{bmatrix} \tag{36}$$

$$a = \operatorname{col}[I_{C_1}, I_{R_x}, I_{R_\pi}, I_{C_\mu}, I_{C_2}, V_{R_B}, V_{R_E}, V_{C_\pi}, V_{C_E}, V_B, V_{R_c}, V_{R_L}] \tag{37}$$

$$b = \operatorname{col}[V_{C_1}, V_{R_x}, V_{R_\pi}, V_{C_\mu}, V_{C_2}, I_{R_B}, I_{R_E}, I_{C_\pi}, I_{C_E}, I_{g_m}, I_{R_c}, I_{R_L}] \tag{38}$$

The vector r and the matrix $Z(s, r)$ are

$$r = \operatorname{col}\left[\frac{1}{C_1}, R_X, R_\pi, \frac{1}{C_\mu}, \frac{1}{C_2}, \frac{1}{R_B}, \frac{1}{R_E}, C_\pi, C_E, g_m, \frac{1}{R_c}, \frac{1}{R_L}\right] \tag{39}$$

$$Z(s, r) = \operatorname{diag}\left[\frac{1}{sC_1}, R_X, R_\pi, \frac{1}{sC_\mu}, \frac{1}{sC_2}, \frac{1}{R_B}, \frac{1}{R_E}, sC_\pi, sC_E, g_m, \frac{1}{R_c}, \frac{1}{R_L}\right] \tag{40}$$

Finally, the connection matrices are

$$[L_{11} \quad L_{12}] = \begin{bmatrix} 0 & 0 & 0 & 0 & 0 & 1 & 1 & 0 & 1 & 0 & 1 & 1 & 0 \\ 0 & 0 & 0 & 0 & 0 & 0 & 1 & 0 & 1 & 0 & 1 & 1 & 0 \\ 0 & 0 & 0 & 0 & 0 & 0 & 1 & -1 & 1 & -1 & 0 & 0 & 0 \\ 0 & 0 & 0 & 0 & 0 & 0 & 0 & 0 & 0 & 1 & 1 & 1 & 0 \\ 0 & 0 & 0 & 0 & 0 & 0 & 0 & 0 & 0 & 0 & 0 & 1 & 0 \\ -1 & 0 & 0 & 0 & 0 & 0 & 0 & 0 & 0 & 0 & 0 & 0 & 1 \\ -1 & -1 & -1 & 0 & 0 & 0 & 0 & 0 & 0 & 0 & 0 & 0 & 1 \\ 0 & 0 & 1 & 0 & 0 & 0 & 0 & 0 & 0 & 0 & 0 & 0 & 0 \\ -1 & -1 & -1 & 0 & 0 & 0 & 0 & 0 & 0 & 0 & 0 & 0 & 1 \\ 0 & 0 & 1 & 0 & 0 & 0 & 0 & 0 & 0 & 0 & 0 & 0 & 0 \\ -1 & -1 & 0 & -1 & 0 & 0 & 0 & 0 & 0 & 0 & 0 & 0 & 1 \\ -1 & -1 & 0 & -1 & -1 & 0 & 0 & 0 & 0 & 0 & 0 & 0 & 1 \end{bmatrix} \tag{41}$$

$$[L_{21} \quad L_{22}] = \begin{bmatrix} -1 & -1 & 0 & -1 & -1 & 0 & 0 & 0 & 0 & 0 & 0 & 0 & 1 \\ 0 & 0 & 0 & 0 & 0 & 1 & 1 & 0 & 1 & 0 & 1 & 1 & 0 \\ 0 & 0 & 0 & 0 & 0 & 0 & 1 & 0 & 1 & 0 & 0 & 0 & 0 \end{bmatrix} \tag{42}$$

The right inverse for L_{21} computed using the LINPACK [16] routine SSVDC is

$$L_{21}{}^{-R} = \begin{bmatrix} -0.25 & 0 & 0 \\ -0.25 & 0 & 0 \\ 0 & 0 & 0 \\ -0.25 & 0 & 0 \\ -0.25 & 0 & 0 \\ 0 & 0.333 & -0.333 \\ 0 & 0 & 0.5 \\ 0 & 0 & 0 \\ 0 & 0 & 0.5 \\ 0 & 0 & 0 \\ 0 & 0.333 & -0.333 \\ 0 & 0.333 & -0.333 \end{bmatrix} \tag{43}$$

A basis for the null space of L_{21} in matrix form is

$$V = \begin{bmatrix} 1 & 1 & 0 & 0 & 0 & 0 & 0 & 0 & 0 \\ -1 & 0 & 0 & 0 & 0 & 0 & 0 & 0 & 0 \\ 0 & 0 & 1 & 0 & 0 & 0 & 0 & 0 & 0 \\ 0 & -1 & 0 & 1 & 0 & 0 & 0 & 0 & 0 \\ 0 & 0 & 0 & -1 & 0 & 0 & 0 & 0 & 0 \\ 0 & 0 & 0 & 0 & 0 & 0 & 0 & 0 & 1 \\ 0 & 0 & 0 & 0 & 0 & 1 & 0 & 0 & 0 \\ 0 & 0 & 0 & 0 & 1 & 0 & 0 & 0 & 0 \\ 0 & 0 & 0 & 0 & 0 & -1 & 0 & 0 & 0 \\ 0 & 0 & 0 & 0 & 0 & 0 & 1 & 0 & 0 \\ 0 & 0 & 0 & 0 & 0 & 0 & 0 & 1 & -1 \\ 0 & 0 & 0 & 0 & 0 & 0 & 0 & -1 & 0 \end{bmatrix} \tag{44}$$

For this circuit $M = N = 12$, $p = 9$, and using complex test frequencies $q = 2$. All parameters have nominal values of unity. The test frequencies are $s_1 = j1.4$ and $s_2 = j2$. If one solves the fault diagnosis equation for this circuit using measurements corresponding to the nominal value of the parameters, the r subvector of the solution will be the nominal values. Call the values of the α vector part of this solution the nominal values for the ambiguity vectors $\boldsymbol{\alpha}_i$. These are handy for initializing the N-R iteration. For this example the

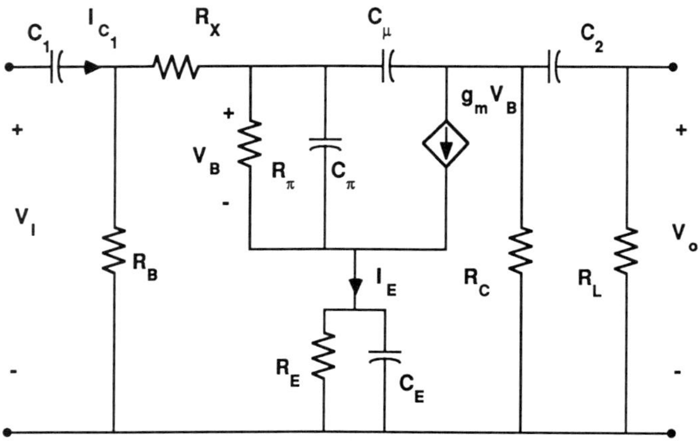

Figure 11.4 Twelve-parameter fault diagnosis example.

nominal values for the ambiguity vectors $\boldsymbol{\alpha}_1$ and $\boldsymbol{\alpha}_2$ are

$$\boldsymbol{\alpha}_1 = \begin{bmatrix} 0.72545e-01 \\ 0.26209e+00 \\ 0.92251e-01 \\ 0.18192e+00 \\ -0.39387e-01 \\ 0.64166e-01 \\ 0.92251e-01 \\ 0.16710e+00 \\ 0.26166e+00 \end{bmatrix} + j \begin{bmatrix} -0.42669e+00 \\ 0.28641e-01 \\ 0.28133e-01 \\ -0.38153e-01 \\ 0.12915e+00 \\ -0.98703e-01 \\ 0.28133e-01 \\ 0.11155e+00 \\ 0.21033e+00 \end{bmatrix} \tag{45}$$

$$\boldsymbol{\alpha}_2 = \begin{bmatrix} -0.86316e-01 \\ 0.29425e+00 \\ 0.10092e+00 \\ 0.17635e+00 \\ -0.21282e-01 \\ 0.35081e-01 \\ 0.10092e+00 \\ 0.19156e+00 \\ 0.31972e+00 \end{bmatrix} + j \begin{bmatrix} -0.48784e+00 \\ 0.80346e-01 \\ 0.10641e-01 \\ -0.11167e-01 \\ 0.20184e+00 \\ -0.13916e+00 \\ 0.10641e-01 \\ 0.97295e-01 \\ 0.21512e+00 \end{bmatrix} \tag{46}$$

Next the parameter vector r was changed to

$$r = \text{col}(2., 1.2, 0.9, 0.9, 1.1, 0.8, 1., 1.1, 2., 0.9, 1.2, 1.1) \tag{47}$$

The small variations from unity represent normal production variations for "good" components, while the larger variations for the first and ninth components represent failures. This perturbed parameter vector r (representing an actual circuit under test) was used to compute the following test outputs:

$$y^M(s_1) = \begin{bmatrix} -0.18299e-01 \\ 0.24554e+00 \\ 0.73848e-01 \end{bmatrix} + j \begin{bmatrix} 0.44648e-01 \\ 0.55346e+00 \\ 0.15117e+00 \end{bmatrix} \tag{48}$$

$$y^M(s_2) = \begin{bmatrix} 0.62142e-02 \\ 0.41992e+00 \\ 0.10101e+00 \end{bmatrix} + j \begin{bmatrix} 0.67445e-01 \\ 0.68044e+00 \\ 0.19389e+00 \end{bmatrix} \tag{49}$$

These test outputs and the nominal data were the input to a diagnosis program using the N-R scheme. The program used the nominal data for the first estimate of the solution. The program used 12 iterations and 31.5 seconds on the VAX 11/780 to compute the estimates of the circuit parameters, all within 0.11% of the actual values. A modification of the program implementing the modified algorithm discussed previously required eight iterations and 23.3 seconds on the same computer.

7 CONCLUSION

This chapter has provided details of the tableau approach for multifrequency fault diagnosis of linear circuits. The system characterization for the method requires that "connection" information and "component" information remain separate. For this we use the component connection model, although other equivalent methods for circuit description suffice. To assist the reader in applying the approach to other models we have detailed the derivation of the fault diagnosis equations. The key here is the unique method used to characterize the ambiguity associated with measurements at a single test frequency. The result is a large but sparse set of fault diagnosis equations. Most significant is the fact that these equations maintain a fixed polynomial order regardless of system size and in many cases they are quadratic. This fact motivated the presentation of the details of the modified Newton-Raphson algorithm and the inclusion of some computer code which demonstrates their implementation. The theory presented includes a means for determining the diagnosability of a network with simple limits on test frequency requirements. The three-parameter example (with solution program) is a simple vehicle for illustration of the method. The larger example provides sufficient detail that one can set it up independently and check results.

Finally, these results can be extended to the case where there is a bound on the number of simultaneous faults. In this case the fault diagnosis equations of (20) are the same but the solution algorithm is modified to account for the limited fault assumption. Details can be found in Refs. [8, 17].

APPENDIX

This appendix contains a simple Fortran 77 program which implements the solution to the three-parameter fault diagnosis example. Although the example is small and would not really benefit from any exploitation of the known quadratic form, a subroutine is included which will use a fourth-order interpolant to compute λ. The inverse in (27) was precomputed and included as data in this subroutine.

```
c     The use of real*8 and integer*2 is for consistency with the
c     subroutine library provided on our system from which the left-
c     inverse and polynomial root finding routines come.
c     You must provide equivalents of these from your own system
c     library.
c
      real*8 r(3), a(2), jf(6,5), f(6), d(5), dmag, eps/.00001/
c     set up measurement data
      real*8 s1/1.0/, s2/10.0/, yms1(2)/1.091,.7273/, yms2(2)/2.4,.4/
      common/meas/ s1, s2, yms1, yms2
      integer*2 m/6/,n/5/,irank,inc(5),ifail
      real*8 aijmax(5), u(6,6), du(5), wd(6), tol/0.0001/, lambda
c      --------------- key variables ---------------
c     r(i)            parameter vector
c     a(i)            alpha1(s1) and alpha1(s2)
c     jf(i,j)         the jacobian JF(x) or its left inverse
c     f(i)            the vector function F(x)
c     s1,s2           test frequency #1 and #2  (Note u=1.0 for both)
c     yms1(i), yms2(i)   measured output at s1 and s2
c
      write(*,*) 'Enter the starting value for the r-s:'
      read(*,*) (r(i),i=1,3)
      write(*,*) 'Enter the starting value for the alpha-s:'
      read(*,*) (a(i),i=1,2)
100    continue
c     set up the Jacobian JF(x)
      call make_jf(jf,r,a)
c     set up F(x)
      call make_f(f,r,a)
      do 30 i=1,6
30     f(i)=-f(i)
```

```
c     The following subroutine (f01blf) is from the Numerical Algorithms
c     Group (NAG) Subroutine library. It computes the left inverse of the
c     Jacobian, JF. You must supply an equivalent routine.
      call f01blf(m,n,tol,jf,m,aijmax,irank,inc,wd,u,m,du,ifail)
c     jf is now the left inverse of JF. Now find d the search direction.
      do 50 i=1,5
      d(i)=0.0
      do 50 j=1,6
50     d(i)=d(i)+f(j)*jf(j,i)
      dmag=0.0
      do 60 i=1,3
60     dmag=dmag+d(i)*d(i)
      if(dmag.lt.eps) stop
c
      lambda=1.0
c     lambda=1 for the standard N-R method
c     call interpo_f(lambda,r,a,d)      uncomment to exploit quad form of F(x)
      a(1)=a(1)+lambda*d(1)
      a(2)=a(2)+lambda*d(2)
      r(1)=r(1)+lambda*d(3)
      r(2)=r(2)+lambda*d(4)
      r(3)=r(3)+lambda*d(5)
c
      write(*,'(a3,3f9.4)') 'r: ',(r(i),i=1,3)
      go to 100
      end
c
      subroutine make_f(f,r,a)
      real*8 f(6), r(3), a(2)
      real*8 s1, s2, yms1(2), yms2(2)
      common/meas/ s1, s2, yms1, yms2
c     s1 part
      f(1)= (1.-yms1(2))*r(1)-yms1(1)
      f(2)= r(2)*(yms1(1)-a(1))/s1 - yms1(2)
      f(3)= yms1(2)*r(3)-a(1)
c     s2 part
      f(4)= (1.-yms2(2))*r(1)-yms2(1)
      f(5)= r(2)*(yms2(1)-a(2))/s2 - yms2(2)
      f(6)= yms2(2)*r(3)-a(2)
      return
      end
c
      subroutine make_jf(jf,r,a)
      real*8 jf(6,5), r(3), a(2)
      real*8 s1, s2, yms1(2), yms2(2)
      common/meas/ s1, s2, yms1, yms2
c
      do 10 i=1,6
      do 10 j=1,5
10     jf(i,j)=0.0
      jf(2,1)= -r(2)/s1
      jf(3,1)= -1.0
      jf(5,2)= -r(2)/s2
      jf(6,2)= -1.0
      jf(1,3)= 1.-yms1(2)
```

```
      jf(4,3)= 1.-yms2(2)
      jf(2,4)= (yms1(1)-a(1))/s1
      jf(5,4)= (yms2(1)-a(2))/s2
      jf(3,5)= yms1(2)
      jf(6,5)= yms2(2)
      return
      end

c
      subroutine interpo_f(lambda,r_in,a_in,d)
c     computes lambda for the N-R iteration by exploiting the fact that
c     the fault diagnosis equations are quadratic.
      integer*2 n, ifail
      real*8 lambda, r_in(3), a_in(2), d(5)
      real*8 lam(5) /0.0,0.25,0.5,0.75,1.0/, r(3), a(2)
      real*8 f(6), g(5), c(5), rez(4), imz(4), tol
      real*8 vandinv(5,5) /
     &   10.666667, -42.666667,  64.000000, -42.666667,  10.666667,
     &  -26.666667,  96.000000,-128.000000,  74.666667, -16.000000,
     &   23.333333, -69.333333,  76.000000, -37.333333,   7.333333,
     &   -8.333333,  16.000000, -12.000000,   5.333333,  -1.000000,
     &    1.000000,   0.000000,   0.000000,   0.000000,   0.000000/
c     compute 5 sample points of the 4th order polynomial which is the
c     square of |f| along the search direction d
c     g(i) = |f(x+lam(i)*d)|**2     lam(i)= 0, .25, .5, .75, 1
      do 10 i=1,5
      a(1)=a_in(1)+lam(i)*d(1)
      a(2)=a_in(2)+lam(i)*d(2)
      r(1)=r_in(1)+lam(i)*d(3)
      r(2)=r_in(2)+lam(i)*d(4)
      r(3)=r_in(3)+lam(i)*d(5)
      call make_f(f,r,a)
      g(i)=0.0
      do 10 j=1,6
10     g(i)=g(i)+f(j)*f(j)
c     find the coefficients, c(i), of g by c=vandinv*g
      do 20 i=1,5
      c(i)=0.0
      do 20 j=1,5
20     c(i)=c(i)+vandinv(i,j)*g(j)
c     find coefficients of the 1st derivative of g
      do 30 i=1,4
30     c(i)=float(5-i)*c(i)
c     the following subroutine (c02aef) is from the Numerical Algorithms
c     Group (NAG) Subroutine library.  It computes the zeros of the poly-
c     nomial  c(1)*x**(n-1) + c(2)*x**(n-2) + ...
      tol=0.000001
      n=4
      call c02aef(c,n,rez,imz,tol,ifail)
c     at this point the roots (rez+j*imz) should be checked to
c     insure proper behavior of the algorithm.  Here we simply grab
c     the first positive real root
      lambda=1.0
      do 40 i=1,3
```

```
      if((abs(imz(i)).lt.tol).and.(rez(i).gt.0.0)) then
         lambda=rez(i)
         return
         endif
40    continue
      return
      end
```

REFERENCES

1. M. N. Ransom and R. Saeks, Fault isolation via term expansion, *Proc. 3rd Pittsburgh Symp. Modeling and Simulation*, Univ. of Pittsburgh, vol. 4, pp. 224–228, 1973.
2. R. Saeks, S. P. Singh, and R. W. Liu, Fault isolation via component simulation, *IEEE Trans. Circuit Theory*, vol. CT-19, pp. 634–640, Nov. 1972.
3. S. P. Singh and R. W. Liu, Existence of state equation representation of linear large-scale dynamical systems, *IEEE Trans. Circuit Theory*, vol. CT-20, pp. 239–246, May 1973.
4. D. J. Rose and R. A. Willoughby, eds., *Sparse Matrices and Their Applications* (Proc. Symp. on Sparse Matrices and Their Applications, Sept. 9–10, 1971, IBM Thomas J. Watson Research Center, Yorktown Heights, N.Y.), Plenum, New York, 1972.
5. H. Trauboth and W. McCallum, *MARSYAS Users Manual*, Tech. Rep. A1-34812, Computation Laboratory, NASA/Marshall Space Flight Center, 1973.
6. N. Sen and R. Saeks, Fault diagnosis for linear system via multifrequency measurements, *IEEE Trans. Circuits Syst.*, vol. CAS-26, pp. 490–496, July 1979.
7. R. DeCarlo and C. Gordan, Tableau Approach to AC-multifrequency Fault Diagnosis, *Proc. IEEE Int. Symp. Circuits Syst.*, May 1981.
8. L. Rapisarda, Multifrequency Analog Fault Diagnosis for Linearized Circuits, Ph.D. Dissertation, School of Electrical Engineering, Purdue Univ., May 1983 (Purdue Univ., School of Electrical Engineering Tech. Rep. TR-EE-83-17, May 1983).
9. L. Rapisarda and R. DeCarlo, Analog multifrequency fault diagnosis, *IEEE Trans. Circuits Syst.*, vol. CAS-30, pp. 223–234, April 1983.
10. G. Strang, *Linear Algebra and Its Application*, Academic Press, New York, 1976.
11. G. Birkhoff and S. MacLane, *A Survey of Modern Algebra*, Macmillan, New York, 1965.

12. N. Navid and A. N. Willson, A theory and an algorithm for analog circuit fault diagnosis, *IEEE Trans. Circuits Syst.*, vol. CAS-26, pp. 440–457, April 1979.
13. R. A. DeCarlo and R. Saeks, *Interconnected Dynamical Systems*, Marcel Dekker, New York, 1981.
14. V. C. Klema and A. J. Laub, The singular value decomposition and some applications, *IEEE Trans. Autom. Control*, vol. AC-25, no. 2, April 1980.
15. IMSL—International Mathematical and Statistical Libraries, IMSL Inc., Houston, Texas.
16. LINPACK—Simultaneous Linear Algebraic Equation Package, Argonne National Laboratories, Argonne, Illinois.
17. Rapisarda and R. DeCarlo, Fault diagnosis in the tableau context with the assumption of limited simultaneous faults, *Proc. 1984 IEEE Int. Symp. Circuits Syst.*, Montreal, May 1984.

12
Computational Approaches to Fault Dictionary

P. M. Lin

School of Electrical Engineering,
Purdue University
West Lafayette, Indiana

Y. S. Elcherif

Department of Electronic and Communication Engineering,
Cairo University
Giza, Egypt

1 INTRODUCTION

The problem of analog circuit fault diagnosis first attracted researchers' attention in the 1960s [1, 2] and became a flourishing research activity in the 1970s [3]. Progress has been slow. Today the field is still in its infancy, as there is not yet any user-oriented publicly available computer program for circuit diagnosis purposes such as those for circuit simulation purposes. Nevertheless, the importance of the diagnosis problem is now widely recognized. Traditionally, the study of circuit theory has centered on two aspects only—analysis and synthesis. To these, we may now add the third equally important aspect, namely diagnosis.

Depending on whether circuit simulations take place before or after the testing process, analog circuit diagnosis methods are classified into two main categories: the simulation-before-test (SBT) approach and the simulation-after-test (SAT) approach. The SAT approach has received far more attention in recent years than the SBT approach. Early efforts in the SAT approach concentrated on *parameter identification techniques* [4–11]. Most of the techniques developed are, strictly speaking, applicable only to linear circuits

[4–8] (or the linearized model of a nonlinear circuit at some operating point), although some are applicable to genuinely nonlinear circuits as well [9–11]. In some special cases the parameter identification problem may be reduced to the solution of a system of linear equations [13, 14]. In general, however, one has to cope with the solution of systems of nonlinear equations that are not *explicitly* given but are implied by the circuit constraint equations [Kirchhoff's current and voltage laws (KCL and KVL) and branch *V-I* relations]. A great deal of research effort has been aimed at making the solution process more efficient [15–17]. For example, in Ref. [17], a technique is presented where the nonlinearity encountered need only be of second degree or lower in each unknown parameter (see also Chapter 11 of this volume). Even so, the *numerical* difficulty is still tremendous when large circuits (in the hundreds of nodes range) are considered. Further simplification is possible by assuming that only a few elements can be faulty simultaneously [11].

The present trend in the SAT approach is *not* to solve for parameter values but to simulate the circuit under different conditions and then use some decision algorithm to locate the faulty components (the parameter values are not found) [10–12]. This branch of the SAT approach may be called the *fault verification techniques*. The approach appears very promising. Whether it will eventually lead to some practical diagnosis programs remains to be seen. A good review of recent advances in SAT techniques may be found in Ref. [18].

The essence of a fault dictionary is as follows. For each fault, its symptom or signature (usually the voltages of some test nodes) is determined through software simulation and stored in the dictionary. Given a faulty circuit, one makes test measurements and then compares the result with those stored in the dictionary to identify the fault. Thus the fault dictionary is an SBT approach. The fault dictionary method actually dated back long before the advent of digital computers. For example, service manuals accompanying electronic equipment usually contain a section on "troubleshooting," where a step-by-step testing procedure is described, together with a table of symptoms and possible causes. That is in essence a fault dictionary approach. In theory, one can compile a fault dictionary manually. But with the use of digital computers the whole process can be automated. As a result, the fault dictionary can be made much more comprehensive and easier to use. In the SAT approach, a great amount of computing power is required after the testing process. In sharp contrast, the SBT approach requires a negligible amount of computing power after the test process to locate the faults. However, a comparable or even greater amount of computing power is needed before the test process in order to compile the fault dictionary.

It is well known that the fault dictionary approach is incapable of diagnosing soft failures, that is, element value drifts. As a result, most of the

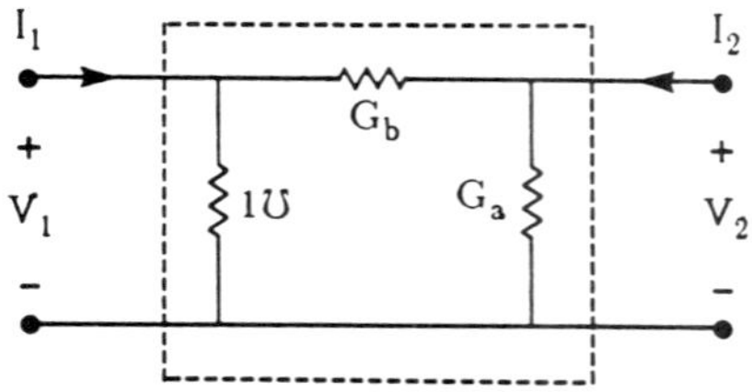

Figure 12.1 Catastrophic failures may lead to numerical difficulty.

recent research activities in fault diagnosis have been in the realm of simulation after test. However, the fault dictionary will remain a very valuable part of an overall fault diagnosis scheme for the following reasons:

1. Catastrophic failures (i.e., open circuits and short circuits, also called "hard failures") usually cause numerical difficulty in the parameter identification techniques. A simple example will illustrate this point. Consider the 2-port consisting of three conductances as shown in Figure 12.1. Suppose that we wish to determine the values of G_a and G_b by measuring two z-parameters, z_{11} and z_{22}. The relationships among these four variables are

$$z_{11} = \frac{G_a + G_b}{G_a + G_b + G_a G_b} \tag{1a}$$

$$z_{22} = \frac{1 + G_b}{G_a + G_b + G_a G_b} \tag{1b}$$

or, equivalently,

$$z_{11}(G_a + G_b + G_a G_b) - G_a - G_b = 0 \tag{2a}$$

$$z_{22}(G_a + G_b + G_a G_b) - 1 - G_b = 0 \tag{2b}$$

Now suppose that the measured results are $z_{11} = 0.5$ ohm and $z_{22} = 0.5$ ohm. By *inspection* of Figure 12.1, we expect the solutions to be $G_a = 1$ mho and $G_b \to \infty$. The latter corresponds to a catastrophic fault of conductance G_b short-circuited. However, in an automated fault diagnosis procedure, Eq. (2) will be solved by some iterative algorithm, say the well-known Newton algorithm. In the present case, no matter what the initial guesses $G_a^{(0)}$ and $G_b^{(0)}$ are, the first iteration always leads to $G_a^{(1)} = 1$. Then the Jacobian matrix

$$\mathbf{J}(G_a, G_b) = \begin{bmatrix} 0.5G_b - 0.5 & 0.5G_a - 0.5 \\ 0.5G_b + 0.5 & 0.5G_a - 0.5 \end{bmatrix}$$

is always singular at $\mathbf{G}^{(1)}$. Therefore the Newton process will always abort after one iteration, regardless of the initial guess of the solution. This example, of course, is contrived and drastic. Nevertheless, it brings out the nasty nature of determining hard failures by the parameter identification technique. In general, if a resistor characterized by its conductance G becomes short-circuited, then the true solution should be $G \rightarrow \infty$. Now if an iterative algorithm is used to solve the nonlinear equations, the computer program, seeing the ever-increasing values of G, might misinterpret the phenomena as a divergence of the algorithm and terminate (possibly giving the result of the last iteration). One has then to judge whether a convergence problem or a short circuit has occurred.

2. The fault dictionary approach is well suited for diagnosing short circuits and open circuits. Although the initial effort to compile the fault dictionary is quite demanding, that task is done once for all.

3. Statistics show that short circuits and open circuits account for about 70–80% of the faults in analog equipment [19].

It is reasonable to believe that a sound fault diagnosis strategy should incorporate both the SBT and SAT approaches. The fault dictionary is first used to locate hard failures. For 70–80% of the cases, this approach will be adequate. For the remaining cases of soft failures, we rely on the SAT approach or a combination of both approaches.

This chapter is organized as follows. Section 2 is a brief review of an existing fault dictionary approach. Section 3 gives a synopsis of some new techniques to be used in the fault dictionary. Some details of these techniques are described in Sections 4 to 8. Digital computer implementation and a complete video amplifier example are described in Section 9.

2 REVIEW OF AN EXISTING FAULT DICTIONARY APPROACH

Various types of inputs have been proposed for the fault dictionary method. These include the DC [19], AC [20–24], and piecewise constant inputs [25]. Unfortunately, most of these methods either are limited to linear networks [20–22] or have not progressed beyond the feasibility study stage [24, 25]. At present the DC fault dictionary is the only one that is used in practice with some degree of success. For this reason we shall in this chapter confine ourselves to the DC fault dictionary.

In order to appreciate the significance of the new approaches, it is necessary first to review what is being done currently in DC fault dictionary. We use the video amplifier example of Ref. [19] as a vehicle to explain all phases of the DC fault dictionary approach. We then (in Section 3) point out where the difficulties lie and describe new techniques for overcoming these difficulties.

The DC fault dictionary approach consists of two distinct stages:

Stage 1: Pretest analysis to compile the fault dictionary.

In this stage the analog circuit is simulated by a digital computer program under nominal as well as all preselected catastrophic faults. Judiciously chosen DC input voltages are applied. The induced DC voltages at a selected set of test nodes are calculated. These voltages are then stored in the automatic test equipment (ATE) and constitute the fault dictionary.

Stage 2: Posttest analysis to identify the fault.

In this stage, measurements of test node voltages have been made on the circuit, and the measured values are compared with those stored in the fault dictionary. First, a fault detection algorithm is applied to determine whether the circuit is faulty at all. If the answer is affirmative, then the fault is identified by the application of some fault isolation algorithm (e.g., minimum sum of squared errors, as in [19]). Some details follow.

2.1 Pretest Analysis

As an example, consider the video amplifier circuit of Ref. [19] whose schematic diagram is reproduced here as Figure 12.2. The amplifier has 9 transistors (Q1 through Q9), 7 diodes (D1 through D7), 4 zener diodes (DZ1 through DZ4), 45 resistors (R1 through R45), and 4 indictors (L1 through L4). The amplifier is constructed with discrete components. There are 43 nodes (excluding the common ground). Not all of these nodes are accessible (otherwise the fault diagnosis problem would be trivial [6]).

If the catastrophic faults of *all* components, single faults as well as multiple faults, are considered, the number of combinations will be enormous. Thus, as the very first step, the engineer must come up with a reasonable fault list, based on the engineer's experience and the past failure history of the circuit. Strictly for the purpose of illustration, a total of 20 faults have been selected in [19]; all are associated with semiconductor devices, as they are more likely to go wrong than passive components. Adopting the abbreviations B, base; C, collector; E, emitter; O, open; and S, short, we have the following fault list (fault number—fault condition):

> 1-Q1BES, 2-Q2CES, 3-Q2BO, 4-Q3BES, 5Q3BO, 6-Q4BES, 7-Q4BO, 8-Q5BES, 9-Q5BO, 10-Q6BES, 11-Q6BCS, 12-Q6BO, 13-DZ1O, 14-DZ1S, 15-DZ2O, 16-DZ2S, 17-DZ3O, 18-DZ3S, 19-DZ4O, 20-D24S

The next step is to select test nodes among the accessible nodes. Discrete-component circuits have most nodes accessible. Next in line are the printed circuit boards. Finally, the integrated circuit chips have the least number of nodes accessible for testing. Even if the accessibility of nodes presents no

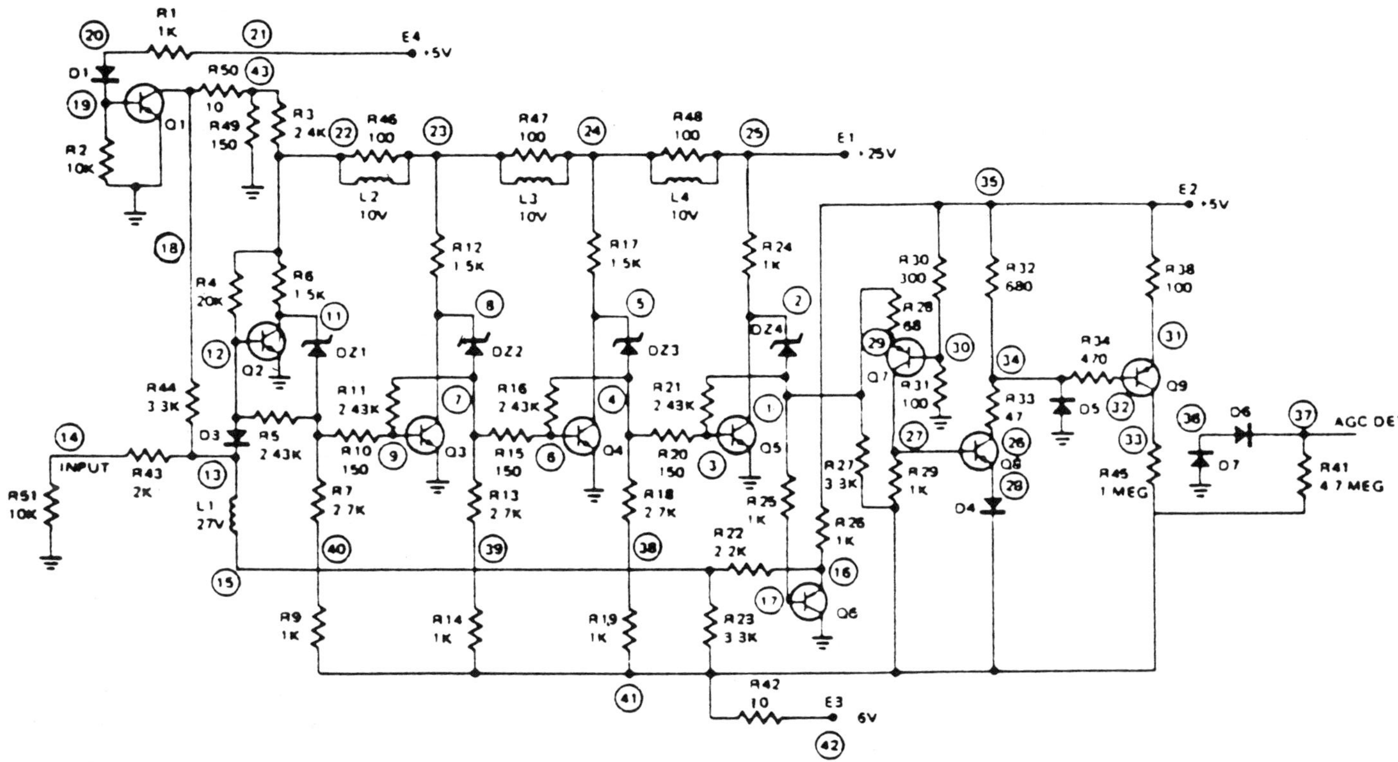

Figure 12.2 Video amplifier example used in Ref. [19].

problem, it is highly important to use as few test nodes as possible, in view of the cost of making test node connections.

In the absence of any better guidelines one may *initially* choose all or most of the accessible nodes as the test nodes. Later, after circuit simulations under all fault conditions have been carried out, a suitable fault isolation algorithm may be executed to reduce the number of test nodes and yet maintain a satisfactory fault isolation.

In the present video amplifier circuit, 10 test nodes are chosen initially. They are nodes 2, 5, 8, 11, 16, 18, 26, 27, 33, and 36, again all associated with semiconductor devices.

In general, the nominal and fault circuits must be simulated under more than one *input combination* in order to achieve adequate separation of faults. Each input combination is also called an *input vector*. At present, no algorithm is available for selection of the input vectors. Trial and error, guided by knowledge of the particular circuit, seems to be the only avenue at this time. The selection of stimuli is initially made by the engineer and expanded if detection (separation from the nominal case) and isolation (separation among fault cases) requirements are not met. For the present example, two input vectors have been used. If we let

$$\text{VIN} = (\text{V14, V25, V35, V42, V21})$$

then the two chosen input vectors are (in volts)

$$\text{VIN1} = (30, 25, 5, -6, 5)$$

and

$$\text{VIN2} = (-30, 25, 5, -6, 5)$$

Note that only the first entry, ± 30 V, represents the externally applied DC input.

As there are 21 circuit conditions (1 nominal and 20 faulty) and 2 input vectors, a total of $21 \times 2 = 42$ circuit simulations must be carried out to determine the 10 selected test node voltages. In Ref. [19], the program SYSCAP is used. Of course, one can use any other suitable CAD programs such as SPICE2 [26] and ASTAP [27]. The data to be gathered from these simulations will be $21 \times 2 \times 10 = 420$ voltage values. These values will be processed by the fault isolation algorithm described below to eliminate the unnecessary test nodes. The voltage values corresponding to the retained test nodes then constitute the fault dictionary.

Before describing the fault isolation algorithm, it is necessary to introduce the concept of an *ambiguity set*. Consider a hypothetical case of a circuit with two test nodes and six faults. Suppose that the use of a CAD program on this circuit yields the results shown in Table 12.1. These voltage values are

Table 12.1 Voltages of Two Test Nodes of a Hypothetical Circuit

	NOM	F1	F2	F3	F4	F5	F6
V1	5.5	9.0	6.8	6.4	6.6	5.1	2.0
V2	4.0	8.0	5.0	5.2	7.8	7.6	3.0

obtained under the assumption of exact element values. In reality, the value of any element may vary within some tolerance range. If the *measured* value of V1 is 5.4 volts, we really cannot be certain whether the circuit is under nominal, or fault 5 condition. All we can say is that when V1 = 5.4 volts, the circuit is under either nominal or fault 5 condition. Thus in this case, NOM and F5 form what is called an *ambiguity set*. Following Ref. [19], we may reasonably define the voltage of an ambiguity set to have a range of ± 0.7 volt about its center value and stipulate that different ambiguity set voltage ranges do not overlap. When we speak of an ambiguity set, we refer to the circuit conditions that produce voltages within the same ambiguity set voltage range. In the present example, test node 1 has four ambiguity sets and test node 2 has three ambiguity sets, which are listed in Table 12.2. Examination of Table 12.2 shows that fault F4 cannot be isolated from F2 and F3 if we use test node 1 only. Similarly, F4 cannot be isolated from F1 and F5 if we use test node 2 only. However, if both test nodes 1 and 2 are used then F4 can be isolated. This is because F4 is the only fault that occurs in both ambiguity sets (1, 2) and (2, 2). On the other hand, faults F2 and F3 cannot be isolated even if both test nodes are used.

To obtain maximum isolation, the ambiguity sets must be manipulated to determine which faults can be isolated and what nodes will provide the greatest degree of isolation. In Ref. [19], two ground rules are used:

Table 12.2 Tabulation of Ambiguity Sets

(Node, ambiguity set)	Circuit condition	Voltage range
(1, 1)	NOM, F5	4.6–6.0
(1, 2)	F2, F3, F4	5.7–7.1
(1, 3)	F1	8.3–9.7
(1, 4)	F6	1.3–2.7
(2, 1)	NOM, F6	2.8–4.2
(2, 2)	F1, F4, F5	7.1–8.5
(2, 3)	F2, F3	4.4–5.8

Rule 1: Any ambiguity set which has a single fault within it uniquely defines that fault at that test node.

Rule 2: Ambiguity sets whose intersection or symmetric difference results in a single fault also uniquely define the fault.

Consider again the above hypothetical example. F1 and F6 each can be uniquely defined by measuring voltage V1 only, according to rule 1. NOM (nominal case) and F5 each can be isolated by measuring both V1 and V2, according to rule 2.

Let us return to the video amplifier example. At each of 10 test nodes and for each of the input vectors, the ambiguity sets are determined. The complete tabulation of the ambiguity sets for all nodes is given as Table 1 in Ref. [19].

After applying the two rules described above to these ambiguity sets, it is found that only five test nodes (nodes 11, 8, 2, 5, and 16) are needed for the isolation of 19 of the 20 preselected faults. The two faults that cannot be uniquely identified are faults 10 and 12. In general, to achieve a higher degree of isolation, we have to use more test nodes or more input vectors. This is, however, unnecessary in the present case since faults 10 and 12 are on the same replaceable component, transistor Q6. If either fault 10 or fault 12 has occurred, then transistor Q6 has to be replaced anyway.

The fault dictionary now consists of the DC nodal voltages at the five test nodes for two inputs under each of the 21 circuit conditions (1 nominal and 20 faulty circuits). This represents a total of 210 ($5 \times 2 \times 21$) voltage values to be stored in the fault dictionary on the ATE. A portion of the fault dictionary corresponding to faults 4, 10, 14 and the nominal circuit is given in Table 12.3.

This completes the pretest compilation of the fault dictionary.

Table 12.3 Portion of a Fault Dictionary

	Input					
Fault	V14	V11	V8	V5	V2	V16
F4	−30	5.32	5.99	0.09	6.95	0.02
	30	0.15	5.99	0.09	6.95	0.03
F10	−30	5.93	0.09	5.93	0.12	3.07
	30	0.20	5.97	0.09	6.91	4.22
F14	−30	1.70	0.08	5.92	0.12	3.11
	30	0.13	6.00	0.09	6.95	4.03
NOM	−30	5.90	0.08	5.95	0.12	3.09
	30	0.18	5.95	0.09	6.93	4.10

Table 12.4 Measurement Results of a Faulty Circuit

	Input				
V14	V11	V8	V5	V2	V16
−30	1.82	0.07	6.38	0.09	2.31
−30	0.11	6.46	0.07	6.73	0.13

2.2 Posttest Analysis

Now suppose that a faulty circuit has been tested and the following measured data in Table 12.4 have been obtained.

We shall illustrate the posttest calculations required to isolate the fault. Let SSD(FJ) denote the sum of squared deviations corresponding to fault FJ, that is,

$$\text{SSD(FJ)} \triangleq \sum(\text{measured node voltage} - \text{calculated node voltage for fault FJ})^2$$

where the summation is over all test nodes and all input vectors. Then after the SSD(FJ) have been calculated for all faults, the one leading to the smallest value is considered to be the fault that has occurred. For the present case, we have (from the previous tables)

$$\begin{aligned}\text{SSD(F4)} &= [(1.82 - 5.32)^2 + (0.07 - 5.99)^2 + (6.38 - 0.09)^2 \\ &\quad + (0.09 - 6.95)^2 + (2.31 - 0.02)^2] \\ &\quad + [(0.11 - 0.15)^2 + (6.46 - 5.99)^2 + (0.07 - 0.09)^2 \\ &\quad + (6.73 - 6.95)^2 + (0.13 - 0.03)^2] \\ &= 139.16 + 0.28 \simeq 139\end{aligned}$$

Similarly, using the data shown in the two previous tables, we find

$$\text{SSD(F10)} = 35$$

$$\text{SSD(F14)} = 1.2$$

$$\text{SSD(NOM)} = 34$$

If the SSD values for all other faults are also calculated (data not shown in [19]), the final result is as follows (Table 3 of [19], third row):

Fault	1	2	3	4	5	6	7	8	9	10
SSD	18	129	189	139	167	120	117	70	74	35

Fault	11	12	13	14	15	16	17	18	19	20
SSD	21	35	300	1.2	196	40	143	40	104	36

Since the minimum value of SSD is 1.2 and occurs for FJ = 14, we conclude that the measured data indicate the occurrence of fault 14.

This completes the description of an existing fault dictionary approach [19].

3 SYNOPSIS OF NEW APPROACHES

The DC fault dictionary approach [19] described in the preceding section has been successful for medium-size circuits, for example, the video amplifier circuit in Ref. [19]. When larger circuits are considered, the first difficulty encountered is the enormous amount of pretest computation. For every possible hard failure, a DC analysis of the nonlinear circuit must be performed, using a circuit simulator such as SPICE2, SYSCAP, or ASTAP. All of these programs use Newton's algorithm (with some modification) to solve systems of nonlinear algebraic equations.

Our aim in the pretest stage is to find a new way of performing DC analysis which is faster than the use of Newton's algorithm, possibly at some loss of the accuracy of calculated node voltages.

In the existing DC fault dictionary approach [19], the posttest analysis consists of the calculations of many SSD (sums of squared deviations).

Our aim in the posttest stage is to find a new method such that the identification of a fault requires practically no arithmetic operations. A mere dictionary "lookup" operation should be enough to identify the fault. This requirement is motivated by two practical considerations. (1) With such a simple posttest procedure, the DC dictionary approach can be used in the field (on board a ship, for example) by a technician, who has only to make measurements and then look up the fault dictionary. No computation is needed. (2) Hardware can be constructed with a microprocessor chip and relatively simple decision-making circuitry such that when the measurement data are received, the fault condition of the circuit will be displayed automatically, eliminating even the human operation of fault dictionary lookup.

To achieve the two aims stated above, we have attacked the problem with techniques quite different from those in Ref. [19]. The following is a brief summary of the distinct features of our new approaches.

1. Model all nonlinearities by piecewise linear characteristics [28].
2. Use switches (instead of resistances as in [29] and several other papers) to represent open circuits and short circuits.

3. Solve the piecewise linear resistive network containing switches by the use of n-port theory [30] and Lemke's complementary pivot algorithm [31].
4. Use multilevel logic operations to reduce the number of test nodes and to generate integer fault codes for the fault dictionary.

These will now be explained briefly in Sections 4 to 8.

4 MODELING OF PIECEWISE LINEAR RESISTIVE NETWORKS WITH IDEAL DIODES

In the DC fault dictionary approach, capacitances are treated as open circuits and inductances as short circuits. The resultant network is a nonlinear resistive network. The nonlinear I-V characteristics encountered are usually associated semiconductor devices. As is well known, a nonlinear curve can be approximated by a piecewise linear (hereafter abbreviated PWL) curve to any desired accuracy by increasing the number of straight-line segments and hence the number of breakpoints. In many applications, including the present case of DC fault analysis, a three-segment or even a two segment approximation to a diode I-V curve is adequate.

Of course, nonlinear characteristics need not occur in two-terminal elements only. However, it was clearly demonstrated in Ref. [28] that models for nonlinear circuits can be constructed in such a way that all nonlinearities are associated with two-terminal nonlinear resistors. In this chapter, we assume that all nonlinearities are associated with two-terminal resistors.

Before the days of digital computers, the PWL approach was considered a very powerful means for understanding the behavior of electronic circuits and for analyzing the same manually. With the advent of high-speed digital computers and with the demand for more accurate analysis results, the PWL approach gave way to the Newton iterative approach, because the exact nonlinear characteristics are used in the latter. Because of the repeated evaluation of the Jacobian matrix, the Newton procedure is in general more time-consuming than the PWL approach.

In our present study of fault diagnosis, we have a situation where the demand for accuracy is less severe than in the usual circuit simulation. This is because of the safety margins provided by the ambiguity sets. To illustrate this point, consider the hypothetical case described in Section 2.1. Under fault 5, the exact voltage of node 1 is V1 = 5.1, and F5 belongs to ambiguity set (1, 1), which has a range from 4.6 to 6.0 volts. Now suppose that, due to model inaccuracies or the limited accuracy of the computer, the calculated value of V1 becomes 5.5 volts (8% relative error). No harm is done! F5 still belongs to ambiguity set (1, 1), and the fault isolation process goes on just as before. It is important, however, to avoid very large errors that might change the constituents of the ambiguity sets.

Once the characteristics of all nonlinear resistors have been approximated by PWL segments, they can be modeled with ideal diodes, linear resistors, DC independent voltage sources, and current sources. An ideal diode here is defined as a two-terminal element that behaves as an open circuit when reverse-biased and as a short circuit when forward-biased. The technique for modeling the most general PWL *I*-*V* curves (negative slope segments allowed) may be found in Ref. [28].

5 THE COMPLEMENTARY PROBLEM AND A METHOD OF SOLUTION

Piecewise linear resistive networks have been under continuous research for over two decades. More than a dozen solution techniques are now available (see Chapter 7 of [30]). Out of these, we have selected the complementary pivot method to be implemented in our fault diagnosis program. This choice is strictly due to the fact that a subroutine using Lęmke's algorithm to solve the complementary problem is readily available.

The general case of an *n*th-order complementary problem [31] is to find vectors **w** and **z** such that

$$\mathbf{w} = \mathbf{M}\mathbf{z} + \mathbf{q} \tag{5.1a}$$

$$\mathbf{w} \geqslant \mathbf{0}, \qquad \mathbf{z} \geqslant \mathbf{0} \tag{5.1b}$$

$$\mathbf{w}^t\mathbf{z} = 0 \tag{5.1c}$$

where the matrix **M** is a square matrix of order n and **w**, **z**, **q** are all n-vectors. **M** and **q** are given, while **w** and **z** are unknowns to be found. For example, the following is a complementary problem of order 3:

$$\begin{bmatrix} w_1 \\ w_2 \\ w_2 \end{bmatrix} = \begin{bmatrix} -2 & -14 & 4 \\ -4 & -4 & 2 \\ 4 & 4 & -2 \end{bmatrix} \begin{bmatrix} z_1 \\ z_2 \\ z_3 \end{bmatrix} + \begin{bmatrix} -4 \\ -6 \\ 10 \end{bmatrix} \tag{5.2a}$$

$$\mathbf{w} \geqslant \mathbf{0}, \qquad \mathbf{z} \geqslant \mathbf{0} \tag{5.2b}$$

$$\mathbf{w}^t\mathbf{z} = w_1z_1 + w_2z_2 + w_3z_3 = 0 \tag{5.2c}$$

If $\mathbf{q} \geqslant \mathbf{0}$, then obviously one solution to the complementary problem (5.1) is $\mathbf{w} = \mathbf{q}$ and $\mathbf{z} = \mathbf{0}$. But this may not be the only solution. In fact, a complementary problem may have no solution, a unique solution, several solutions, or infinitely many solutions. Here we shall content ourselves with knowing what the complementary problem is and that a computer subroutine (implementing Lemke's algorithm) is available for solving this problem. Readers interested in more details of this technique should refer to Refs. [31–33] and also Chapter 3 of this volume. In the next section, we shall describe how this technique is used in DC fault dictionary [34].

6 PRETEST ANALYSIS USING SWITCHES AND THE COMPLEMENTARY PIVOT METHOD

In the pretest analysis stage, the basic problem is the determination of DC node voltages under various fault conditions and DC input stimuli. Usually this is done with the aid of some circuit simulation program, such as SPICE2 or SYSCAP.

We shall now present a new approach to the pretest analysis, making use of the techniques described in Sections 4 and 5 as well as the multiport formulation algorithms [30, Chapter 6]. We assume that the test nodes, the input stimuli, and the list of catastrophic failures are given. Our only concern in this section is the rapid determination of test node voltages under various circuit conditions.

6.1 Use of Switches

By catastrophic failures we refer to open circuits and short circuits. One method for representing these two conditions is by way of the element value. Suppose that a resistance R_j has a nominal value of 1000 ohms. Then $R_j = \infty$ indicates an open circuit and $R_j = 0$ indicates a short circuit.

In our new approach, however, we use switches to represent open circuits and short circuits. Refer to Figure 12.3. The switch S_1 is normally closed (N.C.). Opening S_1 signifies that R_1 becomes an open circuit. The switch S_2 is normally open (N.O.). Closing S_2 signifies that R_2 becomes a short circuit. A fixed change in any parameter value can also be modeled by a switch. For

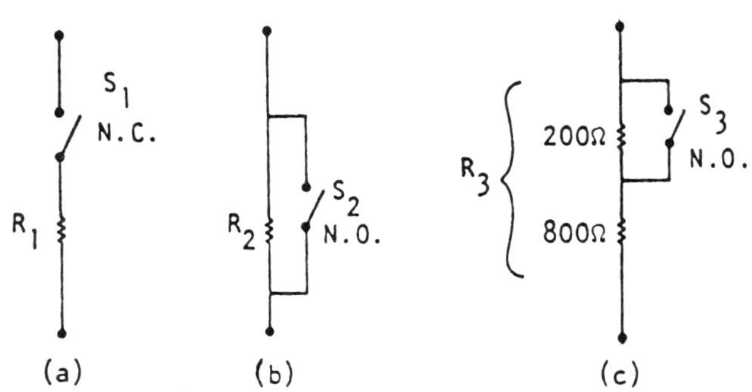

Figure 12.3 Hard failures represented by switches.

example, in Figure 12.3c, S_3 is N.O. and R_3 has a nominal value of 1000 Ω. Closing S_3 means that the value of R_3 is changed from 1000 to 800 Ω. Since these are not physical switches, but merely mathematical models representing fault conditions, we shall call them "fault switches" to distinguish them from real switches.

6.2 Formulation of Multiport Constraint Equation

With DC stimuli, with all nonlinearities approximated by piecewise linear curves, and with hard failures represented by switches, the networks under consideration can be modeled with linear resistors, controlled sources, DC independent sources, switches, and ideal diodes. Let there be t test nodes whose voltages are to be calculated. It is convenient to view the voltages $\mathbf{v}_t$ as those associated with t zero-valued independent current sources ($\mathbf{i}_t \equiv 0$). Let there be d ideal diodes and m fault switches. Extract these elements to form a $(t + m + d)$-port N as shown in Figure 12.4 with appropriate notation for the voltages and currents.

Using the technique described in Ref. [30], we can obtain a set of $(t + m + d)$ independent constraint equations in $2(t + m + d)$ port variables for the multiport. Before stating this equation it is necessary to introduce additional notation. For the m fault switches, there are 2^m combinations of switch conditions, only one of which represents the nominal circuit while the others represent faults (single as well as multiple faults). For any switch j,

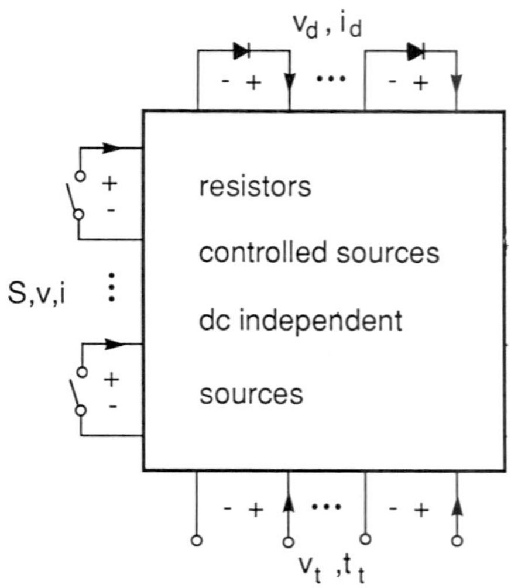

Figure 12.4 Formation of a resistive n-port.

either $i_j \equiv 0$ or $v_j \equiv 0$. Therefore, under any particular switch condition, m variables out of $(\mathbf{v}, \mathbf{i})$ will be identically zero. We may therefore partition $\mathbf{v}$ and $\mathbf{i}$ as follows (subscript NO stands for normally open and NC for normally closed).

$$\mathbf{v} = \begin{bmatrix} \mathbf{v}_{NO} \\ \mathbf{v}_{NC} \end{bmatrix} = \begin{bmatrix} \mathbf{v}_{NO} \\ \mathbf{0} \end{bmatrix}, \qquad \mathbf{i} = \begin{bmatrix} \mathbf{i}_{NO} \\ \mathbf{i}_{NC} \end{bmatrix} = \begin{bmatrix} \mathbf{0} \\ \mathbf{i}_{NC} \end{bmatrix}$$

For the circuit under normal conditions, the hybrid equation for the multiport then expresses $(\mathbf{v}_{NO}, \mathbf{i}_{NC}, \mathbf{v}_t, \mathbf{v}_d)$ in terms of $(\mathbf{i}_{NO}, \mathbf{v}_{NC}, \mathbf{i}_t, \mathbf{i}_d)$ in the following form:

$$\begin{bmatrix} \mathbf{v}_{NO} \\ \mathbf{i}_{NC} \end{bmatrix} = -\mathbf{C}_{14} \begin{bmatrix} \mathbf{i}_{NO} \\ \mathbf{v}_{NC} \end{bmatrix} - \mathbf{C}_{15}\mathbf{i}_t - \mathbf{C}_{16}\mathbf{v}_d + \mathbf{f}_1 \tag{6.1a}$$

$$\mathbf{v}_t = -\mathbf{C}_{24} \begin{bmatrix} \mathbf{i}_{NO} \\ \mathbf{v}_{NC} \end{bmatrix} - \mathbf{C}_{25}\mathbf{i}_t - \mathbf{C}_{26}\mathbf{v}_d + \mathbf{f}_2 \tag{6.1b}$$

$$\mathbf{i}_d = -\mathbf{C}_{34} \begin{bmatrix} \mathbf{i}_{NO} \\ \mathbf{v}_{NC} \end{bmatrix} - \mathbf{C}_{35}\mathbf{i}_t - \mathbf{C}_{36}\mathbf{v}_d + \mathbf{f}_3 \tag{6.1c}$$

where the $\mathbf{f}_i$ $(i = 1, 2, 3)$ are due to the DC independent sources inside the multiport. See [30, Chapter 6] for a discussion of the conditions under which the hybrid representation (6.1) exists.

6.3 Calculation of Test Node Voltages

Two different cases of using Eq. (6.1) will now be considered.

1. *Analysis of the nominal circuit.* Since $\mathbf{i}_{NO} \equiv \mathbf{0}$, $\mathbf{v}_{NC} \equiv \mathbf{0}$, $\mathbf{i}_t \equiv \mathbf{0}$, the corresponding columns in Eq. (6.1) may be discarded. Since the variables $(\mathbf{v}_{NO}, \mathbf{i}_{NC})$ are not needed for the fault dictionary, Eq. (6.1a) may also be discarded. The equation then simplifies to

$$\begin{bmatrix} \mathbf{1} & \mathbf{0} & \mathbf{C}_{26} \\ \mathbf{0} & \mathbf{1} & \mathbf{C}_{36} \end{bmatrix} \begin{bmatrix} \mathbf{v}_t \\ \mathbf{i}_d \\ \mathbf{v}_d \end{bmatrix} = \begin{bmatrix} \mathbf{f}_2 \\ \mathbf{f}_3 \end{bmatrix} \tag{6.2}$$

From Eq. (6.2), one may write the following two equations:

$$\mathbf{v}_t = -\mathbf{C}_{26}\mathbf{v}_d + \mathbf{f}_2 \tag{6.3}$$

and

$$\mathbf{i}_d = -\mathbf{C}_{36}\mathbf{v}_d + \mathbf{f}_3 \tag{6.4}$$

Equation (6.4) together with the ideal diode constraints $\mathbf{v}_d \geqslant \mathbf{0}$, $\mathbf{i}_d \geqslant \mathbf{0}$, $\mathbf{v}_d{}^t\mathbf{i}_d = 0$ forms a complementary problem which may be solved by use of

Lemke's complementary pivot algorithm. After $\mathbf{v}_d$ has been found, we calculate the test node voltage vector $\mathbf{v}_t$ by use of Eq. (6.3).

2. *Analysis of fault circuits.* Some normally open switches may now be closed, and some normally closed switches may now be open. Let $\mathbf{x}$ denote the voltages of the closed switches and the currents of the open switches of S. Let $\mathbf{y}$ denote the complementary variables of $\mathbf{x}$ (i.e., if x_j is v_j, then y_j is i_j, and vice versa). Then obviously $\mathbf{x} \equiv \mathbf{0}$. Equation (6.1) may be rewritten with $\mathbf{x}$ taking the place of $(\mathbf{i}_{\mathrm{NO}}, \mathbf{v}_{\mathrm{NC}})$ and $\mathbf{y}$ taking the place of $(\mathbf{v}_{\mathrm{NO}}, \mathbf{i}_{\mathrm{NC}})$. This of course calls for some *interchanges* between the columns of $(\mathbf{i}_{\mathrm{NO}}, \mathbf{v}_{\mathrm{NC}})$ and the corresponding columns of $(\mathbf{v}_{\mathrm{NO}}, \mathbf{i}_{\mathrm{NC}})$. Such operations, however, require only routine bookkeeping. No additional information other than Eq. (6.1) is needed. The new equation will be of the following form:

$$\begin{bmatrix} \mathbf{D}_{11} & \mathbf{0} & \mathbf{0} & \mathbf{D}_{14} & \mathbf{C}_{15} & \mathbf{C}_{16} \\ \mathbf{D}_{21} & \mathbf{1} & \mathbf{0} & \mathbf{D}_{24} & \mathbf{C}_{25} & \mathbf{C}_{26} \\ \mathbf{D}_{31} & \mathbf{0} & \mathbf{1} & \mathbf{D}_{34} & \mathbf{C}_{35} & \mathbf{C}_{36} \end{bmatrix} \begin{bmatrix} \mathbf{y} \\ \mathbf{v}_t \\ \mathbf{i}_d \\ \mathbf{x} \\ \mathbf{i}_t \\ \mathbf{v}_d \end{bmatrix} = \begin{bmatrix} \mathbf{f}_1 \\ \mathbf{f}_2 \\ \mathbf{f}_3 \end{bmatrix} \tag{6.5}$$

Since $\mathbf{x} \equiv \mathbf{0}$, $\mathbf{i}_t \equiv \mathbf{0}$, the corresponding columns in Eq. (6.5) may be discarded. This leads to the following simplified equation:

$$\begin{bmatrix} \mathbf{D}_{11} & \mathbf{0} & \mathbf{0} & \mathbf{C}_{16} \\ \mathbf{D}_{21} & \mathbf{1} & \mathbf{0} & \mathbf{C}_{26} \\ \mathbf{D}_{31} & \mathbf{0} & \mathbf{1} & \mathbf{C}_{36} \end{bmatrix} \begin{bmatrix} \mathbf{y} \\ \mathbf{v}_t \\ \mathbf{i}_d \\ \mathbf{v}_d \end{bmatrix} = \begin{bmatrix} \mathbf{f}_1 \\ \mathbf{f}_2 \\ \mathbf{f}_3 \end{bmatrix} \tag{6.6}$$

For almost all practical circuits, the square submatrix $\mathbf{D}_{11}$ is nonsingular. Pivoting on $\mathbf{D}_{11}$, we obtain from Eq. (6.6)

$$\mathbf{v}_t = (-\mathbf{C}_{26} + \mathbf{D}_{21}\mathbf{D}_{11}^{-1}\mathbf{C}_{16})\mathbf{v}_d + (\mathbf{f}_2 - \mathbf{D}_{21}\mathbf{D}_{11}^{-1}\mathbf{f}_1) \tag{6.7}$$

$$\mathbf{i}_d = (-\mathbf{C}_{36} + \mathbf{D}_{31}\mathbf{D}_{11}^{-1}\mathbf{C}_{16})\mathbf{v}_d + (\mathbf{f}_3 - \mathbf{D}_{31}\mathbf{D}_{11}^{-1}\mathbf{f}_1) \tag{6.8}$$

Equation (6.8) together with the ideal diode constraints $\mathbf{v}_d \geqslant \mathbf{0}$, $\mathbf{i}_d \geqslant \mathbf{0}$, $\mathbf{v}_d^t\mathbf{i}_d = 0$ forms a complementary problem which may be solved by Lemke's complementary pivot algorithm. After $\mathbf{v}_d$ has been found, $\mathbf{v}_t$ is calculated from Eq. (6.7).

Remarks:

1. The data base required for the compilation of the fault dictionary is the following $(m + d + t) \times (m + d + 1)$matrix.

$$\begin{array}{l} m \text{ rows} \\ t \text{ rows} \\ d \text{ rows} \\ \end{array} \begin{array}{c} \left[\begin{array}{ccc} \mathbf{C}_{14} & \mathbf{C}_{16} & \mathbf{f}_1 \\ \mathbf{C}_{24} & \mathbf{C}_{26} & \mathbf{f}_2 \\ \mathbf{C}_{34} & \mathbf{C}_{36} & \mathbf{f}_3 \end{array}\right] \\ m \text{ col} \quad d \text{ col.} \quad 1 \text{ col.} \end{array} \tag{6.9}$$

A very comprehensive list of hard failures may be considered initially to set up the data base given by (6.9). Later on, if only a subset of the faults are deemed likely, then only a portion of (6.9) needs to be considered.

2. In actual computer implementation, Eqs. (6.7) and (6.8) will be derived from Eq. (6.6) by row echelon reduction instead of finding $\mathbf{D}_{11}^{-1}$ explicitly.

6.4 Simple Example

A numerical example will now be given to illustrate the procedures and notation. The circuit is deliberately chosen to be simple so that all steps can be verified without the aid of a digital computer.

Figure 12.5a shows a circuit in the normal operating condition. Suppose that the faults consist of R_1 shorted (F_1), R_1 open (F_2), and less likely, R_2 open (F_3), and R_2 changing from 1 to 0.5 Ω (F_4).

The first step is to model these faults with switches S_1, S_2, $\hat{S}_1$, and $\hat{S}_2$ as shown in Figure 12.5b, with less likely faults indicated by circumflex. Under the normal condition, we have S_1, $\hat{S}_1$ open and S_2, $\hat{S}_2$ closed. It is desired to determine the test node voltage v_t corresponding to each of these faults.

The four fault switches, two ideal diodes, and one test node pair are extracted to form a 7-port. A straightforward circuit analysis leads to the following equation corresponding to Eq. (6.1). (Note that $m = 4$, $t = 1$, and $d = 2$. Voltage and current notation is shown in Figure 12.5b.)

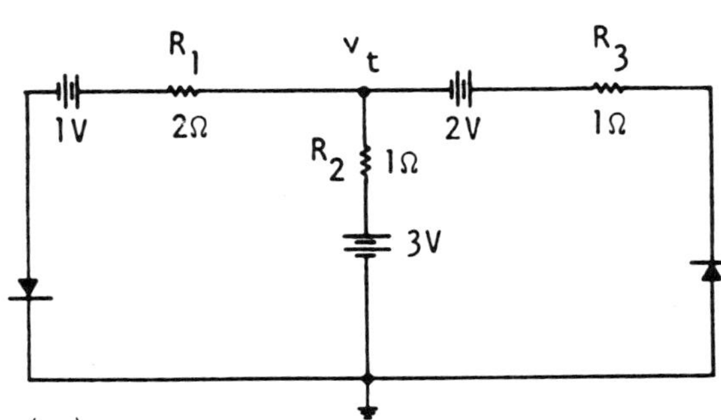

(a)

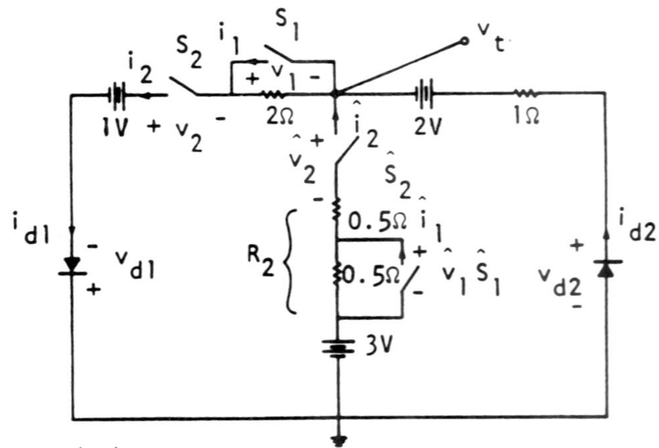

(b)

Figure 12.5 A simple circuit example.

$$
\left[\begin{array}{c|ccccccc}
 & -0.35 & 0.3 & 0.2 & 0.1 & -0.2 & 0.1 & -0.2 \\
 & 0.3 & 0.6 & 0.4 & 0.2 & 1.6 & 0.2 & -0.4 \\
 & -0.2 & -0.4 & 0.4 & -0.8 & -0.4 & -0.8 & -0.4 \\
1_7 & -0.1 & -0.2 & -0.8 & -0.4 & -0.2 & -0.4 & -0.2 \\
 & -0.2 & -0.4 & 0.4 & 0.2 & -0.4 & 0.2 & -0.4 \\
 & -0.1 & -0.2 & -0.8 & -0.4 & -0.2 & -0.4 & -0.2 \\
 & 0.2 & 0.4 & -0.4 & -0.2 & 0.4 & -0.2 & -0.6
\end{array}\right]
\begin{bmatrix} \hat{v}_1 \\ \hat{i}_2 \\ v_1 \\ i_2 \\ v_t \\ i_{d1} \\ i_{d2} \\ \hat{i}_1 \\ \hat{v}_2 \\ i_1 \\ v_2 \\ i_t \\ v_{d1} \\ v_{d2} \end{bmatrix}
= \begin{bmatrix} -1.2 \\ -2.4 \\ -0.4 \\ -0.2 \\ 0.6 \\ -0.2 \\ -2.6 \end{bmatrix} \qquad (6.10)
$$

For the fault F_1, we have $(S_1, S_2, \hat{S}_2)$ closed and $\hat{S}_1$ open. The equation corresponding to (6.6) is

$$\begin{bmatrix} 0.4 & 0 & 0 & 0 & 0 & -0.8 & -0.4 \\ -0.8 & 1 & 0 & 0 & 0 & -0.4 & -0.2 \\ 0.4 & 0 & 1 & 0 & 0 & 0.2 & -0.4 \\ -0.8 & 0 & 0 & 1 & 0 & -0.4 & -0.2 \\ -0.4 & 0 & 0 & 0 & 1 & -0.2 & -0.7 \end{bmatrix} \begin{bmatrix} i_1 \\ i_2 \\ v_t \\ i_{d1} \\ i_{d2} \\ v_{d1} \\ v_{d2} \end{bmatrix} = \begin{bmatrix} -0.4 \\ -0.2 \\ 0.6 \\ -0.2 \\ -2.6 \end{bmatrix} \tag{6.11}$$

Observe that first column in (6.11) is obtained from column 10 for i_1 in Eq. (6.10). Elementary row operations are now applied to Eq. (6.11) to reduce it to Eq. (6.12).

$$\begin{bmatrix} 1 & 0 & 0 & 0 & 0 & -0.2 & -0.1 \\ 0 & 1 & 0 & 0 & 0 & -2 & -1 \\ 0 & 0 & 1 & 0 & 0 & 1 & 0 \\ 0 & 0 & 0 & 1 & 0 & -2 & -1 \\ 0 & 0 & 0 & 0 & 1 & -1 & -1 \end{bmatrix} \begin{bmatrix} i_1 \\ i_2 \\ v_t \\ i_{d1} \\ i_{d2} \\ v_{d1} \\ v_{d2} \end{bmatrix} = \begin{bmatrix} -1 \\ -1 \\ 1 \\ -1 \\ -3 \end{bmatrix} \tag{6.12}$$

From (6.12), we obtain the following equation corresponding to Eq. (6.8):

$$\begin{bmatrix} i_{d1} \\ i_{d2} \end{bmatrix} = \begin{bmatrix} 2 & 1 \\ 1 & 1 \end{bmatrix} \begin{bmatrix} v_{d1} \\ v_{d2} \end{bmatrix} + \begin{bmatrix} -1 \\ -3 \end{bmatrix} \tag{6.13}$$

This equation together with $\mathbf{i}_d \geqslant \mathbf{0}$, $\mathbf{v}_d \geqslant \mathbf{0}$, $\mathbf{v}_d{}^t\mathbf{i}_d = 0$ forms the complementary problem. Solution by Lemke's complementary pivot algorithm gives $i_{d1} = 2$, $v_{d1} = 0$, $i_{d2} = 0$, and $v_{d2} = 3$.

The test node voltage v_t, given by Eq. (6.7), is obtained from Eq. (6.12):

$$v_t = v_{d1} + 1 = -0 + 1 = 1$$

The values of v_t for other faults are determined in like manner.

7 FAULT ISOLATION AND REDUCTION OF THE NUMBER OF TEST NODES

In Section 2, we described the concept of ambiguity set and two rules used (as in [19]) to obtain maximum isolation and to reduce the number of test nodes. We shall continue to use the ambiguity set concept as defined in Ref. [19]. But our method for manipulating the ambiguity sets is quite different from and more systematic than the two rules used in [19]. Instead of describing our method in general terms, we shall illustrate it with a specific (although hypothetical) example.

7.1 Construction of the Table of Ambiguity Sets

Suppose that for a given circuit the preselected fault list consists of eight faults designated F1 through F8. The nominal circuit condition is designated F0 or NOM. One input vector and four test nodes (V1, V2, V3, V4) have been chosen. The test node voltages have been determined by the method of Sections 6 or by the use of a circuit simulation program. The origin of the data is immaterial for the intended fault isolation. The voltages are given in Table 12.5.

For each test node we can define its ambiguity sets, voltage ranges, and circuit conditions. This process becomes very clear if we present the information in Table 12.5 in the form of plots as shown in Figure 12.6. Circuit

Table 12.5 Calculated Voltages of All Test Nodes

	F0	F1	F2	F3	F4	F5	F6	F7	F8
V1	5.0	7.0	7.4	7.3	7.2	9.6	9.7	9.8	5.2
V2	9.0	5.0	6.0	6.4	6.2	5.1	5.2	5.3	9.2
V3	9.5	6.0	6.1	6.2	8.0	6.3	6.4	5.3	4.0
V4	5.0	5.1	5.2	8.8	6.0	6.1	9.0	5.3	6.2

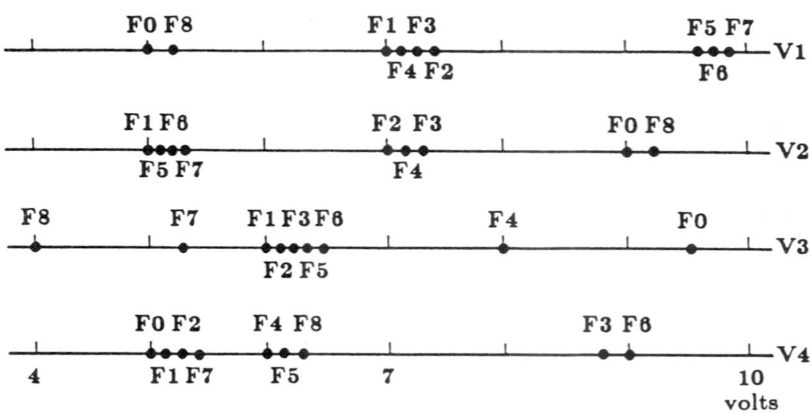

Figure 12.6 Formation of ambiguity sets.

Table 12.6 Ambiguity Sets' Contents and Voltage Ranges

(Node, ambiguity set)	Circuit conditions	Voltage range
(1, 1)	F0, F8	4.4–5.9
(1, 2)	F1, F2, F3, F4	6.4–7.8
(1, 3)	F5, F6, F7	9.0–10.4
(2, 1)	F1, F5, F6, F7	4.5–5.6
(2, 2)	F2, F3, F4	5.7–6.9
(2, 3)	F0, F8	8.4–9.8
(3, 1)	F8	3.3–4.4
(3, 2)	F7	4.6–5.7
(3, 3)	F1, F2, F3, F5, F6	5.8–6.9
(3, 4)	F4	7.3–8.7
(3, 5)	F0	8.7–10.2
(4, 1)	F0, F1, F2, F7	4.5–5.5
(4, 2)	F4, F5, F8	5.7–6.8
(4, 3)	F3, F6	8.2–9.6

conditions that belong to the same ambiguity set correspond to the points in Figure 12.6 that form a "cluster." With the aid of Figure 12.6, we can easily construct Table 12.6 for ambiguity sets.

Note that node 3 has five ambiguity sets, while nodes 1, 2, and 4 each have three ambiguity sets.

The range of each ambiguity set in Table 12.6 is determined in the following manner. First, the center of each cluster is taken to be the average of the two extreme values of the cluster. Next a range of ± 0.7 volt from the center is *tentatively* set. After the *tentative* ranges for all ambiguity sets have been calculated, a check is made to see whether the ranges of any two ambiguity sets (of the same test node) overlap. If so, both ranges are reduced by an equal amount, until a gap or 0.1 or 0.2 volt is obtained. After such revisions, the ranges are accepted for use. As an example, consider ambiguity sets (3, 2) and (3, 3) in Table 12.6. The second ambiguity set of node 3 has only one value of 5.3 volts (corresponding to F7), which is then also the center value. Therefore, ambiguity set (3, 2) has a *tentative range* from 4.6 to 6.0 volts. The third ambiguity set of node 3 has two extreme values, 6.0 and 6.4 (corresponding F1 and F6, respectively), and hence a center value of 6.2 volts. Therefore ambiguity set (3, 3) has a *tentative range* from 5.5 to 6.9. These two ranges overlap. We decrease the upper boundary of set (3, 2) from 6.0 to 5.7 and increase the lower boundary of set (3, 3) from 5.5 to 5.8. Each range is reduced by 0.3 volt, and a gap of 0.1 volt has been created. This explains how the range from 5.8 to 6.9 is obtained for ambiguity set (3, 3). Similar adjustments are made for all ambiguity set ranges.

7.2 Fault Isolation by Intersection of Ambiguity Sets

Suppose that one ambiguity set of some test node VJ contains only one circuit condition FK; then whether that circuit condition has occurred can be determined by measuring node voltage VJ only. In this case, we say that fault FK has been isolated. For example, let the measured value of V3 for the hypothetical circuit be 8.2 volts. Then Table 12.6 indicates that the value belongs to ambiguity set (3, 4). Since this set has only one element, namely F4, the circuit must be under the condition of fault 4.

On the other hand, if we measure one node voltage only and obtain V3 = 6.5 volts, we will not be able to isolate the fault. Table 12.6 indicates that 6.5 volts belongs to ambiguity set (3, 3), and the circuit may be under any one of the following conditions: F1, F2, F3, F5, or F6.

Let us see how the use of additional test nodes can help in isolating the faults. We shall disregard rule 1 but carry out rule 2 of Ref. [19] (see also Section 2) more systematically by constructing an "ambiguity sets intersection table" as shown in Table 12.7. To avoid verbosity, we simply say "intersection of VJ and VK" when we really mean the intersection of ambiguity sets of these nodes. In Table 12.7 the row headings contain ambiguity sets of nodes 3, whereas the column headings contain those of node 4. Each (i, j) block of the matrix contains the result of intersection of ambiguity sets $(3, i)$ and $(4, j)$, with $\varnothing$ denoting a null set. For example, the content of the (3, 1) block is determined as follows:

$$\text{amb. set } (3, 3) \cap \text{amb. set } (4, 1) = \{F1, F2, F3, F5, F6\} \cap \{F0, F1, F2, F7\} = \{F1, F2\}$$

Table 12.7 Intersection of Ambiguity Sets of V3 and V4

	V4		
V3	F0, F1, F2, F7	F4, F5, F8	F3, F6
F8	∅	F8	∅
F7	F7	∅	∅
F1, F2, F3, F5, F6	F1, F2	F5	F3, F6
F4	∅	F4	∅
F0	F0	∅	∅

We note that this intersection yields a total of seven ambiguity sets: {F8}, {F7}, {F4}, {F0}, {F5}, {F1, F2}, {F3, F6}. In particular, F5 has been isolated with the addition of test node 4. For example, if the measured values are V3 = 6.5 volts and V4 = 6.2 volts, then the circuit condition belongs to ambiguity sets (3, 3) *and* (4, 2), according to Table 12.7. But Table 12.7 shows that the only fault which occurs in both ambiguity set (3, 3) *and* (4.2) is F5. Therefore we conclude that the circuit is under condition F5.

With two test nodes V3 and V4, we have isolated faults F4, F5, F7, and F8—a 50% isolation. We note that F1 has not been separated from F2, nor has F3 been separated from F6. More test nodes must be used to achieve a higher percentage of isolation.

Suppose that we decide to add test node V1 with the hope of resolving the ambiguity in {F1, F2} and also in {F3, F6}. The effect of adding V1 can be seen from Table 12.8. An ambiguity set with only one element is called a *singleton*. The intersection of a singleton with another ambiguity set is trivially simple—either a null set or the singleton itself. To save space, operations involving singletons are not shown in detail in the intersection tables (except in Table 12.7). Observe that in Table 12.8 F3 and F6 have been isolated, but F1 and F2 have not. Let us further add test node 2. The intersection operation is shown in Table 12.9. The faults F1 and F2 are now

Table 12.8 Intersection of (V3, V4) with V1

	V1		
(V3, V4)	F0, F3	F1, F2, F3, F4	F5, F6, F7
F1, F2	∅	F1, F2	∅
F3, F6	∅	F3	F6
5 singletons		5 singletons	

Table 12.9 Intersection of (V3, V4, V1) with V2

	V2		
(V3, V4, V1)	F1, F5, F6, F7	F2, F3, F4	F0, F8
F1, F2	F1	F2	∅
7 singletons		7 singletons	

Table 12.10 Intersection of (V3, V4) with V2

	V2		
(V3, V4)	F1, F5, F6, F7	F2, F3, F4	F0, F8
F1, F2	F1	F2	∅
F3, F6	F6	F3	∅
5 singletons		5 singletons	

isolated. This indicates that if we use all of the four test nodes, we can have 100% fault isolation. But the result does not imply that one *must* use all four test nodes to achieve 100% isolation. For example, if the node to be added after (V3, V4) is V2 instead of V1, we will have the intersection table shown in Table 12.10. The result indicates that 100% fault isolation can also be achieved without test node 1.

7.3 Reduction of the Number of Test Nodes

In the general case, the determination of a *minimum* set of test nodes to achieve the highest percentage (not always 100%) of isolation is a very time-consuming process for large circuits. It can be shown that the computation time is not polynomial-bound. Fortunately, for practical applications, we need not insist on getting the *theoretical minimum* number of test nodes. Any *near-minimum* solution will serve our purpose if the solution is simple. In other words, a heuristic method might be more useful for solving practical problems.

We present two heuristic procedures for reducing the number of test nodes.

Procedure 1

Step 1. Select the node that has the largest number of ambiguity sets. If a tie occurs, arbitrarily select one among them.

Step 2. Select the next node whose intersection with previously selected nodes will result in the *largest number* of ambiguity sets. In case of a tie, arbitrarily select one.

Step 3. If the number of the resultant ambiguity sets is equal to the number of circuit conditions (number of faults + 1, the one being for the nominal case), stop. Otherwise go to step 2.

Consider the previous example of Table 12.6. Node 3 is selected first, because it has five ambiguity sets, the largest among V1, V2, V3, and V4.

Next, one node from V2, V3, and V4 is to be selected. The intersection of V3 with V4 yields a total of seven ambiguity sets (see Table 12.7). Similarly, $V3 \cap V1$ yields six sets, and so does $V3 \cap V2$. Therefore V4 is chosen as the second test node. The third test node is to be selected from V1 and V2. Now $(V3 \cap V4) \cap V2$ yields nine ambiguity sets (see Table 12.10), whereas $(V3 \cap V4) \cap V1$ yields only eight sets (see Table 12.8). Therefore V2 is chosen. With V3, V4, V2 chosen as the test nodes, 100% fault isolation is achieved. Test node V1 is seen to be redundant.

Procedure 1 will often lead to a *near-optimum* selection of test nodes (in fact, an optimum selection in the previous example). But even this procedure may be too time-consuming for large circuits. This is because that in step 2 every node has to be intersected with the previously selected group of nodes. Therefore, a further simplified procedure is given below.

Procedure 2

Step 1. Select the node that has the largest number of ambiguity sets. If a tie occurs, arbitrarily select one among them.

Step 2. In the remaining nodes, *tentatively* select one having the largest number of ambiguity sets. If a tie occurs, pick any one among them. Now obtain the intersection of this node, VJ, with the previous selected group of nodes. If the intersection increases the total number of ambiguity sets, then select VJ as a test node. Otherwise, disregard VJ.

Step 3. If the number of resultant ambiguity sets is equal to the number of circuit conditions, stop. Otherwise, to go step 2.

Let us illustrate procedure 2 with the previous example of Table 12.6. In step 1, we select V3 since it has five ambiguity sets, the largest among V1, V2, V3, V4. Each of the remaining nodes, V1, V2, and V4, has three ambiguity sets. According to step 2, we may arbitrarily pick one. Suppose that node 1 is picked. The intersection $V3 \cap V1$ has six ambiguity sets, one more than that of V3 alone. Therefore, V1 is selected as the second test node. The third test node is to be arbitrarily selected from V2 and V4. Suppose that we tentatively pick V2. The intersection $V2 \cap (V3 \cap V1)$ has seven ambiguity sets, one more than $(V3 \cap V4)$. Therefore V2 is selected as the third test node. There is a total of nine circuit conditions (one nominal plus eight faulty conditions). Since $7 < 9$, we go through step 2 another time and include V4 as the fourth test node. As shown previously, with V1, V2, V3, and V4 all selected as test nodes, we achieve 100% fault isolation. But this clearly is not an optimum solution, since three test nodes, V3, V4, and V2, will achieve the same goal.

In most cases procedure 2 will produce a satisfactory solution to the reduction of test nodes. Since its computational effort is much less than that of procedure 1, we have implemented procedure 2 in our present digital computer program.

In Ref. [19], a distinction is made between "fault detection" and "fault isolation." In our present approach, this distinction requires no additional computational effort. We include the nominal circuit (designated by F0 or NOM) in the ambiguity set manipulations. Separation of a fault FJ from NOM amounts to fault detection, while separation among faults is the usual fault isolation.

What happens if all test nodes have been used and still less than 100% fault isolation is achieved? In this case, the first question to be investigated is whether further fault isolation is necessary. If several unseparated faults belong to the same shop replaceable unit (SRU), then further isolation is really unnecessary, since the whole unit has to be replaced anyway.

Suppose that further fault isolation is necessary. Then there are two avenues open to solve the problem:

1. Increase the number of test nodes. Usually, an engineer's familiarity and experience with the circuit may help in the selection of additional test nodes. In the absence of such experience, we may initially choose all *accessible nodes* as the test nodes and use procedure 1 or procedure 2 described above to eliminate unnecessary nodes.
2. Use more input vectors; that is, test the circuit under more input conditions. Very little work has been reported in the literature about the design of stimuli for fault isolation. This is a topic on which much research needs to be done.

Assume that additional input vectors have been decided on. Then the ambiguity set manipulations will have to be modified slightly. Our strategy (as implemented in the digital computer program) is to consider first each node separately. The ambiguity sets of each node under different input vectors are "intersected" to obtain the "all-input ambiguity sets." After such all-input ambiguity sets have been obtained for all nodes, they are processed according to procedure 1 and procedure 2 to select the desired test nodes. The details of implementing such a scheme may be found in Ref. [35].

8 INTEGER-CODE FAULT DICTIONARY AND POSTTEST FAULT IDENTIFICATION

8.1 Compilation of the Fault Dictionary

Once the test nodes have been selected using procedure 1 or procedure 2 described in Section 7, we can determine a unique integer code for each circuit condition. For this purpose we need only the ambiguity sets table as given by Table 12.6. Each fault FJ belongs to exactly one ambiguity set of every test node. This information can be tabulated as shown in Table 12.11

Table 12.11 Integer Codes for All Faults

Circuit condition	Integer code		
	V3	V4	V2
F0	5	1	3
F1	3	1	1
F2	3	1	2
F3	3	3	2
F4	4	2	2
F5	3	2	1
F6	3	3	1
F7	2	1	1
F8	1	2	3

for the hypothetical example of Table 12.6. We assume that V3, V4, and V2 have been selected as the test nodes. As an illustration, consider the code 312 for F2. This means that F2 is in the third ambiguity set of V3, the first set of V4, and the second set of V2. Other codes are interpreted in the same manner.

As pointed out in Section 7.1, fault F4 can be identified by measuring voltage V3 alone, since F4 is the only element in ambiguity set (3, 4). Thus, we could have given F4 an integer code of the form 4XX, where X means "don't care." The code 4XX for F4 implies that measurements of V4 and V2 are unnecessary (don't care) for the identification of F4. For the same reason, the alternative codes in Table 12.12 could have been assigned to all faults (other possibilities exist).

At first glance, it looks as though the use of Table 12.12 is preferable to Table 12.11, because some measurements (don't care) need not be done. But in our work we have preferred Table 12.11 for two reasons:

1. Once the test connections are available, taking additional voltage readings involves very little additional effort.
2. The use of Table 12.11 provides more certainty about fault location than the use of Table 12.12.

The integer codes in Table 12.11 may now be arranged in the dictionary order (ascending numbers) as shown in Table 12.13, which is what we call an integer-code fault dictionary. Since the rightmost column has only one fault for each code, 100% fault isolation has been achieved. Had we used only two test nodes V3 and V4, the fault dictionary in Table 12.14 would have resulted.

Table 12.12 Integer Fault Codes Including "Don't Care"

	Integer code		
Circuit condition	V3	V4	V2
F0	5	X	X
F1	3	1	1
F2	3	1	2
F3	3	3	2
F4	4	X	X
F5	3	2	X
F6	3	3	1
F7	2	X	X
F8	1	X	X

Table 12.13 Fault Dictionary Using Test Nodes V3, V4, and V2

Fault code			
V3	V4	V2	Faults
1	2	3	F8
2	1	1	F7
3	1	1	F1
3	1	2	F2
3	2	1	F5
3	3	1	F6
3	3	2	F3
4	2	2	F4
5	1	3	F0

Table 12.14 shows that F1 and F2 are not isolated, nor are F3 and F6. As mentioned earlier, further isolation may not be necessary if the unseparated faults are located within the same "shop replaceable unit."

The fault dictionary setup for the multiple input vectors case is discussed in Ref. [35].

Table 12.14 Fault Dictionary Using Test Nodes V3 and V4

Fault code		
V3	V4	Faults
1	2	F8
2	1	F7
3	1	F1, F2
3	2	F5
3	3	F3, F6
4	2	F4
5	1	F0

8.2 Posttest Fault Identification by Dictionary Lookup

In Section 2 we reviewed the fault dictionary approach of Ref. [19]. The fault dictionary consists of the calculated voltages of all test nodes under all fault conditions. After the test on a faulty circuit has been made, the posttest analysis to identify the fault involves the calculation of many sums of squared deviations.

The most attractive feature of the integer-code fault dictionary is that no arithmetic operations are needed after test. We only have to look up the dictionary to identify the fault (or group of faults). Since the dictionary entries are arranged in a prescribed order (ascending integers in the present case), the looking-up operation becomes very simple. We will now illustrate the procedure with a specific example.

Let us continue with the hypothetical example of Table 12.6. Suppose that a test on the faulty circuits yields the following readings:

$$V3 = 6.2, \qquad V4 = 8.5, \qquad V2 = 6.0 \quad \text{volts}$$

Referring to Table 12.6, we see that the reading of V3 falls in ambiguity set 3, V4 in set 3, and V2 in set 2. Therefore, the circuit condition has an integer code 332. Now refer to the fault dictionary, Table 12.13. There is only one fault associated with the code 332. Therefore we conclude that fault F3 has occurred.

What happens if the voltage reading of some test node does not fall in any of its ambiguity set ranges? If we use the fault dictionary approach of Ref.

[19], there is a danger of being led to a wrong conclusion. This is because one of the faults, although not the actual fault, may produce a minimum SSD (see Section 2.3) small enough for us to believe that it has occurred. In contrast, using the present approach, we will not draw any conclusion about the circuit condition—a case of "no decision." Such a situation indicates that either the fault list (of hard failures) is not comprehensive enough or the fault is not a hard failure. The former case can be remedied by expanding the fault list and recompiling the fault dictionary. The latter case of soft failures requires some SAT approach for diagnosis.

9 COMPUTER IMPLEMENTATION AND VIDEO AMPLIFIER CIRCUIT EXAMPLE

The techniques described in Sections 4 to 8 have been implemented as a FORTRAN program called HAFDIC [36] (hard fault dictionary) which runs on CDC6500. After preparing the piecewise linear circuit model (with switches), the user enters the circuit information *interactively* through a terminal. The program is currently dimensioned to handle networks up to the size of a video amplifier and requires a memory of about 30K. For a total of 20 preselected hard failures, the execution time for compiling the integer code fault dictionary is typical on the order of 5 seconds.

We shall illustrate the use of HAFDIC with a video amplifier circuit, from the very beginning of specifying hard failures to the final product of an integer-code fault dictionary.

Figure 12.7a shows the schematic diagram of a video amplifier. The engineer, based on experience, preselects 16 faults for detection. The list of faults is given in Table 12.15. Note that the nominal case is just one of the many circuit conditions and is listed as case 1 in Table 12.15.

The piecewise linear models for transistors Q1 and Q2 are next obtained, with the fault conditions Q1BES, Q2BES, Q1BO, Q2BO represented by switches. For analysis purpose, the circuit schematic is replaced by the piecewise linear model shown in Figure 12.7b. The 11 independent current sources in Figure 12.7b actually have zero values. They are required by the n-port theory to facilitate the calculation of the test nodes voltages. Initially, 11 test nodes are chosen, and they are the nodes numbered 2, 6, 7, 9, 11, 12, 13, 14, 18, 19, and 21.

The method used to analyze the piecewise linear network is explained in Section 6. In Table 12.16 we show a portion of the computer output that contains all test node voltages under all fault conditions.

Next, the ambiguity sets at each test node are determined using an algorithm similar to that described in Section 7. The computer output is a

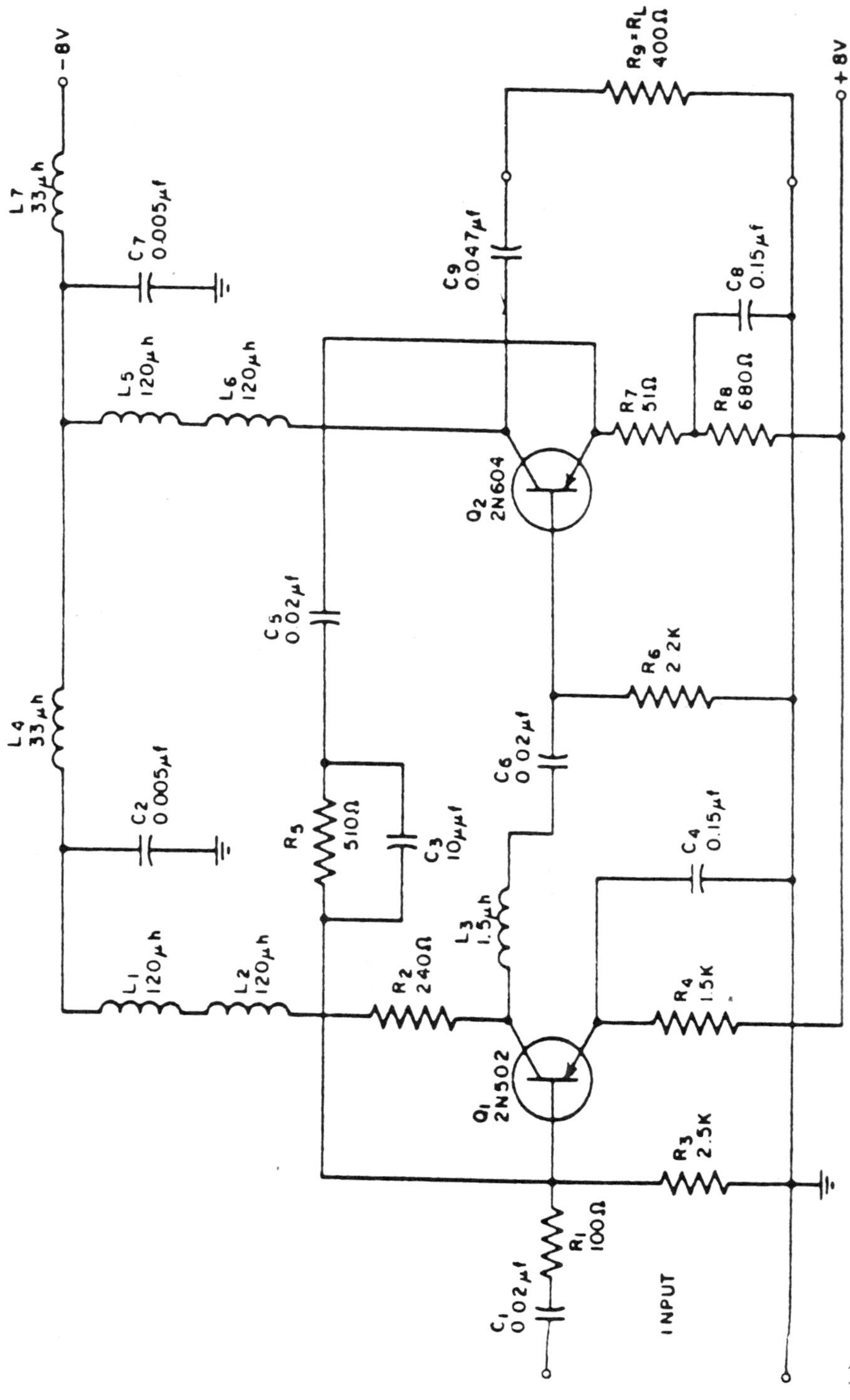
-8V
L7
33μh
C7
0.005μf
L5
120μh
L6
120μh
L4
33μh
C2
0.005μf
L1
120μh
L2
120μh
C5
0.02μf
R5
510Ω
C3
10μμf
R2
240Ω
C9
0.047μf
Q2
2N604
C6
0.02μf
L3
1.5μh
Q1
2N502
C1
0.02μf
R1
100Ω
INPUT
R3
2.5K
R4
1.5K
C4
0.15μf
R6
2.2K
R7
51Ω
R8
680Ω
C8
0.15μf
R9 = RL
400Ω
+8V

(a)

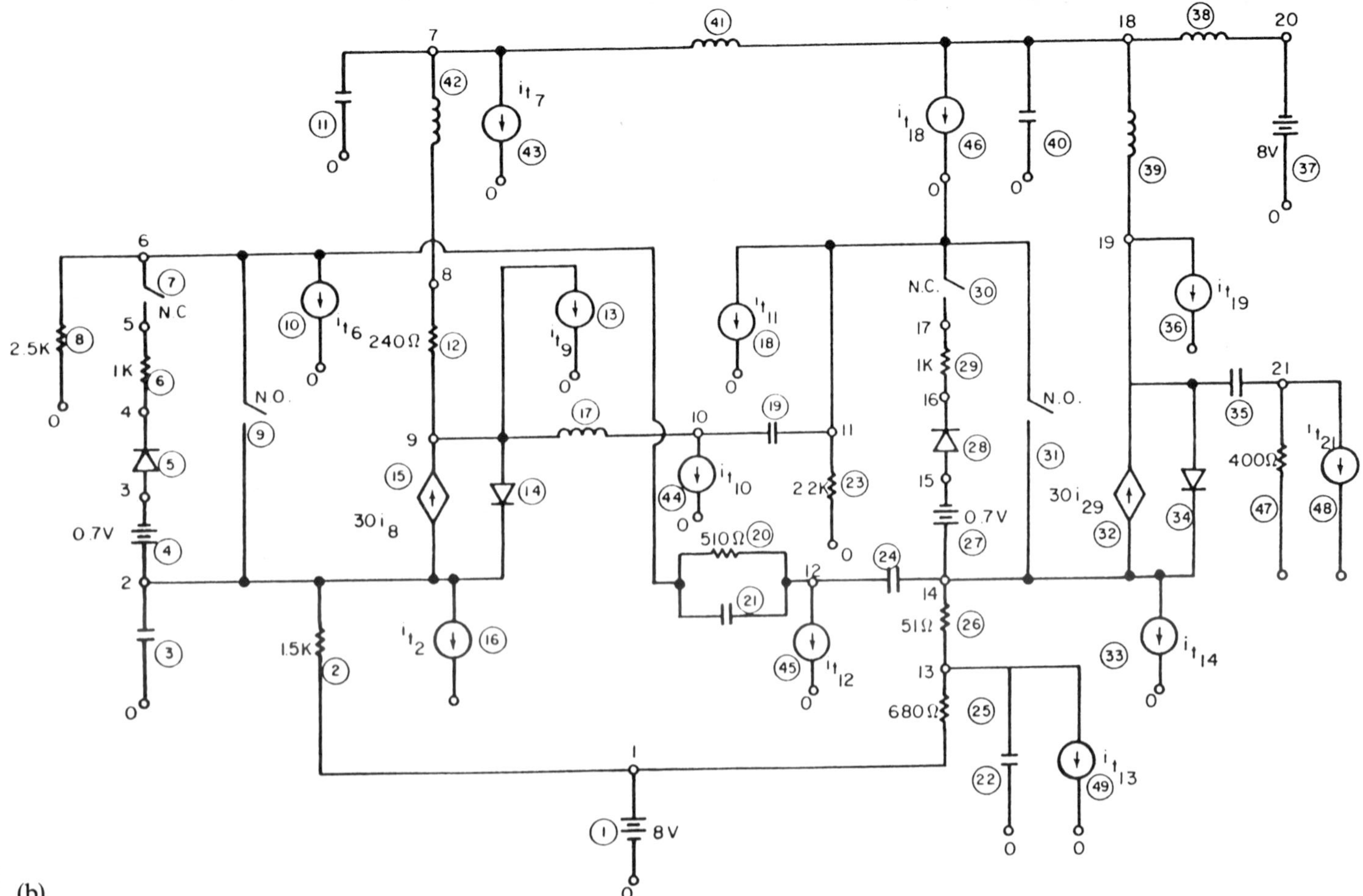

(b)

Figure 12.7 A video amplifier and its PWL model for fault analysis.

Table 12.15 Definition of Faults

Number	Description
1	Nominal case
2	L1 and/or L2 open
3	L4 open
4	L3 open
5	L7 open
6	L5 and/or L6 open
7	Q1 base open
8	Q2 base open
9	C4 shorted
10	C6 shorted
11	C3 shorted
12	C5 shorted
13	C8 shorted
14	C9 shorted
15	Q1, B to E shorted
16	Q2, B to E shorted

Table 12.16 Node Voltages for All Faults

	F1	F2	F3	F4	⋯
V2	1.21	5.81	5.18	1.21	
V6	3.65	3.65	3.65	3.65	
V7	−8.00	−8.00	−5.81	−8.00	
V9	−6.95	5.81	5.81	−6.95	
⋮					

table of ambiguity set ranges. The portion for test node 2 is shown in Table 12.17. Similar tables are printed out by the computer for all test nodes.

As shown in Table 12.17, there are six ambiguity sets for node 2. Ambiguity set 2 is from 5.11 to 6.51 volts and contains F2, F3, and F5.

The algorithm described in Section 7 is used to process the above tables with the aim of reducing the number of test nodes to near minimum. The computer output from this algorithm shows that in the present case only five test nodes voltages are necessary: V2, V11, V13, V7, and V21. The algorithm

Table 12.17 Ambiguity Sets for Node 2

Ambiguity set	Voltage range	Fault cases
1	0.51–1.91	1, 4, 6, 8, 10, 11, 13, 14, 16
2	5.11–6.51	2, 3, 5
3	7.30–8.00	7
4	−0.70–0.70	9
5	1.48–2.88	12
6	4.30–5.70	15

at the same time generates the integer codes for all faults. These computer-generated codes are then sorted in ascending order to form the fault dictionary as shown in Table 12.18.

To illustrate the use of this fault dictionary, suppose that the video amplifier becomes faulty with the following measured node voltages:

$$V2 = 1.2, \quad V13 = 8.0, \quad V11 = 0.5, \quad V7 = -8.0, \quad V21 = -8.0 \text{ volts}$$

Table 12.18 Fault Dictionary for the Video Amplifier

Fault code (V2, V11, V13, V7, V21)	Fault number
1 1 1 1 1	1, 4, 11
1 1 1 1 2	14
1 2 2 1 1	6
1 1 4 1 1	16
1 3 1 1 1	8
1 4 3 1 1	10
1 5 1 1 1	13
2 1 1 1 1	2
2 1 1 2 1	3
2 2 2 2 1	5
3 1 1 1 1	7
4 1 1 1 1	9
5 1 1 1 1	12
6 1 1 1 1	15

Referring to Table 12.17, we find that the fault is in ambiguity set 1 for node 2. Similarly, referring to the remaining tables (not shown here, but given in [35]), we find the fault is in set 3 for node 13, set 1 for node 11, set 1 for node 7, and set 1 for node 21. Hence the integer code is 13111. Now referring to Table 12.18, we find that this corresponds to fault number 8. Further referring to Table 12.15, we see that the fault has been determined as F8, that is, transistor Q2 base open.

10 CONCLUDING REMARKS

DC fault diagnosis has been found quite useful for identifying hard failures, which account for about 80% of failures in analog electronic equipment [19]. In order to enhance the capability of the DC fault dictionary approach, we have in this chapter presented some new techniques (first appeared in references [34] and [37]):

1. Model all nonlinearities by piecewise linear characteristics.
2. Use switches to represent open circuits and short circuits.
3. Solve the piecewise linear resistive network containing switches by the use of multiport theory and Lemke's complementary pivot algorithm.
4. Use multilevel logic to reduce the number of test nodes and to generate an integer-code fault dictionary.

A digital computer program HAFDIC [36] has been written to implement these techniques. The program employs full matrix technique and can adequately handle medium-size circuits such as the video amplifier circuit shown in Section 9. The program, however, cannot handle circuits having more than one DC solution at the nominal or any faulty situation (e.g., bistable multivibrators).

Although the feasibility of the new approach has been established, much research remains to be done before user-oriented software and hardware can be produced to handle larger circuits (at least one order of magnitude larger than the video amplifier circuit of Section 9). Listed below are several topics we consider important for future studies.

1. Investigate the use of sparse matrix techniques in all phases of the computation in order to handle larger circuits.
2. Investigate the construction of piecewise linear macro models for shop replaceable units.
3. Devise more effective fault isolation algorithms. This study naturally includes the selection of test nodes, the determination of ambiguity sets, and the design of input stimuli.
4. Investigate the nondeterministic aspects of DC fault diagnosis. This study will consider the device parameters as random variables. At present, the only precaution we have against measurement inaccuracies and device

parameter variation is to widen the gaps between adjacent ambiguity sets. Apparently, a more elegant theory and a more powerful computational technique are needed. Some preliminary results on the probabilistic aspect of the problem have been reported recently in Refs. [38, 39].

REFERENCES

1. R. S. Berkowitz, Conditions for network-element-value solvability, *IRE Trans. Circuit Theory*, vol. CT-9, pp. 24–29, March 1962.
2. S. D. Bedrosian and R. S. Berkowitz, Solution procedure for single element-kind networks, *IRE Int. Conv. Rec.*, pt. 2, pp. 16–24, March 1962.
3. Special Issue on Automatic Analog Fault Diagnosis, *IEEE Trans. Circuits Syst.*, vol. CAS-26, July 1979.
4. N. David and A. N. Wilson, A theory and an algorithm for analog circuit fault diagnosis, *IEEE Trans. Circuits Syst.*, vol. CAS-26, pp. 440–457, July 1979.
5. N. Sen and R. Saeks, Fault diagnosis for linear systems via multifrequency measurements, *IEEE Trans. Circuits Syst.*, vol. CAS-26, pp. 457–465, July 1979.
6. T. N. Trick, W. Mayeda, and A. A. Sakla, Calculation of parameter values from node voltage measurements, *IEEE Trans. Circuits Syst.*, vol. CAS-26, pp. 466–474.
7. T. Ozawa and Y. Kajitani, Diagnosability of linear active networks, *IEEE Trans. Circuits Syst.*, vol. CAS-26, pp. 485–489, July 1979.
8. R. W. Lin and V. Visvanathan, Sequentially linear fault diagnosis, *IEEE Trans. Circuits Syst.*, vol. CAS-26, pp. 490–496, July 1979.
9. V. Visvanathan and A. Sangiovanni-Vincentelli, Diagnosability of nonlinear circuits and systems—Part I: The dc case, *IEEE Trans. Circuits Syst.*, vol. CAS-28, pp. 1093–1102, Nov. 1981.
10. J. F. M. Theeuwen and J. A. G. Jess, A new approach to the biasing problem and the fault location of nonlinear electronic circuits, *IEEE Trans. Circuits Syst.*, vol. CAS-29, pp. 125–135, March 1982.
11. C. C. Wu, K. Nakajima, C. L. Wei, and R. Saeks, Analog fault diagnosis with failure bounds, *IEEE Trans. Circuits Syst.*, vol. CAS-29, pp. 277–284, May 1982.
12. R. M. Biernacki and J. W. Bandler, Multiple-fault location of analog circuit, *IEEE Trans. Circuits Syst.*, vol. CAS-28, pp. 361–367, May 1981.
13. T. Ozawa, S. Shinoda and M. Yamada, An equivalent-circuit transformation and its application to network-element-value calculations, *IEEE Trans. Circuits Syst.*, vol. CAS-30, pp. 432–441, July 1983.

14. J. A. Starzyk and J. W. Bandler, Design of tests for parameter evaluation within remote inaccessible faulty subnetworks, *Proc. IEEE Int. Symp. Circuits Syst.*, Newport Beach, Calif., pp. 1106–1109, May 1983.
15. Z. F. Huang, C.-S. Lin, and R.-W. Liu, Node-fault diagnosis and a design of testability, *IEEE Trans. Circuits Syst.*, vol. CAS-30, pp. 257–265, May 1983.
16. M. N. S. Swany, L. M. Roytman, and E. Plotkin, Multifrequency approach to fault diagnosis, *Int. J. Circuit Theory Appl.*, pp. 105–109, April 1984.
17. L. Rapisarda and R. A. DeCarlo, Analog multifrequency fault diagnosis, *IEEE Trans. Circuits Syst.*, vol. CAS-30, pp. 223–234, April 1983.
18. J. W. Bandler and A. E. Salama, Fault diagnosis of analog circuits, *Proc. IEEE*, vol. 73, pp. 1279–1325, Aug. 1985.
19. W. Hochwald and J. D. Bastian, A dc approach for analogue fault dictionary determination, *IEEE Trans. Circuits Syst.*, vol. CAS-26, pp. 523–529, July 1979.
20. A. Pahwa and R. A. Rohrer, Band faults: Efficient approximation to fault bands for the simulation before fault diagnosis of linear circuits, *IEEE Trans. Circuits Syst.*, vol. CAS-29, pp. 82–88, Feb. 1982.
21. S. Seshu and R. Waxman, Fault isolation in conventional linear systems—a feasibility study, *IEEE Trans. Reliabil.*, vol. R-15, pp. 11–16, 1966.
22. J. H. Maenpaa, C. J. Stehman, and W. J. Stahl, Fault isolation in conventional linear systems, a progress report, *IEEE Trans. Reliabil.*, vol. R-18, pp. 12–14, 1969.
23. C. Morgan and D. R. Towill, Application of the multiharmonic Fourier filter to nonlinear system fault location, *IEEE Trans. Instrum. Meas.*, vol. IM-26, pp. 164–169, 1977.
24. K. Nadesalingam and D. R. Towill, Frequency domain fault detection and diagnosis in hybrid control systems: a feasibility study, *IEEE Trans. Instrum. Meas.*, vol. IM-27, pp. 193–199, 1978.
25. H. H. Schreiber, Fault dictionary based upon stimulus design, *IEEE Trans. Circuits Syst.*, vol. CAS-26, pp. 529–537, 1979.
26. L. W. Nagel, SPICE2: A computer program to simulate semiconductor circuits, Memo ERL-M520, Electronic Research Laboratory, Univ. of California, Berkeley, May 1975.
27. *ASTAP General Information Manual*, GH20-1271-0, IBM Corp., 1973.
28. L. O. Chua, *Introduction to Nonlinear Network Theory*, McGraw-Hill, New York, 1969.
29. R. E. Tucker and L. P. McNamee, Computer-aided design application to fault detection and isolation techniques, *Proc. 1977 IEEE Int. Symp. Circuits Syst.*, pp. 684–687, April 1977.

30. L. O. Chua and P. M. Lin, *Computer-Aided Analysis of Electronic Circuits: Algorithms and Computational Techniques*, Prentice-Hall, Englewood Cliffs, N.J., 1975.
31. D. T. Phillips, A. Ravindran, and J. J. Solberg, *Operations Research: Principle and Practice*, Wiley, New York, 1976.
32. W. M. G. van Bokhoven, and J. A. G. Jess, Some new aspects of P- and P_0-matrices and their application to networks with ideal diodes, *Proc. 1978 IEEE Int. Symp. Circuits Syst.*, pp. 806–810, 1978.
33. S. N. Stevens and P. M. Lin, Analysis of piecewise linear resistive network using complementary pivot theory, *IEEE Trans. Circuits Syst.*, CAS-28, pp. 429–441, May 1981.
34. P. M. Lin, DC fault diagnosis using complementary pivot theory, *Proc. 1982 Int. Symp. Circuits Syst.*, pp. 146–149, May 1982.
35. Y. S. Elcherif and P. M. Lin, An isolation algorithm for the analog fault dictionary, School of Electrical Engineering, Purdue Univ., Tech. Rep. TR-EE 82-30, Nov. 1982.
36. Y. S. Elcherif and P. M. Lin, Fault diagnosis of nonlinear analog circuits. Vol. V, HAFDIC: A program for generating a hard fault dictionary, School of Electrical Engineering, Purdue Univ., Tech. Rep. to Office of Naval Research, April 1983.
37. P. M. Lin and Y. S. Elcherif, Analogue Circuits fault dictionary—New approaches and implementation, *Int. J. Circuit Theory Appl.*, pp. 149–172, April 1985.
38. V. Visvanathan, E. Szeto, and A. Tits, A robust simulation-before-test technique for dc analog fault diagnosis, *Proc. 1984 Int. Symp. Circuits Syst.*, pp. 689–692, May 1984.
39. V. Visvanathan and L. S. Milor, An efficient algorithm to determine the image of a parallelepiped under a linear transformation, *Proc. 2nd Ann. Symp.* on Computational Geometry, Yorktown Heights, N.Y., June 1986.

13
Decomposition Approaches to Fault Location

Takao Ozawa

Department of Electrical Engineering, Kyoto University, Kyoto, Japan

1 INTRODUCTION

It is well known that decomposition approaches to network analysis are very effective in reducing the amount of computation when the size of the network to be analyzed becomes large. In many cases of network diagnosis we can assume that faulty elements are localized within a small portion of the network and the remaining part is fault-free. Then, decomposition of networks into smaller subnetworks seems to bring about very attractive results, although the techniques used in network diagnosis may be different from those used in network analysis.

Using the component connection model, Wu et al. [1] presented a fault location algorithm for an analog system. In this model the system under test is constituted by interconnected components or subsystems. At each step of testing, components in the network are partitioned into two groups, group 1 and group 2, and it is assumed that all components in group 1 are fault-free or good and faults are localized in group 2. Using the measurement data and the nominal characteristics of components in group 1, the inputs and outputs of components in group 2 are calculated (it is assumed that this is possible). The components in group 2 whose calculated inputs and outputs are consistent with their nominal characteristics are considered good, since it is very unlikely that the effects of two independent analog failures will cancel each other. On the other hand, if the calculated and nominal characteristics are inconsistent, no decision can be made, since the inconsistency may be due to faulty components in group 1 or to those in group 2. The components found good are moved to group 1, and this test step is repeated. The technique used here, that is, making assumptions on faults and checking their validity, is called fault verification.

The decomposition approach proposed by Salama et al. [2] for fault location in a large-scale network is also based on fault verification. A network is decomposed into subnetworks at accessible nodes by hypothetically breaking the connection to the nodes. For each subnetwork its terminal currents (the currents flowing into it) are computed from its terminal voltages (the voltages at the accessible nodes) assuming that it is fault-free, or, in other words, using its nominal element or parameter values (it is assumed that this is possible). The validity of the assumption is tested by applying Kirchhoff's current law (KCL) at accessible nodes. A test at an accessible node is passed if the computed terminal currents satisfy KCL at this node, and all the subnetworks connected to the node are fault-free. If KCL is not satisfied and the test is failed, at least one of the subnetworks connected to the node is faulty. The pass-or-fail results of different tests are analyzed, using logical diagnostic functions, to identify the faulty subnetwork(s).

Salama et al. propose that the decomposition for fault location be hierarchical [2]. The original network is decomposed into a rather small number of subnetworks, and the subnetwork which contains the fault is identified. The faulty subnetwork is further decomposed into smaller sub-subnetworks and the faulty sub-subnetwork is sought. The process is repeated until the fault is localized in the smallest possible portion of the network. The logical fault analysis at each stage of repetition involves only a small number of subnetworks or sub-subnetworks, and therefore the computational effort needed to determine the location of the fault is small. On the other hand, the parameters of subnetworks, sub-subnetworks, and so on are necessary for computing the terminal currents, and a great amount of computation would be needed. They can be computed before actual testing and stored in memory, and therefore this approach would be attractive in the case of on-line testing where a quick fault analysis is needed.

The actual element values may deviate from their nominal values within prescribed tolerance bounds. In most cases it is not possible to calculate all the actual element values from measurements performed on the normal network (if this is possible, all the element values of the faulty network can also be calculated and the faulty element can be determined). Assuming that some of the terminal currents are measurable, Salama et al. derive an underdetermined system of equations which relate the terminal current deviations to the element value deviations. The weighted least-squares solution of the equations gives the conditional expected values of element value deviations.

The diagnosability in the above decomposition approach was considered by Ozawa et al. [3]. The network is said to be n-diagnosable if, under the assumption that the network contains at most n faulty subnetworks, all the faulty subnetworks can be located. A diagnostic matrix is constructed from the incidence or connection matrix of subnetworks to accessible nodes. A theorem for n-diagnosability is given.

One can easily notice the similarity between the two approaches described above. The components in the component connection model used in the first approach may be subnetworks obtained by the nodal decomposition in the second approach. Although components are divided into two groups in the first approach, not all the components in group 1 but only adjacent ones, in general, are involved in the calculation of the inputs and outputs of components in group 2. Not all the inputs and outputs of components in group 2 can be calculated, either. Calculating them and comparing them with those obtained from the nominal characteristics may be equivalent to the process of calculating the inputs and outputs of components in groups 1 and 2 using the nominal characteristics and checking their consistency.

It should be noted that in principle hard faults (i.e., open and/or short faults) as well as soft faults (element value deviations) can be handled by the decomposition approaches, since the topology of the faulty circuit is not used in them.

Since the model used in the second approach is directly connected with electrical networks, we will give details of this approach in the following sections. One of the problems in fault verification is that of deciding whether or not the assumption made on faults is valid. The decision criterion must be established considering element value deviations and measurement errors. The decision algorithm must be efficient to locate faults in large-scale networks. Some new investigations of this problem are presented in Section 3.

2 NODAL DECOMPOSITION APPROACH

2.1 Diagnostic Procedure

Let N be the network under test. Direct measurement of currents is not possible in most cases of network diagnosis except perhaps at the inputs (exciting points) or outputs of the network. Therefore we assume voltage measurement only and say nodes in N are accessible if their voltages are measurable. The nodal decomposition is decomposition of N into subnetworks by hypothetically breaking the connections (not actually cutting connecting wires) at accessible nodes in such a way that there is no mutual coupling between any two subnetworks. The number of resultant subnetworks is denoted by n. For simplicity, we assume that all the accessible nodes can be the nodes of decomposition and there are m accessible nodes.

Example 1 An example of the nodal decomposition is illustrated in Figure 13.1. Suppose we have nodes of decomposition 1, 2, 3, 4 and 0 (the ground) for the filter circuit shown in Figure 13.1a. It is decomposed into six subcircuits as shown in Figure 13.1b.

The terminal voltages of subnetworks obtained by the nodal decomposition are equal to the voltages of the accessible nodes where the terminals are connected in the original network. We assume that the terminal currents of subnetworks can be computed from their terminal voltages and the excitation. As will be shown in Example 2 below, our method may work even

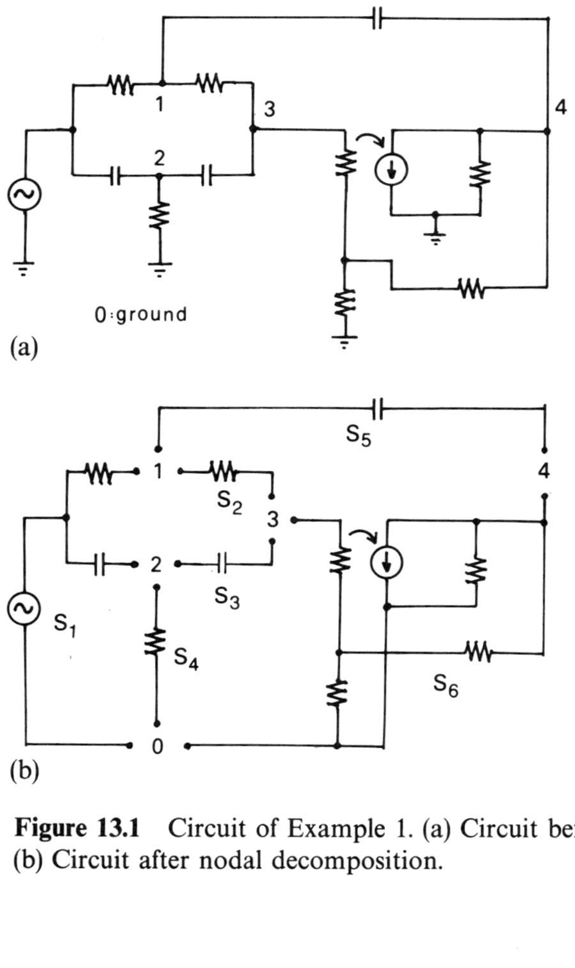

Figure 13.1 Circuit of Example 1. (a) Circuit before nodal decomposition. (b) Circuit after nodal decomposition.

if this assumption does not hold for some subnetworks. At present we assume it for simplicity of discussion. Then the major diagnostic steps become as follows.

DIAG

Step 1. Perform the nodal decomposition of N.

Step 2. Compute terminal currents of the resultant subnetworks using their measured terminal voltages, the known exciting voltages and currents, and *nominal* element or parameter values.

Step 3. Test whether or not the computed terminal currents satisfy KCL at accessible nodes in N. It is assumed that if a subnetwork is faulty, the tests at the accessible nodes where its terminals are connected are all failed. From the test result point of view it is assumed that if KCL is satisfied at an accessible node, all the subnetworks connected to this node in N are good; otherwise, at least one of these subnetworks is faulty.

Step 4. Locate faulty subnetworks from the test results obtained at step 3.

The tests in step 3 are called the KCL tests. The relation between the test results and faulty subnetworks as stated above is based on the assumption that the effects of two independent analog faults do not cancel each other.

Example 2 The nominal circuit is shown in Figure 13.2a. Nodes of decomposition are a, ~~b~~, c, and e, and then each subcircuit consists of one element. The faulty circuit is shown in Figure 13.2b. Resistor r_3 is faulty and is now 3 Ω instead of its nominal value of 1 Ω. The measured node voltages will be $v_a = 12$ V, $v_b = 8$ V, $v_c = 2$ V. Using these voltages and nominal element values, we get $i_1 = 4$ A, $i_2 = 2$ A, $i_3 = 6$ A, and $i_4 = 2$ A. For the subcircuit consisting of the voltage source it is not possible to calculate its terminal currents from its terminal voltages. We can, however, apply KCL to this subcircuit and we see that we must have $i_1 = i_2 + i_4$. This equation is satisfied by the calculated currents. KCL is not satisfied, however, at nodes b and c.

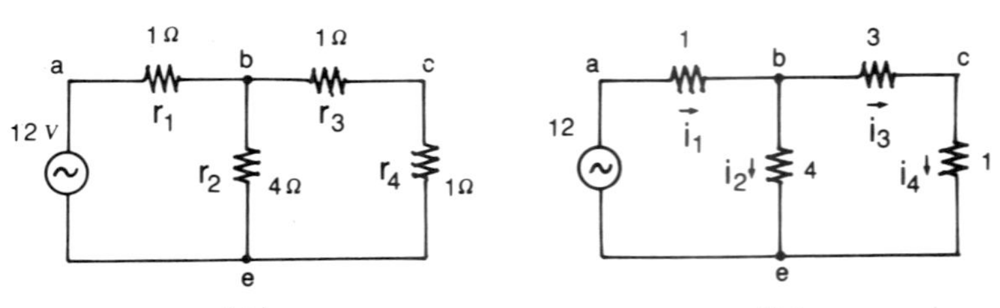

Figure 13.2 Circuit of Example 2. (a) Nominal circuit. (b) Faulty circuit.

Thus we conclude that the subcircuits connected to nodes a and e (the voltage source can be regarded as a short circuit) are good; that is, resistors r_1, r_2, and r_4 are good. Resistor r_3 is connected to nodes b and c, where the KCL tests are failed, and thus it is faulty. Note that the computed currents $i_1 = 4$ A, $i_2 = 2$ A, and $i_4 = 2$ A of good resistors agree with the actual currents flowing in the faulty network. Therefore KCL equations containing these currents only must be satisfied.

Suppose N is in the sinusoidal steady state. If a subnetwork is linear and does not contain exciting sources, its terminal currents can be computed from its terminal voltages using its indefinite admittance matrix. In general, the amount of computation necessary to get this matrix grows rapidly as the size of the subnetwork becomes large. Besides, the effect of faults on the terminal currents becomes less detectable. Therefore it is advantageous to deal with subnetworks as small as possible.

2.2 Diagnosability

Obviously, diagnostic procedure DIAG given above works only if there is a limit on the number of faulty subnetworks. This situation is the same as that with other approaches based on fault verification. Therefore let us define diagnosability of network N as follows.

***t*-diagnosability** Network N is said to be t-diagnosable if, under the assumption that N contains at most t faulty subnetworks, all the faulty subnetworks can be located.

We will derive a theorem on t-diagnosability for DIAG. Let K be the connection matrix of subnetworks to accessible nodes, that is, the matrix whose rows and columns correspond to the accessible nodes and subnetworks, respectively, and whose i–j element is 1 if subnetwork s_j is connected to accessible node n_i and 0 otherwise. Let us represent the results of the KCL tests by 1 and 0: the test at node n_i is denoted by τ_i, and $\tau_i = 0$ if KCL is satisfied; $\tau_i = 1$ if KCL is not satisfied. We first consider 1-diagnosability.

Suppose there is only one faulty subnetwork, and subnetwork s_j is faulty. Then KCL is not satisfied by the computed terminal currents at the accessible nodes to which s_j is connected, but it is satisfied at the others [refer to eq. (8) in Section 3.1]. Therefore the results of the KCL tests agree with the 0–1 pattern of column j of K. In other words, K is identical to a conventional diagnostic matrix for a single fault, its rows corresponding to tests made for subnetworks. Let $D_1 := K$. Obviously, N is 1-diagnosable if and only if the columns of D_1 are all distinct.

Example 1 continued For the nodal decomposition of Figure 13.1b we get $K = D_1$ as given in Table 13.1, where column j corresponds to subnetwork s_j. The columns of D_1 are all distinct, and the circuit is 1-diagnosable.

If the 0–1 patterns of columns j and k are the same, we say that subnetworks s_j and s_k are parallel. A fault in parallel subnetworks cannot be localized within a subnetwork from measurements of voltages only.

The above discussion of 1-diagnosability can easily be extended to t-diagnosability for $t = 2, 3$, and so on. Let D_t be the matrix whose rows correspond to accessible nodes and thus to the KCL tests and whose columns correspond to all possible combinations of t subnetworks. A column of D_t is the union (logical OR) of the t columns of $D_1 = K$ corresponding to these t subnetworks it represents. We can easily see that if these t subnetworks are faulty, the results of the KCL tests agree with the 0–1 patterns of the column. Hence we have the following theorem.

Theorem 1 Network N is t-diagnosable if and only if the columns of matrix

$$D := [D_1 \quad D_2, \quad \ldots, \quad D_t] \tag{1}$$

are all distinct.

Example 1 continued For the nodal decomposition of Figure 13.1b we get D_2 as given in Table 13.2, where column j–k corresponds to the combination of subnetworks s_j and s_k. Columns 1–2 and 1–3, for example, have the same 0–1 pattern, and thus N is not 2-diagnosable.

Let us regard a column of D as the binary representation of an integer. Then the distinctness of the columns of D can be checked by sorting the

Table 13.1 $K = D_1$

	1	2	3	4	5	6
$n_1(\tau_1)$	1	1	0	0	1	0
$n_2(\tau_2)$	1	0	1	1	0	0
$n_3(\tau_3)$	0	1	1	0	0	1
$n_4(\tau_4)$	0	0	0	0	1	1
$n_0(\tau_0)$	1	0	0	1	0	1

Table 13.2 D_2

	1–2	1–3	1–4	1–5	1–6	2–3	2–4	2–5	2–6	3–4	3–5	3–6	4–5	4–6	5–6
n_1	1	1	1	1	1	1	1	1	1	0	1	0	1	0	1
n_2	1	1	1	1	1	1	1	0	0	1	1	1	1	1	0
n_3	1	1	0	0	1	1	1	1	1	1	1	1	0	1	1
n_4	0	0	0	1	1	0	0	1	1	0	1	1	1	1	1
n_0	1	1	1	1	1	0	1	0	1	1	0	1	1	1	1

integers obtained from the 0–1 patterns of the columns. Many efficient sorting algorithms are known [4]. Therefore t-diagnosability can easily be checked, if t is not so large. For a fixed value of t a set of subnetworks or subnetwork combinations such that the fault can be localized within the set but cannot be further localized within a subnetwork or subnetwork combination in the set is called a t-diagnosable set. We can get t-diagnosable sets by finding the columns of D which have the same 0–1 patterns. Again, a sorting algorithm can be used.

2.3 Fault Location Algorithm

In general, we can expect the following when the size of network N or the number of elements in N becomes large. (1) The number of accessible nodes increases (perhaps in proportion to the size of N). (2) The number of subnetworks obtained by the nodal decomposition increases (perhaps in proportion to the size of N). (3) The number of subnetworks connected to an accessible node is limited within a certain range (perhaps less than 10). (4) The number of terminals of a subnetwork is limited within a certain range. (5) Faults are localized within a rather small portion of N, and only a small number of subnetworks are faulty. Then the number of tests whose results are fail is small compared with the total number of KCL tests or subnetworks. The number t of faulty subnetworks, however, is not known.

In view of the above observation, we define the fault region R as a set of subnetworks all of whose terminals are connected to accessible nodes where KCL tests fail. We can say R is the smallest set of subnetworks within which faults cannot be further localized if the value of t is not known. Let F be the set of the accessible nodes for which the results of KCL tests are fail. R is the set of the subnetworks whose terminals are all connected to nodes in F. R can be determined by the algorithm FAULTREG below. In FAULTREG f_j is the number of the accessible nodes connected to s_j and, at the same time, belonging to F. Initially $f_j = 0$. The number of terminals of s_j is denoted by t_j.

FAULTREG

Step 1. For each node n_i in F repeat the following.
If subnetwork s_j is connected to node n_i, set $f_j := f_j + 1$.
Step 2. For f_j not equal to 0 repeat the following.
If $f_j = t_j$, then include s_j in R.

For a large network it would be better to have, instead of a two-dimensional array for K, a linked list of the subnetworks which are connected to the same accessible nodes. If the total number of subnetworks is not so large, we can prepare a linear array for f_j's. Otherwise it would be better to prepare a binary search tree or AVL tree [4] for nonzero f_j's only. The key for the search in such a tree is j, and the location of key j is sought in step 1.

If only one subnetwork is faulty, the subnetwork in R such that the number of terminals is equal to $|F|$† is faulty.

Example 1 continued Suppose $\tau_1 = \tau_2 = \tau_3 = 1$, and $\tau_4 = \tau_0 = 0$. Then $f_1 = 2$, $f_2 = 2$, $f_3 = 2$, $f_4 = 1$, $f_5 = 1$, and $f_6 = 1$. We get $R = \{s_2, s_3\}$ by checking the numbers of terminals belonging to the subnetworks.

Once the faulty subnetwork is identified, and if the size of the subnetwork is small, it is rather easy to find the faulty element in it. For example, techniques for element value calculation from multiexcitation measurements can be used [5–10].

3 FAULT LOCATION FOR PRACTICAL NETWORKS

3.1 Decision Criterion for KCL Tests

Although the approach introduced in the preceding section is simple in principle and efficient in computation, it has a problem in common with many other fault location techniques based on fault verification. The problem is that KCL at step 3 of DIAG is never exactly satisfied. The terminal currents of a subnetwork are computed using *nominal element values*, but the actual element values may deviate from their nominal values within tolerance bounds. Therefore the computed terminal currents do not agree, in general, with the actual terminal currents even if the subnetwork is fault-free, and KCL is not satisfied. It may also happen that one of the terminal currents at an accessible node (terminal currents from different subnetworks) is much smaller than the others. Even if this small current changes considerably in ratio because of faults, its contribution to the KCL equation at the accessible node may be smaller than the changes which are caused by element value deviations in the other terminal currents and which can be considered normal. There are some errors in the voltage measurements. Therefore we have to establish some pass-or-fail decision criterion to be used in the KCL tests for an actual network. In the following we will give some heuristic solutions to this problem.

The network which contains elements in tolerance bounds but which is regarded as normal is called the perturbed network. The nominal, faulty, and perturbed networks are denoted by N^n, N^f, and N^p, respectively.

---

†In general $|S|$ is the cardinality of set S.

In the following we consider a linear network in the sinusoidal steady state. Let I_j, V_j, and U_j be the vectors of terminal currents, terminal voltages, and exciting voltages and/or currents of subnetwork s_j, respectively. Also, let Y_j and H_j be the indefinite admittance matrix and the matrix of transfer functions from the excitation to the terminal currents, respectively. The vectors and matrices for nominal, faulty, and perturbed networks are identified by superscripts n, f, and p, respectively.

For the terminal currents of N^n and N^f we have

$$I_j^n = Y_j^n V_j^n + H_j^n U_j \tag{2}$$

$$I_j^f = Y_j^f V_j^f + H_j^f U_j \tag{3}$$

respectively.

Let A_j be the incidence matrix of subnetwork s_j to the accessible nodes; that is, A_j is the matrix which has m rows corresponding to the accessible nodes and whose i–k element is 1 if the kth terminal of s_j is connected to node n_i, and 0 otherwise. [Each column of A_j has only one 1, and the union (logical OR) of all columns of A_j becomes column j of K.] Then the KCL equations at the accessible nodes can be written as

$$\sum_{j=1}^{n} A_j I_j^n = 0 \tag{4}$$

$$\sum_{j=1}^{n} A_j I_j^f = 0 \tag{5}$$

for the nominal and faulty networks, respectively. For the KCL tests applied to the faulty network we compute the following residual current vector:

$$J^f := \sum_{j=1}^{n} A_j (Y_j^n V_j^f + H_j^n U_j) \tag{6}$$

at the accessible nodes. Using Eqs. (6), (3), and (5), we get

$$J^f = \sum_{j=1}^{n} A_j [(Y_j^n - Y_j^f) V_j^f + (H_j^n - H_j^f) U_j] \tag{7}$$

Suppose there is no element value deviation. Then from Eq. (7) we see that if subnetwork s_j is faulty and $Y_j^f \neq Y_j^n$ and/or $H_j^f \neq H_j^n$, in general it gives rise to nonzero residual currents at accessible nodes where its terminals are connected. Test τ_i is fail if the element of J^f corresponding to node n_i is nonzero, and pass otherwise. Thus D_1 becomes identical to K.

Next let us consider the perturbed network. The terminal currents of subnetwork s_j in the perturbed network are given by

$$I_j^p = Y_j^p V_j^p + H_j^p U_j \tag{8}$$

and the KCL equations at the accessible nodes are

$$\sum_{j=1}^{n} A_j I_j^p = 0 \tag{9}$$

The residual current vector for the perturbed network is computed from

$$J^p = \sum_{j=1}^{n} A_j(Y_j^n V_j^p + H_j^n U_j) \tag{10}$$

Using Eqs. (2) and (4), we get

$$J^p = \sum_{j=1}^{n} A_j[Y_j^n(V_j^p - V_j^n)] \tag{11}$$

If we can measure node voltages of the perturbed network, we can compute J^p from Eq. (10) or Eq. (11) and use the result in the KCL tests for the faulty network. Let j_i^f and j_i^p be the elements of J^f and J^p, respectively, corresponding to node n_i. Then we set

$$\begin{aligned} \tau_i &= 1 \qquad \text{if} \quad \|j_i^f - j_i^p\| > c_i\|j_i^p\|^{\dagger} \\ \tau_i &= 0 \qquad \text{otherwise} \end{aligned} \tag{12}$$

where c_i is a constant representing tolerance and should be chosen properly, considering the size of subnetworks and so forth.

Example 2 continued Suppose perturbed element values of the circuit in Figure 13.2a are $r_1 = 1.05\,\Omega$, $r_2 = 4.30\,\Omega$, $r_3 = 0.90\,\Omega$, and $r_4 = 0.95\,\Omega$, as given in Figure 13.3a. Let v_j be the voltage of r_j for $j = 1, 2, 3, 4$. Then we get

$$v_a = 12.0\text{ V}, \quad v_b = v_2 = 6.623\text{ V}, \quad v_c = v_4 = 3.401\text{ V},$$
$$v_1 = 5.377\text{ V}, \quad v_3 = 3.222\text{ V}$$

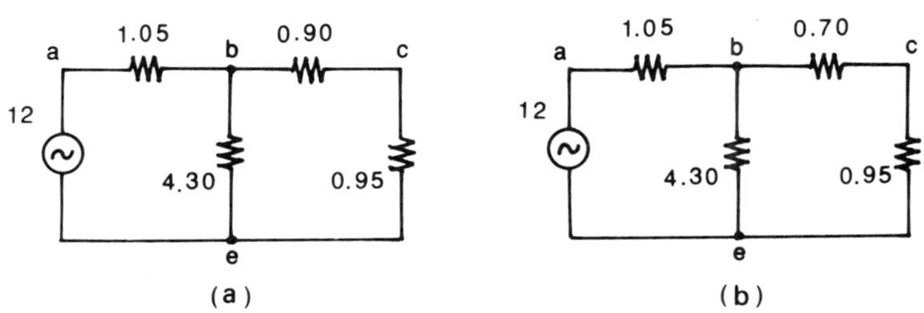

Figure 13.3 Circuit of Example 2. (a) Perturbed circuit. (b) Faulty circuit.

---

† $\|x\|$ is the effective value of x.

and from these voltages we can compute

$$j_{ae}{}^p = 5.377 - 1.656 - 3.401 = 0.320 \text{ A}$$

$$j_b{}^p = -5.377 + 1.656 + 3.222 = -0.499 \text{ A}$$

$$j_c{}^p = -3.222 + 3.401 = 0.179 \text{ A}$$

Now if r_3 becomes faulty and $r_3 = 0.70\ \Omega$ as given in Figure 13.3b, then we get

$$v_a = 12.0 \text{ V}, \qquad v_b = v_2 = 6.381 \text{ V}, \qquad v_c = v_4 = 3.674 \text{ V},$$

$$v_1 = 5.619 \text{ V}, \qquad v_3 = 2.707 \text{ V}$$

and we can compute

$$j_{ae}{}^f = 5.619 - 1.595 - 3.674 = 0.350 \text{ A}$$

$$j_b{}^f = -5.619 + 1.595 + 2.707 = -1.317 \text{ A}$$

$$j_c{}^f = -2.707 + 3.674 = 0.967 \text{ A}$$

Since the size of the circuit is small, we can choose small values for c_{ae}, c_b, and c_c, say $c_{ae} = c_b = c_c = 0.5$. Then $\tau_{ae} = 0$, $\tau_b = 1$, and $\tau_c = 1$ and r_3 is identified as faulty.

If V_j^p is not known, it is rather difficult to estimate J^p. Therefore we propose the following approach. Since the perturbed network is normal, we can expect that its performance is close to nominal, and thus $V_j^p \simeq V_j^n$ in general. Then, neglecting the second-order perturbation, we get from Eqs. (8) and (2) the vector of terminal current deviations

$$\Delta I_j := I_j^p - I_j^n \simeq [(Y_j^n - Y_j^p)V_j^n + (H_j^n - H_j^p)U_j] \tag{13}$$

Equation (13) shows that ΔI_j can be estimated from a sensitivity analysis of subnetworks. The terminal current deviations due to element or parameter value deviations are computed with the terminal voltages and the excitation held constant. This can be done by the well-known method using the adjoint network [11, 12]. Let $\|m_i{}^p\|$ be the maximum absolute value (effective value) among the terminal current deviations at node n_i. Then a decision criterion for KCL tests is

$$\begin{aligned} \tau_i &= 1 \qquad \text{if} \quad \|j_i{}^f\| > c_i\|m_i{}^p\| \\ \tau_i &= 0 \qquad \text{otherwise} \end{aligned} \tag{14}$$

3.2 Modified Fault Location Algorithm

If the test criterion stated in the preceding section is used, faulty terminal currents at node n_i which are smaller than $c_i\|j_i^p\|$ or $c_i\|m_i^p\|$ are considered normal, and the test result τ_i may become zero. Likewise, if τ_i becomes 1, it is probably due to terminal currents whose nominal values are large. Therefore it is reasonable to neglect small nominal terminal currents in locating faulty subnetworks, and the connection of a terminal to n_i is not considered if its nominal current is smaller than $c_i\|j_i^p\|$ or $c_i\|m_i^p\|$. The connection matrix K and the number of terminals t_j are modified accordingly, and the new matrix and number of terminals are denoted by K^* and t_j^*, respectively.

In spite of the above modification, erroneous test results can arise, since the decision criterion (12) or (14) is based only on reasonable estimation. Also, the effect of the fault on some terminal currents may be small. Then the test result 1 may arise when it should be 0, or vice versa. In most cases we can assume that only one subnetwork is faulty, and it is reasonable to compute the Hamming distance† between the test results and 0–1 patterns of the connection matrix to find the most probably faulty subnetwork. Thus we have the following algorithm.

FAULTSUB

Step 1. For each node n_i in F repeat the following.
If subnetwork s_j is connected to n_i (K^* is used), set $f_j := f_j + 1$.

Step 2. For f_j not equal to 0 compute

$$d_j^* := (t_j^* - f_j) + (|F| - f_j) = t_j^* + |F| - 2f_j \tag{15}$$

Step 3. Subnetwork s_j which gives the smallest values of d_j^* is considered faulty.

4 CONCLUDING REMARKS

The nodal decomposition approach presented in Section 2 can easily be modified if some of the terminal currents are measurable or known; that is, the measured or known current values are substituted in the KCL equations in such a case. In DIAG the KCL tests are performed at accessible nodes. Obviously, however, KCL can be applied to cutsets in N, as is illustrated by Example 2, and then the KCL tests are modified accordingly.

---

†The Hamming distance between two 0–1 vectors is the number of bits which do not agree at the corresponding positions of two vectors.

Note that only measurement data obtained by a particular network excitation are used in the KCL tests. If measurements on the network with different excitations are possible, for example, if multifrequency measurements are possible, more reliable decisions can be made. The terminal currents may change as the excitation is varied, and small terminal currents at one excitation may become large at another. Thus matrix K^* changes depending on the excitation. The effect of the fault on terminal currents may also change. Thus we will get different computed values of d_j^*. Applying statistical techniques to the results obtained with different excitations, we can determine the subnetwork which is most probably faulty.

REFERENCES

1. C.-C. Wu, K. Nakajima, C.-L. Wey, and R. Saeks, Analog fault diagnosis with failure bounds, *IEEE Trans. Circuits Syst.*, vol. CAS-29, pp. 277–284, 1982.
2. A. E. Salama, J. A. Starzyk, and J. W. Bandler, A unified decomposition approach for fault location in large analog circuits, *IEEE Trans. Circuits Syst.*, vol. CAS-31, pp. 609–622, 1984.
3. T. Ozawa, J. W. Bandler, and A. E. Salama, Diagnosability in the decomposition approach for fault location in large analog networks, *IEEE Trans. Circuits Syst.*, vol. CAS-32, pp. 415–416, 1985.
4. D. E. Knuth, *The Art of Computer Programming*; vol. 3, Addison-Wesley, Reading, Mass., 1975.
5. L. Rapisarda and R. A. DeCarlo, Analog multifrequency fault diagnosis, *IEEE Trans. Circuits Syst.*, vol. CAS-30, pp. 223–234, 1983.
6. N. Navid and A. N. Willson, Jr., A theory and an algorithm for analog fault diagnosis, *IEEE Trans. Circuits Syst.*, vol. CAS-26, pp. 441–457, 1979.
7. T. Ozawa, S. Sinoda, and M. Yamada, An equivalent-circuit transformation and its application to network-element-value calculation, *IEEE Trans. Circuits Syst.*, vol. CAS-30, pp. 432–441, 1983.
8. T. Ozawa and M. Yamada, Conditions for determining parameter values in a linear active network from node voltage measurements, *1981 IEEE Int. Symp. Circuits Syst. Proc.*, pp. 274–277, 1981.
9. T. Ozawa and M. Yamada, Conditions for network-element-value determination by multifrequency measurements, *1982 IEEE Int. Symp. Circuits Syst. Proc.*, pp. 1156–1159, 1982.
10. J. A. Starzyk, R. M. Biernacki, and J. W. Bandler, Evaluation of faulty elements within linear subnetworks, *Int. J. Circuit Theory Appl.*, vol. 12, pp. 23–37, 1984.

11. R. K. Brayton and R. Spence, *Sensitivity and Optimization*, Elsevier, Amsterdam, 1980.
12. J. Vlach and K. Singhal, *Computer Methods for Circuit Analysis and Design*, Van Nostrand-Reinhold, New York, 1983.

14

Optimization Techniques for Modeling, Diagnosis, and Tuning

John W. Bandler and Qi-jun Zhang

McMaster University
Hamilton, Ontario, Canada

1 INTRODUCTION

This chapter deals with the application of optimization techniques for modeling, diagnosis, and tuning (MDT) of electrical circuits. A conventional interpretation of such techniques for modeling and diagnosis is the determination of appropriate network parameters leading to the best match between circuit responses and measured data. When the measurements are insufficient to evaluate all network elements, the most likely faults may be located. Otherwise, if the measurements are sufficient, parameter identification is initiated, resulting in a circuit model whose performance best fits the measurement data in the presence of uncertainties and noise. Closely related is the tuning problem, which has been approached mostly from the optimization point of view. Existing software for mathematical programming can be readily exploited in this case.

Our presentation is tutorial but designed to be helpful for a state-of-the-art understanding. We first review circuit-oriented optimization methods with emphasis on aspects important in MDT. A general formulation of circuit diagnosis as an optimization problem is introduced. It is followed by a detailed investigation into three specific formulation cases. Optimization methods for modeling and tuning are presented and compared with those for diagnosis. Illustrative examples are provided.

2 CIRCUIT-ORIENTED OPTIMIZATION TECHNIQUES

Optimization methods have played an important role in computer-aided design of circuits and systems [1–9]. Recent advances in this area produced successful results that would have been prohibitively labor-intensive with other techniques [10]. Typical circuit design objectives are to satisfy or to exceed design specifications as much as possible. The MDT problems, however, are usually oriented either toward (response) data fitting or toward "parameter fitting" or a combination of both. The parameter fitting can be interpreted as forcing parameters to approach a desired pattern. Such a pattern is constructed to best represent

1. An estimation of the parameters, e.g., results from a deliberate perturbation of the circuit (for more measurement information), a projected target parameter point for tuning
2. An assumption of the circuit philosophy, e.g., type of faults, whether catastrophic or soft
3. A criterion for optimality, e.g., the objective for minimum parameter adjustment in tuning

2.1 Introduction to Mathematical Programming

An optimization problem can be stated as

$$\underset{\boldsymbol{\phi}}{\text{minimize}}\ U(\boldsymbol{\phi}) \tag{1a}$$

subject to constraints

$$\mathbf{g}(\boldsymbol{\phi}) \geqslant \mathbf{0} \tag{1b}$$

and

$$\mathbf{h}(\boldsymbol{\phi}) = \mathbf{0} \tag{1c}$$

where $\boldsymbol{\phi} \triangleq [\phi_1 \quad \phi_2 \quad \cdots \quad \phi_n]^T$, $\mathbf{g} \triangleq [g_1 \quad g_2 \quad \cdots \quad g_{n_g}]^T$, and $\mathbf{h} \triangleq [h_1 \quad h_2 \quad \cdots \quad h_{n_h}]^T$.

When U, $\mathbf{g}$, and $\mathbf{h}$ are all linear functions of $\boldsymbol{\phi}$, (1) is a linear programming (LP) problem, readily solvable by the simplex method [11], a classical approach being currently challenged by Karmarkar's algorithm [12, 13].

To handle the nonlinear programming (NLP) problem, i.e., the nonlinear case of (1), a variety of methods have been developed. The unconstrained NLP problem can be solved by conjugate direction methods and quasi-Newton methods. The constrained NLP problem can be handled using, e.g., penalty and barrier methods and augmented Lagrangian methods.

A systematic treatment of (1) can be found in many textbooks, e.g., Luenberger [11]. A comprehensive examination of optimization from the circuit design point of view is provided in Refs. [1–9]. In this section, we highlight those aspects of optimization which are relevant to MDT.

2.2 Least *p*th Optimization [14–16]

A frequently encountered objective $U(\boldsymbol{\phi})$ is the pth norm of $\mathbf{f}(\boldsymbol{\phi}) \triangleq [f_1(\boldsymbol{\phi}) \quad f_2(\boldsymbol{\phi}) \quad \cdots \quad f_m(\boldsymbol{\phi})]^T$, that is,

$$U(\boldsymbol{\phi}) = \left(\sum_{i=1}^{m} |f_i(\boldsymbol{\phi})|^p \right)^{1/p}, \qquad p \geqslant 1 \tag{2}$$

The larger the value of p, the more emphasis is being put on $\max\{|f_1|, |f_2|, \ldots, |f_m|\}$. At the solution, large (small) p typically produces many $|f_i|$'s that are equal to $\max\{|f_1|, |f_2|, \ldots, |f_m|\}$ (equal to zero).

The $p = 1$ case of (2) corresponds to the l_1 norm optimization, solvable by the two-stage algorithm of Hald and Madsen [17, 18]. The algorithm combines a first-order method that approximates the solution by successive linear programming with a quasi-Newton method that uses approximate second-order information to solve the system of nonlinear equations arising from the necessary first-order conditions at a solution.

The $p = 2$ case of (2) (least-squares or l_2 approximation) is a problem of wide publicity. Both first-order and second-order methods have been derived for general nonlinear l_2 problems [19, 20]. For certain linear l_2 problems, a closed-form solution is obtainable by invoking generalized matrix inversion [21, 22].

The objective function defined in (2) is used to penalize the modulus of f_i. To penalize the value of f_i, we use the generalized least pth function

$$U(\boldsymbol{\phi}) = \begin{cases} M_f \left(\sum_{i \in K} (f_i(\boldsymbol{\phi})/M_f)^q \right)^{1/q} & \text{if } M_f \neq 0 \\ 0 & \text{if } M_f = 0 \end{cases} \tag{3}$$

where

$$M_f \triangleq \max_{i \in J} f_i(\boldsymbol{\phi})$$
$$J \triangleq \{1, 2, \ldots, m\} \tag{4}$$

and

$$\begin{array}{lll} \text{if } M_f > 0, & \text{then } K = \{i \,|\, f_i \geqslant 0, i \in J\} & \text{and} \quad q = p \\ \text{if } M_f < 0, & \text{then } K = J & \text{and} \quad q = -p \end{array} \tag{5}$$

In the case of $M_f > 0$ ($M_f < 0$), the larger the value of p, the more nearly would we expect the maximum (minimum) $|f_i|$ to be emphasized. Therefore, the minimization of (3) corresponds to the effort to meet (when $M_f > 0$) or to exceed (when $M_f < 0$) a design specification as much as possible.

As $p \to \infty$, the generalized least pth optimization approaches the minimax optimization, the latter being effectively solved by the combined LP and quasi-Newton method of Hald and Madsen [23, 24]. The algorithm is a two-stage one similar to the l_1 optimization algorithm of [17]. Initially, stage 1 is used and at each point $\mathbf{f}$ is approximated by linear functions using first-order information. In stage 2, the quasi-Newton iteration is used to solve a set of nonlinear equations that necessarily hold at a local minimum. Usually, stage 1 is used to obtain fast convergence to the neighborhood of the solution. Stage 2 is used to obtain superlinear final convergence, but several switches between the two stages may take place.

The two-stage algorithms for l_1 and minimax optimizations are computationally practical and have been implemented by Bandler et al. [25, 26].

2.3 Quadratic Programming

In a quadratic programming (QP) problem, the objective function is defined as

$$U(\boldsymbol{\phi}) \triangleq \Lambda + \mathbf{s}^T\boldsymbol{\phi} + \tfrac{1}{2}\boldsymbol{\phi}^T\mathbf{H}\boldsymbol{\phi} \tag{6}$$

where Λ is a scalar, $\mathbf{s}$ is an n-vector, and $\mathbf{H}$ is an $n \times n$ matrix.

The QP problems arise both in their own right and as subproblems within general nonlinear optimization methods. Typically, a QP problem is to minimize the function of (6) subject to linear equality and/or inequality constraints. Such a problem can be solved, e.g., using the iterative methods described by Gill and Murray [27, 28]. The linear inequality constraints are treated using the active-set methods, in which a prediction of the set of constraints that are active at the solution is maintained. This prediction is called the working set and is updated by adding or deleting constraints as the iterations proceed. By treating the working set as equality constraints, the constrained QP problem is transformed into an unconstrained one. The problem is relatively easy to solve if the original $\mathbf{H}$ is positive definite [27].

For unconstrained QP problems, with $\mathbf{H}$ as positive definite, the minimum can be uniquely located in a finite number of steps, using, e.g., Newton's method and the conjugate gradient method.

2.4 MINMAX and MINBOX Approaches in Linearization

Linearization is often used in solving nonlinear programming problems. Hachtel et al. [29] described the MINMAX and MINBOX approaches, where the range of the validity of a linear approximation is specified in the variable domain and the function domain, respectively. Used in nonlinear minimax optimization, the MINMAX approach resembles the conventional way of locating the minimax point of linearized functions subject to a prescribed "box constraint" on $\boldsymbol{\phi}$. The MINIBOX approach, on the other hand, either produces a smallest step $\Delta\boldsymbol{\phi}$ that achieves user-specified levels of improvement in $\mathbf{f}$, or states that the levels are infeasible.

2.5 Gradient and Nongradient Approaches

The use of exact gradient information $\partial U/\partial\boldsymbol{\phi}$ significantly improves the effectiveness of an optimization algorithm. The well-known adjoint network method developed by Director and Rohrer [30, 31] remains a powerful tool for sensitivity calculation. An equivalent but pure algebraic approach has also been studied [32, 33]. For special types of networks, e.g., branched cascaded networks, more effective methods can be derived [34].

Not infrequently, the gradient is difficult or even impossible to obtain. Approximate gradient methods have been developed, in addition to the direct search methods, which do not depend explicitly on evaluation or estimation of gradients. The theoretical background is the Broyden formula [11, 35], which utilizes function values to improve the gradient estimation as the optimization proceeds. This feature has been implemented in nonlinear l_1 and minimax optimization packages [36].

3 GENERAL FORMULATION OF DIAGNOSIS AS OPTIMIZATION PROBLEMS

3.1 Introduction

The analog diagnosis techniques are described here using a single frequency measurement. Such a description offers both conceptual and notational simplicity. Particular mathematical manipulations required for multifrequency cases are illustrated whenever necessary.

Suppose from the circuit under test (CUT) we obtain a set of measurements represented by an n_F-vector $\mathbf{F}^M$. The corresponding responses as functions of circuit parameters $\boldsymbol{\phi} \triangleq [\phi_1 \quad \phi_2 \quad \cdots \quad \phi_n]^T$ are given by $\mathbf{F} \triangleq \mathbf{F}(\boldsymbol{\phi}, \omega)$. For single-frequency cases, $\mathbf{F} \triangleq \mathbf{F}(\boldsymbol{\phi})$ is used for notational convenience. A nominal design of the circuit is characterized by $\boldsymbol{\phi}^0$ and $\mathbf{F}^0$.

When the measurements are insufficient to identify all parameters, e.g., when $n_F < n$, the equation

$$\mathbf{F}^M = \mathbf{F}(\boldsymbol{\phi}^0 + \Delta\boldsymbol{\phi}) \tag{7}$$

is an underdetermined one. An optimization technique can be used to find the most likely $\Delta\boldsymbol{\phi}$ among an infinite number of solutions to (7). Such a problem can be stated as

$$\underset{\Delta\boldsymbol{\phi}}{\text{minimize}}\ U(\Delta\boldsymbol{\phi}) \tag{8a}$$

$$\text{s.t. } \mathbf{h}(\mathbf{F}^M, \Delta\boldsymbol{\phi}) \triangleq \mathbf{F}(\boldsymbol{\phi}^0 + \Delta\boldsymbol{\phi}) - \mathbf{F}^M = \mathbf{0} \tag{8b}$$

where U is an increasing function of $|\Delta\phi_i|$, $i = 1, 2, \ldots, n$.

A convenient approach to solving (8) is to use penalty methods. For example, a least pth formulation is

$$\underset{\Delta\boldsymbol{\phi}}{\text{minimize}} \left(\sum_{i=1}^{n} w_i|\Delta\phi_i|^p + \sum_{i=1}^{n_F} \beta_i|F_i(\boldsymbol{\phi}^0 + \Delta\boldsymbol{\phi}) - F_i^M|^p \right)^{1/p} \tag{9}$$

where w_i, $i = 1, 2, \ldots, n$, and β_i, $i = 1, 2, \ldots, n_F$, are appropriate weighting factors [25].

3.2 Constraint Equation

Suppose the N-node circuit is characterized by its nodal equation

$$\mathbf{YV} = \mathbf{I} \tag{10}$$

where $\mathbf{Y}$, $\mathbf{V}$, and $\mathbf{I}$ are the nodal admittance matrix, voltage vector, and current excitation vector, respectively. We assume, for convenience, that the measurable responses of the CUT, namely $\mathbf{F}$, can be represented by linear combinations of nodal voltages using an $N \times n_F$ matrix $\mathbf{C}$ such that

$$\mathbf{F} = \mathbf{C}^T\mathbf{V} \tag{11}$$

Thus,

$$\mathbf{F} = \mathbf{F}(\boldsymbol{\phi}) = \mathbf{C}^T[\mathbf{Y}(\boldsymbol{\phi})]^{-1}\mathbf{I} \tag{12}$$

To simplify the nonlinear optimization of (8) and (9), researchers have employed two effective formulations, transforming the constraint equation into linear forms by introducing intermediate parameters. These formulations are the current/voltage source substitution model and the component connection model. The former model will be used throughout this chapter. A comprehensive treatment of the latter can be found in Refs. [37–39].

3.3 The Current/Voltage Source Substitution Model [40–45]

Changes in element values can be equivalently characterized by current or voltage sources. Figure 14.1 shows equivalent representations for some typical elements in linear circuits. Without loss of generality, we assume that the changes are represented by current sources only. Let $\Delta\mathbf{I}^b$ be an n-vector containing such sources corresponding to the n variable elements and $\mathbf{Q}$ be

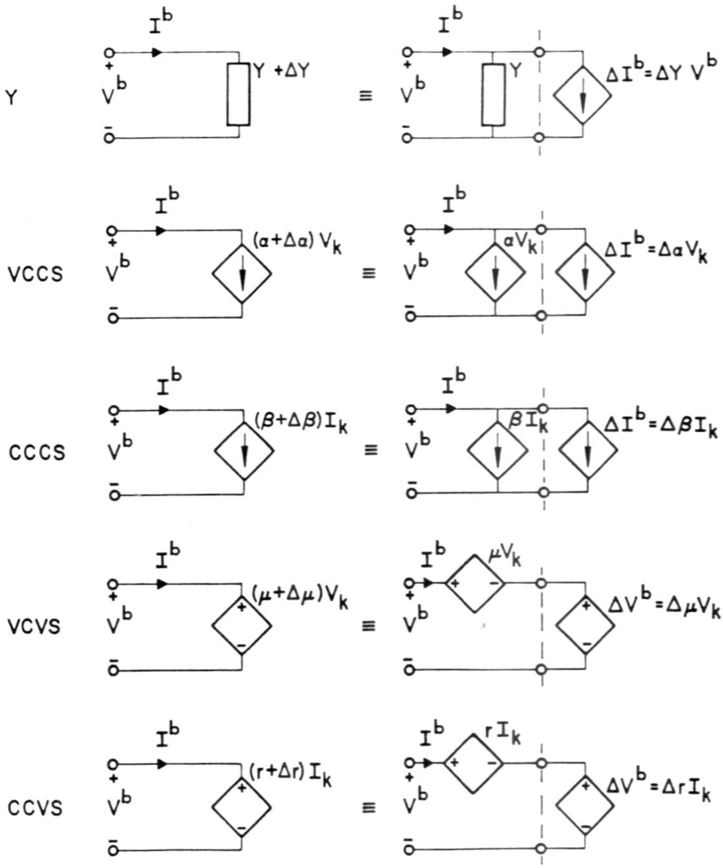

Figure 14.1 Equivalent representation of changes in element values.

an $N \times n$ incidence matrix relating the n branches containing variables to the N nodes of the circuit. By invoking the superposition theorem, we may write

$$\mathbf{Y}(\boldsymbol{\phi}^0)\Delta\mathbf{V} = -\mathbf{Q}\Delta\mathbf{I}^b \tag{13}$$

where $\Delta\mathbf{V}$ is the deviation of actual nodal voltages from their nominal values. Also,

$$\Delta\mathbf{F} \triangleq \mathbf{F} - \mathbf{F}^0 = \mathbf{C}^T\Delta\mathbf{V} = -\mathbf{C}^T[\mathbf{Y}(\boldsymbol{\phi}^0)]^{-1}\mathbf{Q}\Delta\mathbf{I}^b \tag{14}$$

Denote

$$\mathbf{A}' \triangleq -\mathbf{C}^T[\mathbf{Y}(\boldsymbol{\phi}^0)]^{-1}\mathbf{Q} \tag{15}$$

Then we have the constraint equation in linear form as

$$\mathbf{A}'\Delta\mathbf{I}^b = \mathbf{F}^M - \mathbf{F}^0 \tag{16}$$

or in real form as

$$\mathbf{A}\mathbf{x} = \mathbf{b} \tag{17}$$

where

$$\mathbf{A} = \begin{bmatrix} \mathrm{Re}(\mathbf{A}') & -\mathrm{Im}(\mathbf{A}') \\ \mathrm{Im}(\mathbf{A}') & \mathrm{Re}(\mathbf{A}') \end{bmatrix} \tag{18}$$

$$\mathbf{b} = [\mathrm{Re}(\mathbf{F}^M - \mathbf{F}^0)^T \quad \mathrm{Im}(\mathbf{F}^M - \mathbf{F}^0)^T]^T \tag{19}$$

and

$$\mathbf{x} = [\mathrm{Re}(\Delta\mathbf{I}^b)^T \quad \mathrm{Im}(\Delta\mathbf{I}^b)^T]^T \tag{20}$$

To compute $\Delta\boldsymbol{\phi}$ from $\mathbf{x}$, we simulate the network with all components held at nominal values and with additional current excitations $\Delta I_i^b = x_i + jx_{i+n}$, $i = 1, 2, \ldots, n$, connected across corresponding components. After measuring or calculating branch voltages V_i^b, $i = 1, 2, \ldots, n$, the component change is evaluated as

$$\Delta\phi_i = \frac{x_i + jx_{i+n}}{V_i^b}(j\omega)^{-\alpha}, \qquad i = 1, 2, \ldots, n \tag{21}$$

where $\alpha \equiv \alpha_i$, whose value can be 0, 1, or -1 depending on whether the ith component is resistive, capacitive, or inductive [40, 41].

For multifrequency diagnosis, we use $\Delta\boldsymbol{\phi}$ as optimization variables directly. $\mathbf{A}$, $\mathbf{b}$, and $\mathbf{x}$ are redefined accordingly. For example,

$$\mathbf{A}_i = -\mathbf{C}^T[\mathbf{Y}(\boldsymbol{\phi}^0, \omega_i)]^{-1}\mathbf{Q}\ \mathrm{diag}\ \{(j\omega_i)^{\alpha_1}V_1{}^b(\omega_i), \tag{22}$$

$$(j\omega_i)^{\alpha_2}V_2{}^b(\omega_i), \quad \ldots, \quad (j\omega_i)^{\alpha_n}V_n{}^b(\omega_i)\}$$

$$i = 1, 2$$

$$\mathbf{A}'' = \begin{bmatrix} \mathbf{A}_1 \\ \mathbf{A}_2 \end{bmatrix}, \qquad \mathbf{b}'' = \begin{bmatrix} \mathbf{F}^M(\omega_1) - \mathbf{F}^0(\omega_1) \\ \mathbf{F}^M(\omega_2) - \mathbf{F}^0(\omega_2) \end{bmatrix} \tag{23}$$

$$\mathbf{A} = \begin{bmatrix} \mathrm{Re}(\mathbf{A}'') \\ \mathrm{Im}(\mathbf{A}'') \end{bmatrix}, \qquad \mathbf{b} = \begin{bmatrix} \mathrm{Re}(\mathbf{b}'') \\ \mathrm{Im}(\mathbf{b}'') \end{bmatrix} \tag{24}$$

and

$$\mathbf{x} = \Delta\boldsymbol{\phi} \tag{25}$$

where we have assumed that two frequency points are taken. The branch voltages $V_k^b(\omega_i)$, $k = 1, 2, \ldots, n$, are initially assumed. An iterative procedure updates $V_k^b(\omega_i)$ and at the same time computes the changes in $\boldsymbol{\phi}$ [41].

If the nodal equation of (10) is replaced by a hybrid equation, a more general form of (17) can be similarly deduced where both current and voltage sources exist for an equivalent representation of $\Delta\boldsymbol{\phi}$ [40, 41].

3.4 The Component Connection Model [37–39]

We assume that the system topology is described by a matrix relation

$$\begin{bmatrix} \mathbf{u}' \\ \mathbf{F} \end{bmatrix} = \begin{bmatrix} \mathbf{L}_{11} & \mathbf{L}_{12} \\ \mathbf{L}_{21} & \mathbf{0} \end{bmatrix} \begin{bmatrix} \mathbf{v} \\ \mathbf{u} \end{bmatrix} \tag{26}$$

Here, $\mathbf{u}'$ and $\mathbf{v}$ are the component input and output variables, respectively, related by

$$\mathbf{v} = \mathbf{Z}\mathbf{u}' \tag{27}$$

where $\mathbf{Z}$ is the component parameter matrix. The $\mathbf{u}$ and $\mathbf{F}$ in (26) are the system input and output variables related using the system matrix $\boldsymbol{\Gamma}$ as

$$\mathbf{F} = \boldsymbol{\Gamma}\mathbf{u} \tag{28}$$

By introducing intermediate variables $\mathbf{R}$, we have the linear relation

$$\boldsymbol{\Gamma} = \mathbf{L}_{21}\mathbf{R}\mathbf{L}_{12} \tag{29}$$

where $\mathbf{R}$ is related to $\mathbf{Z}$, using

$$\mathbf{R} = (1 - \mathbf{Z}\mathbf{L}_{11})^{-1}\mathbf{Z} \tag{30}$$

It has been shown [39] that for small changes in $\mathbf{Z}$,

$$\Delta\mathbf{Z} \approx \Delta\mathbf{R} \tag{31}$$

As such, $\mathbf{R}$ can be used instead of $\mathbf{Z}$ for optimization. Final results for $\mathbf{Z}$ can be computed using either the exact [i.e., deduced from (30)] or the approximate [i.e., deduced from (31)] relation between $\mathbf{R}$ and $\mathbf{Z}$.

3.5 General Formulation

The intermediate variables $\mathbf{x}$ defined in (20) exhibit a similar pattern to the parameters $\Delta\boldsymbol{\phi}$, since an equivalent source current ΔI^b increases as the corresponding $\Delta\boldsymbol{\phi}$ increases. Also, $\Delta I^b = 0$ if and only if $\Delta\boldsymbol{\phi} = 0$. Now, we can solve the optimization problem with $\mathbf{x}$ as variables and use the solution to find $\Delta\boldsymbol{\phi}$. A simple yet reasonable objective function is the least pth function of

x. A general formulation of diagnosis as an optimization problem is

$$\underset{\mathbf{x}}{\text{minimize}}\, U(\mathbf{x}) \triangleq \left(\sum_{i=1}^{2n} w_i |x_i|^p \right)^{1/p} \tag{32a}$$

$$\text{s.t. } \mathbf{Ax} - \mathbf{b} = \mathbf{0} \tag{32b}$$

where w_i, $i = 1, 2, \ldots, 2n$, are weighting factors and the constraint (32b) is derived from (17)–(20). For the multifrequency case, (22)–(25) can be used to define **A**, **b**, and **x** for the constraint equation (32b). In this case, the objective function U is the weighted least pth function of x_i, $i = 1, 2, \ldots, n$. After solving (32), $\Delta\boldsymbol{\phi}$ can be found using (21) or (25).

4 DIAGNOSIS USING THE LEAST-SQUARES METHOD

The diagnosis technique using least-squares optimization was suggested by Ransom and Saeks [39]. It is based on the assumption that the catastrophic faults have been eliminated and the circuit failure is due to components drifting out of tolerance (as from age, temperature changes, etc.) [39, 42].

The optimization problem can be stated as

$$\underset{\mathbf{x}}{\text{minimize}}\, U(\mathbf{x}) \triangleq \mathbf{x}^T\mathbf{W}\mathbf{x} \tag{33a}$$

$$\text{s.t. } \mathbf{Ax} - \mathbf{b} = \mathbf{0} \tag{33b}$$

where the constraint equation (33b) is defined consistently with (32b). **W** is a diagonal matrix containing weighting factors w_i, $i = 1, 2, \ldots, 2n$. An appropriate choice of the weightings can be such that the U of (33a) approximates

$$\sum_{i=1}^{n} \Delta\phi_i^2$$

under the assumption that $\Delta\phi_i$, $i = 1, 2, \ldots, n$, are quite small. For example [42], for $1 \leqslant i \leqslant n$,

$$\begin{aligned} w_i &= \tfrac{1}{2}(\text{Re}[(j\omega)^{\alpha_i} V_i^b])^{-2} \\ w_{i+n} &= \tfrac{1}{2}(\text{Im}[(j\omega)^{\alpha_i} V_i^b])^{-2} \end{aligned} \tag{34}$$

The solution of the l_2 problem is directly obtained using generalized matrix inversion [21, 22], e.g.,

$$\mathbf{x} = \mathbf{W}^{-1}\mathbf{A}^T(\mathbf{A}\mathbf{W}^{-1}\mathbf{A}^T)^{-1}\mathbf{b} \tag{35}$$

Such a technique using a component connection model has been presented in [39]. The variables **x** consist of elements of the matrix $\Delta\mathbf{R}$. The optimization problem is to minimize the l_2 norm of $\Delta\mathbf{R}$ subject to

$$\Delta \mathbf{\Gamma} = \mathbf{L}_{21} \Delta \mathbf{R} \mathbf{L}_{12} \tag{36}$$

where $\Delta\mathbf{\Gamma}$ is the difference between the measured values and the nominal values of $\mathbf{\Gamma}$. The solution is the generalized inverse of the matrix in (36) [21, 22]. The component connection model is effective here since $\Delta\mathbf{R} \approx \Delta\mathbf{Z}$ under the assumption that no parameters have a significant deviation from nominal.

5 DIAGNOSIS USING THE QUADRATIC PROGRAMMING METHOD

The quadratic programming technique for diagnosis was suggested by Merrill [46]. He considered such a class of situations where a system becomes inoperative due to the failure of one or a few components. He pointed out that because the individual system components are generally highly reliable and well maintained, a diagnosis that implicates many components as having failed is probably not correct. Therefore, contrary to the l_2 optimization technique, the main assumption here is that the difference between the actual and the nominal values for a few elements, which correspond to the faulty elements, is much greater than that for the remaining elements that are nonfaulty.

The optimization problem can be described as

$$\underset{\mathbf{x}}{\text{minimize}}\ U(\mathbf{x}) \triangleq \sum_{i=1}^{2n} w_i \sqrt{|x_i| + \delta} \tag{37a}$$

$$\text{s.t. } \mathbf{Ax} - \mathbf{b} = \mathbf{0} \tag{37b}$$

where the constraint equation (37b) is defined consistently with (32b). The δ under the radical prevents the derivative of the objective function from becoming unbounded.

To solve (37) efficiently, Merrill put the constraint (37b) into the objective function in a quadratic form as a penalty term, applied uniform weightings $w_i = 1$, $i = 1, 2, \ldots, 2n$, and transformed the problem into

$$\underset{\mathbf{y}}{\text{minimize}}\ U(\mathbf{y}) \triangleq \sum_{i=1}^{4n} \sqrt{y_i + \delta} + \frac{1}{2}\beta(\bar{\mathbf{A}}\mathbf{y} - \mathbf{b})^T(\bar{\mathbf{A}}\mathbf{y} - \mathbf{b}) \tag{38a}$$

$$\text{s.t. } \mathbf{y} \geqslant \mathbf{0} \tag{38b}$$

where $\bar{\mathbf{A}} \triangleq [\mathbf{A} \quad -\mathbf{A}]$ and $\mathbf{y}$ is a $4n$-vector related to $\mathbf{x}$ via

$$\begin{aligned} &y_i = x_i \quad \text{and} \quad y_{2n+i} = 0 \qquad \text{if } x_i \geqslant 0 \\ &y_i = 0 \quad \text{and} \quad y_{2n+i} = -x_i \qquad \text{if } x_i < 0 \\ &\quad i = 1, 2, \ldots, 2n \end{aligned} \tag{39}$$

Also, **x** can be calculated from **y** using

$$x_i = y_i - y_{2n+i}, \qquad i = 1, 2, \ldots, 2n \tag{40}$$

Furthermore, the square-root portion of $U(\mathbf{y})$ is linearized at $\mathbf{y} = \mathbf{y}^j$, resulting in

$$U_j(\mathbf{y}) = \Lambda + \mathbf{s}^T\mathbf{y} + \tfrac{1}{2}\mathbf{y}^T\mathbf{H}\mathbf{y} \tag{41}$$

where

$$\mathbf{s} = \tfrac{1}{2}[(y_1{}^j + \delta)^{-1/2} \quad (y_2{}^j + \delta)^{-1/2} \quad \cdots \quad (y_{4n}{}^j + \delta)^{-1/2}]^T - \beta\bar{\mathbf{A}}^T\mathbf{b} \tag{42}$$

and

$$\mathbf{H} = \beta\begin{bmatrix} \mathbf{A}^T\mathbf{A} & -\mathbf{A}^T\mathbf{A} \\ -\mathbf{A}^T\mathbf{A} & \mathbf{A}^T\mathbf{A} \end{bmatrix} \tag{43}$$

The scalar Λ is also a function of β, δ, $\mathbf{y}^j$, and **b**, but as its value is irrelevant to the minimization of $U_j(\mathbf{y})$, it will never actually have to be calculated.

As Merrill indicated, the use of variables **y**, instead of **x**, can eliminate the difficulty of derivative discontinuity of U at $x_i = 0$. The quasi-linearization of U from (38a) to U_j of (41) leads to the natural application of powerful quadratic programming methods [27]. The optimization problem of (38) is solved iteratively by the following steps.

Step 1 $j = 0$, $\mathbf{y}^j = \mathbf{0}$.

Step 2 Compute **s** as a function of $\mathbf{y}^j$ using (42).

Step 3 Minimize $U_j(\mathbf{y})$ of (41), subject to $\mathbf{y} \geqslant \mathbf{0}$, using the quadratic programming method [27]. The solution is defined as $\mathbf{y}^{j+1}$.

Step 4 If $U(\mathbf{y}^{j+1}) \approx U(\mathbf{y}^j)$, then calculate **x** using (40) and stop; otherwise, $j \leftarrow j + 1$ and go to step 2.

6 DIAGNOSIS USING THE LINEAR PROGRAMMING METHOD

Bandler et al. proposed the diagnosis technique using the l_1 norm optimization [40, 41]. The main assumption is similar to that for the quadratic programming approach. However, instead of solving a sequence of quadratic optimization problems, a linear programming problem is formulated, taking advantage of the nature of the l_1 norm as well as the linearity of the constraint equation. A solution to such a problem tends to satisfy the constraint with a minimum number of parameters different from zero. This is consistent with the assumption that a few elements are actually faulty [42, 43].

The optimization problem can be expressed as

$$\underset{\mathbf{x}}{\text{minimize}}\ U(\mathbf{x}) \triangleq \sum_{i=1}^{2n} w_i|x_i| \tag{44a}$$

$$\text{s.t. } \mathbf{Ax} - \mathbf{b} = \mathbf{0} \tag{44b}$$

where the constraint equation (44b) is defined consistently with (32b).

Such a problem can be solved directly using l_1 optimization algorithms, e.g., [17, 25]. It can also be handled by using a regular linear programming solver in a manner similar to that in [47]. Let $\mathbf{y}$ be defined by (39). The problem of (44) is transformed into a standard LP problem as

$$\underset{\mathbf{y}}{\text{minimize}}\ U(\mathbf{y}) \triangleq [w_1 \quad w_2 \quad \cdots \quad w_{2n} \quad w_1 \quad w_2 \quad \cdots \quad w_{2n}]\mathbf{y} \tag{45a}$$

$$\text{s.t. } [\mathbf{A} \quad -\mathbf{A}]\mathbf{y} = \mathbf{b} \tag{45b}$$

$$\mathbf{y} \geqslant \mathbf{0} \tag{45c}$$

At the solution of (45), $\mathbf{x}$ can be calculated from (40).

7 MODELING USING OPTIMIZATION METHODS

In a modeling problem, it is required to find parameter values of an equivalent device model to best fit measurement data. As Hachtel et al. have described [29, 48], the problem is of a type that is frequently encountered by product assurance engineers. These engineers are faced with the fact that the circuits which come off the product line differ from the circuits designed with circuit simulation programs. Consequently, they need device models that agree with on-chip measurements in order to estimate the statistics of the on-chip circuit performance.

7.1 Basic Formulation

Let $\mathbf{f} = \mathbf{f}(\boldsymbol{\phi})$ be an m-vector containing the weighted difference between calculated response $\mathbf{F}(\boldsymbol{\phi}, \omega)$ and measured data $\mathbf{F}^M(\omega)$ in the form

$$w_i(\omega_j)(F_i(\boldsymbol{\phi}, \omega_j) - F_i^M(\omega_j)), \qquad i \in \{1, 2, \ldots, n_F\}, j \in \{1, 2, \ldots, n_\omega\} \tag{46}$$

Due to measurement errors and nonideal effects, $\mathbf{f} = \mathbf{0}$ may not be possible. Therefore, the modeling problem can be stated as

$$\underset{\boldsymbol{\phi}}{\text{minimize}}\ U(\boldsymbol{\phi}) \tag{47a}$$

$$\text{s.t. } \boldsymbol{\phi}_L \leqslant \boldsymbol{\phi} \leqslant \boldsymbol{\phi}_U \tag{47b}$$

where U is an increasing function of $|f_i(\boldsymbol{\phi})|$, $i = 1, 2, \ldots, m$. $\boldsymbol{\phi}_L$ and $\boldsymbol{\phi}_U$ are lower and upper bounds, respectively, for $\boldsymbol{\phi}$.

A reasonable objective function $U(\boldsymbol{\phi})$ can be the least pth function of $\mathbf{f}(\boldsymbol{\phi})$ in the form of (2).

With a small value of p, the objective function tends to accommodate measurements that may contain accidental large errors. Large values of p produce satisfactory results when all measurement errors and nonideal effects are small. Successfully implemented algorithms have used $p = 1$ [25], $p = 2$ [49, 50], and $p = \infty$ [29, 48].

7.2 Limitations of the Basic Formulation

The basic formulation of modeling problems is a traditional approach that is almost entirely directed at achieving the best possible match between measured and calculated responses. This approach has serious shortcomings in two frequently encountered cases. The first case is when the equivalent circuit parameters are not unique with respect to the responses selected and the second is when nonideal effects are not modeled adequately, the latter causing an imperfect match, even if small measurement errors are allowed for. In both cases, a family of solutions for circuit model parameters may exist which produce a reasonable and similar match between measured and simulated responses [51]. Such problems become more difficult to handle with a large number of variables, where a direct optimization is hopeless unless started with accurate estimates of most circuit element values from independent measurements or calculations [49, 52].

Efforts to alleviate those difficulties have been made in several directions. Straightforward approaches include seeking additional independent measurements and/or predetermining some variables. Since both actions reduce the freedom of variables, they can be effectively applied if a further exploitation of physical properties of a given device is permitted. However, when faced with a prescribed set of possible measurements and variables, we can proceed to general approaches such as decomposition and multicircuit measuring.

7.3 Reduction of Model Parameters

Reduction of model parameters may be possible by full investigation of physical properties of the device to be modeled. Such an approach was demonstrated by Curtice and Camisa in a field effect transistor (FET) modeling problem. Using DC and zero-bias measurements, they reduced the number of variables from 16 to 8. The final result of the modeling was reported to be accurate and unique [52].

In laboratory experiments, a repeated trial-and-error procedure may be necessary. Reduction of model variables can be achieved by exploiting the laboratory experience with sample devices. Insensitive variables should be removed at initial stages of an optimization process. Variables tending to reach the upper or lower bounds during the optimization can be fixed in an appropriate manner [29, 48].

7.4 Decomposition Approach

Tsironis and Meierer [49], Kondoh [50] and Bandler and Zhang [10] have suggested decomposing the overall optimization problem of (47) into a sequence of suboptimizations. They illustrated successful FET modeling by properly defining and ordering subsets of parameters and responses. Insensitively related parameters and responses are separated into different subproblems. A series of suboptimizations can provide a good starting point for the overall optimization [49]. It also improves model accuracy and reduces the possibility of stopping at an undesired local minimum.

7.5 Multicircuit Approach

This approach was proposed by Bandler et al. [51]. The l_1-norm objective function was used. Suppose that after taking measurements on a device at a number of frequency points, we make an easy-to-achieve physical adjustment such that one or a few components of $\boldsymbol{\phi}$ are changed in a dominant fashion and the rest remain constant or change slightly. Consider the following optimization problem:

$$\underset{\boldsymbol{\phi}^1, \boldsymbol{\phi}^2}{\text{minimize}} \sum_{k=1}^{2} \sum_{i=1}^{m^k} |f_i^k| + \sum_{j=1}^{n} \beta_j |\phi_j^{\,1} - \phi_j^{\,2}| \tag{48}$$

with superscript k identifying the original network model ($k = 1$) or the model after physical adjustment ($k = 2$). β_j represents an appropriate weighting factor and m^k is an index whose value depends on k; that is, a different number of frequencies may be used for the original and the perturbed model. $\boldsymbol{\phi}^1$ and $\boldsymbol{\phi}^2$ are vectors containing circuit parameters of the original and perturbed networks, respectively.

By adding the second segment to the objective function, we take advantage of the knowledge that only one or a few components of $\boldsymbol{\phi}$ should change dominantly by perturbing a physical component of the device. Therefore, we penalize the objective function for any change in $\boldsymbol{\phi}$. However, by cleverly selecting the l_1 norm, we still allow for one or a few large changes in $\boldsymbol{\phi}$.

Confidence in the validity of the equivalent circuit parameters increases if (1) an optimization using the objective function of (48) results in a reasonable match between calculated and measured responses for both circuits 1 and 2 (original and perturbed) and (2) the examination of the solution reveals changes from $\boldsymbol{\phi}^1$ to $\boldsymbol{\phi}^2$ that are consistent with the physical adjustment; that is, only the expected components have changed significantly. We can build our confidence even more by expanding the technique to more adjustments, that is, formulating the optimization problem as

$$\underset{\boldsymbol{\phi}'}{\text{minimize}} \sum_{k=1}^{n_c} \sum_{i=1}^{m^k} |f_i^k| + \sum_{k=2}^{n_c} \sum_{j=1}^{n} \beta_j^k |\phi_j^1 - \phi_j^k| \tag{49}$$

where n_c circuits and their corresponding sets of responses, measurements, and parameters are considered and the first circuit is the reference model before any physical adjustment. $\boldsymbol{\phi}'$ contains all $\boldsymbol{\phi}^k$, $k = 1, 2, \ldots, n_c$.

8 TUNING USING OPTIMIZATION METHODS

Postproduction tuning is often essential in the manufacturing of electrical circuits. Tolerances on the circuit components, parasitic effects and uncertainties in the circuit model cause deviations in the manufactured circuit's performance, and violation of the design specifications may result. Therefore, postproduction tuning is included in the final stages of the production process to readjust the network performance in an effort to meet the specifications.

Computer-aided designers have approached the tuning problem in two ways, each emphasizing one distinct facet. Before production, at the time of designing a circuit, one can consider tuning as an integral part of the design process [53, 54], the objective being to relax the tolerances on the circuit components and compensate for the uncertainties in the model parameters. The integral design problem is formulated and solved using optimization such that the essential demand of production cost reduction is optimally met. The solution of the design problem provides the manufacturer with the allowed design tolerances and the tunable parameters.

In the final production stages, the manufactured circuit is usually tested to check whether or not it meets design specifications. Tuning is often needed. Here, it is required to implement necessary changes in the tunable parameters to adjust the manufactured circuit to satisfy the design requirements [55].

8.1 Preproduction Tuning [53, 54]

Suppose $\boldsymbol{\varepsilon} \triangleq [\varepsilon_1 \quad \varepsilon_2 \quad \cdots \quad \varepsilon_n]^T$ and $\mathbf{t} \triangleq [t_1 \quad t_2 \quad \cdots \quad t_n]^T$ are vectors containing tolerances and maximum tuning amounts, respectively, for the parameter $\boldsymbol{\phi} \triangleq [\phi_1 \quad \phi_2 \quad \cdots \quad \phi_n]^T$. A nonlinear programming problem integrating design centering, tolerancing, and tuning can be stated as

$$\underset{\boldsymbol{\phi}^0, \boldsymbol{\varepsilon}, \mathbf{t}}{\text{minimize}} \; U(\boldsymbol{\phi}^0, \boldsymbol{\varepsilon}, \mathbf{t}) \tag{50a}$$

$$\text{s.t. } \boldsymbol{\phi} = \boldsymbol{\phi}^0 + \mathbf{E}\boldsymbol{\mu} + \mathbf{T}\boldsymbol{\rho} \in \mathbf{R}_c$$

$$\text{for all } \boldsymbol{\mu}, \quad \boldsymbol{\mu} \in R_\mu$$

$$\text{and some } \boldsymbol{\rho}, \quad \boldsymbol{\rho} \in R_p \tag{50b}$$

where **E** and **T** are $n \times n$ diagonal matrices containing ε_i, $i = 1, 2, \ldots, n$, and t_i, $i = 1, 2, \ldots, n$, respectively, and

$$\boldsymbol{\mu} \triangleq [\mu_1 \quad \mu_2 \quad \cdots \quad \mu_n]^T \tag{51}$$

$$\boldsymbol{\rho} \triangleq [\rho_1 \quad \rho_2 \quad \cdots \quad \rho_n]^T \tag{52}$$

Also, R_c is a constraint region in which all responses satisfy their specifications. R_μ is a group in which $|\mu_i| \leqslant 1, i = 1, 2, \ldots, n$. R_ρ is defined as the region $\{\boldsymbol{\rho} | -1 \leqslant \rho_i \leqslant 1, i = 1, 2, \ldots, n\}$ for two-way tuning and $\{\boldsymbol{\rho} | 0 \leqslant \rho_i \leqslant 1, i = 1, 2, \ldots, n\}$ or $\{\boldsymbol{\rho} | -1 \leqslant \rho_i \leqslant 0, i = 1, 2, \ldots, n\}$ for one-way tuning. The objective function can be an increasing function of $|t_i/\phi_i{}^0|$ and a decreasing function of $|\varepsilon_i/\phi_i{}^0|$, respectively.

8.2 Postproduction Tuning: Problem Formulation

Prior to postproduction tuning, the manufactured circuit is characterized by the actual parameter values given by

$$\boldsymbol{\phi}^a = \boldsymbol{\phi}^0 + \mathbf{E}\boldsymbol{\mu}^a \tag{53}$$

Suppose, for convenience, that the preproduction stage resulted in $t_i > 0$ for $i = 1, 2, \ldots, n_t$ and $t_i = 0$ for $i = n_t + 1, \ldots, n$. Therefore, the tunable parameters are ϕ_i, $i = 1, 2, \ldots, n_t$. A set of circuit performance functions given by

$$\mathbf{F}(\boldsymbol{\phi}, \omega) = \mathbf{F}(\boldsymbol{\phi}^0 + \mathbf{E}\boldsymbol{\mu}^a + \mathbf{T}\boldsymbol{\rho}, \omega) \tag{54}$$

are usually monitored during the tuning process. The desired values for **F**, denoted as $\mathbf{F}^d$, can be either an optimal response or a design specification. Define $\mathbf{f} = \mathbf{f}(\boldsymbol{\phi})$ as an m-vector whose elements are in the form

$$w_{Ui}(\omega_j)(F_i(\boldsymbol{\phi}, \omega_j) - S_{Ui}(\omega_j)) \\ - w_{Li}(\omega_j)(F_i(\boldsymbol{\phi}, \omega_j) - S_{Li}(\omega_j)) \tag{55}$$

where $i \in \{1, 2, \ldots, n_F\}$, $j \in \{1, 2, \ldots, n_\omega\}$, and $\boldsymbol{\phi} \equiv \boldsymbol{\phi}^0 + \mathbf{E}\boldsymbol{\mu}^a + \mathbf{T}\boldsymbol{\rho}$. S_{Ui} and S_{Li} are upper and lower specifications, respectively. w_{Ui} and w_{Li} are weighting factors and are nonnegative. If it is required to match $F_i(\boldsymbol{\phi}, \omega)$ with its desired value $F_i{}^d(\omega)$, one can either use (55) by setting

$$S_{Ui}(\omega) = S_{Li}(\omega) = F_i{}^d(\omega) \tag{56}$$

or define elements of **f** as

$$w_i(\omega_j)|F_i(\boldsymbol{\phi}, \omega_j) - F_i{}^d(\omega_j)| \tag{57}$$

The postproduction tuning can be formulated as the optimization problem

$$\underset{\boldsymbol{\rho}'}{\text{minimize}}\ U(\boldsymbol{\rho}) \tag{58a}$$

$$\text{s.t. } |\rho_j| \leqslant 1, \qquad j = 1, 2, \ldots, n_t \tag{58b}$$

where $\boldsymbol{\rho}'$ is an n_t-vector containing the first n_t elements in $\boldsymbol{\rho}$. The objective function can be a least pth or a generalized least pth function of $\mathbf{f}(\boldsymbol{\phi}^0 + \mathbf{E}\boldsymbol{\mu}^a + \mathbf{T}\boldsymbol{\rho})$, that is, in the forms of (2) and (3), respectively.

8.3 Postproduction Tuning: Functional Approach

Functional tuning is a traditional approach. The tunable parameters are sequentially adjusted until the circuit specifications are met. Here, the network elements are generally assumed unknown.

Let $\mathbf{J}$ be an $m \times n_t$ Jacobian matrix whose (i, j)th element is defined by

$$J_{ij} \triangleq \frac{\partial f_i}{\partial \rho_j} = \frac{\partial f_i}{\partial \phi_j} t_j, \qquad i = 1, 2, \ldots, m, j = 1, 2, \ldots, n_t \tag{59}$$

The least-squares optimization of (58), namely taking $U = \mathbf{f}^T\mathbf{f}$, was proposed by Antreich et al. [56] and Adams and Manaktala [57]. The solution is given by

$$\Delta\boldsymbol{\rho}' = -(\mathbf{J}^T\mathbf{J})^{-1}\mathbf{J}^T\mathbf{f}(\boldsymbol{\phi}^0 + \mathbf{E}\boldsymbol{\mu}^a + \mathbf{T}\boldsymbol{\rho}) \tag{60}$$

The minimax optimization of (58), namely taking $U = \max f_i$, was approximated by Bandler and Salama [43, 55, 58], who solved the following linear programming problem:

$$\underset{\Delta\boldsymbol{\rho}', z}{\text{minimize}}\ z \tag{61a}$$

$$\text{s.t. } f_i(\boldsymbol{\phi}^0 + \mathbf{E}\boldsymbol{\mu}^a + \mathbf{T}\boldsymbol{\rho}) + \sum_{j=1}^{n_t} J_{ij}\Delta\rho_j \leqslant z \tag{61b}$$

$$\rho_{Lj} \leqslant \Delta\rho_j \leqslant \rho_{Uj}, \qquad i = 1, 2, \ldots, m, j = 1, 2, \ldots, n_t$$

$\boldsymbol{\rho}$ is initially set to $\mathbf{0}$. After each solution of (60) or (61), $\boldsymbol{\rho}$ is updated using $\Delta\boldsymbol{\rho}'$. As proposed by Bandler and Salama, simulated sensitivities and the Broyden formula can be used for obtaining and updating $\mathbf{J}$.

8.4 Postproduction Tuning: Deterministic Approach

In contrast to the functional tuning approach, deterministic tuning requires that all circuit parameters $\boldsymbol{\phi}$ and possible parasitic parameters ζ (or its effects) can be either measured or identified. By utilizing this information, the optimization of (58) becomes faster.

A sequential tuning algorithm has been introduced by Lopresti [59]. Let $\mathbf{f}$ be the m-vector defined in (55) or (57). Initially, we set $\boldsymbol{\rho} = \mathbf{0}$ and define

$$\mathbf{f}_1 \triangleq \sum_{i=n_t+1}^{n} \phi_i \frac{\partial \mathbf{f}}{\partial \phi_i} \frac{\Delta \phi_i}{\phi_i} + \sum_i \zeta_i \frac{\partial \mathbf{f}}{\partial \zeta_i} \frac{\Delta \zeta_i}{\zeta_i} \tag{62}$$

which represents the deviation of $\mathbf{f}$ from $\mathbf{f}(\boldsymbol{\phi}^0)$ due to parasitic effects and tolerances in untunable parameters. In the kth iteration, we have

$$\mathbf{f}^{k+1} = \mathbf{f}^k + [J_{1k}\, J_{2k} \cdots J_{mk}]^T \Delta \rho_k, \qquad k = 1, 2, \ldots, n_t \tag{63}$$

By defining U of (58) as a quadratic function of $\mathbf{f}^{n_t+1}$ and adding a term penalizing large changes in $\Delta\boldsymbol{\rho}'$, we obtain an optimal control problem, that is, finding $\Delta\boldsymbol{\rho}'$ such that

$$U = (\mathbf{f}^{n_t+1})^T \mathbf{B} \mathbf{f}^{n_t+1} + \sum_{j=1}^{n_t} \beta_j (\Delta \rho_j)^2 \tag{64}$$

is minimized subject to (63). $\mathbf{B}$ of (64) is a positive semidefinite matrix and $\beta_j > 0$, $j = 1, 2, \ldots, n_t$. A closed-form solution can be obtained in the form

$$\Delta \rho_k = \boldsymbol{\gamma}_k{}^T \mathbf{f}^k \tag{65}$$

where $\boldsymbol{\gamma}_k$ is an m-vector calculated using the Riccatti equation [59].

Instead of using first-order sensitivity information $\mathbf{J}$, which becomes invalid when components of $\Delta\boldsymbol{\rho}'$ are not small enough, Alajajian et al. suggested a large-change sensitivity method for deterministic tuning [60–62]. The resulting equation is

$$[\mathbf{J}^L \quad -\mathbf{f}(\boldsymbol{\phi}^0)] \begin{bmatrix} \Delta\boldsymbol{\rho}' \\ c \end{bmatrix} = -\mathbf{f}(\boldsymbol{\phi}^a) \tag{66}$$

where $\mathbf{J}^L$ is the large-change sensitivity matrix of $\mathbf{f}$ with respect to $\boldsymbol{\rho}'$ and c is an unknown variable.

9 EXAMPLES

In this section, we first present the application of optimization techniques for circuit diagnosis through a simple illustrative example. This is followed by selected problems of practical interest for diagnosis, modeling, and tuning.

9.1 Diagnosis Using Optimization: An Illustrative Example

Consider the passive resistive network of Figure 14.2. Nominal values for elements G_i, $i = 1, 2, \ldots, 5$, are equal to 1. Each element has $\pm 5\%$ tolerance.

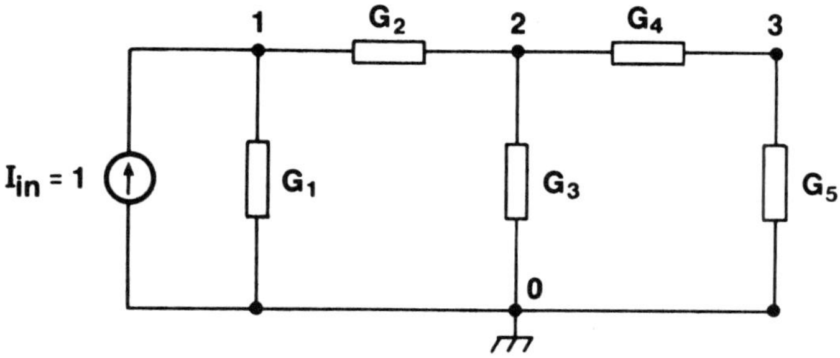

Figure 14.2 Passive resistive circuit as an example for diagnosis using optimization techniques.

The measurable responses are nodal voltages, $\mathbf{F} = [V_1 \quad V_2 \quad V_3]^T$, causing the $\mathbf{C}$ of (11) to be a 3×3 identity matrix. Also for the example, $N = 3$, $n_F = 3$, and $n = 5$. The incidence matrix is given by

$$\mathbf{Q} = \begin{bmatrix} 1 & 1 & 0 & 0 & 0 \\ 0 & -1 & 1 & 1 & 0 \\ 0 & 0 & 0 & -1 & 1 \end{bmatrix} \tag{67}$$

The variable parameters are defined as $\boldsymbol{\phi} = [G_1 \quad G_2 \quad G_3 \quad G_4 \quad G_5]^T$. The nodal admittance matrix at nominal point $\boldsymbol{\phi}^0 = [1 \quad 1 \quad 1 \quad 1 \quad 1]^T$ is

$$\mathbf{Y}(\boldsymbol{\phi}^0) = \begin{bmatrix} 2 & -1 & 0 \\ -1 & 3 & -1 \\ 0 & -1 & 2 \end{bmatrix} \tag{68}$$

For such a circuit, all quantities are real. Therefore, the constraint equations as well as the related definitions (17)–(20) become

$$\mathbf{Ax} = \mathbf{b} \tag{69}$$

where

$$\mathbf{A} = -\mathbf{C}^T[\mathbf{Y}(\boldsymbol{\phi}^0)]^{-1}\mathbf{Q}$$

$$= \frac{-1}{8}\begin{bmatrix} 5 & 3 & 2 & 1 & 1 \\ 2 & -2 & 4 & 2 & 2 \\ 1 & -1 & 2 & -3 & 5 \end{bmatrix} \tag{70}$$

$$\mathbf{b} = \mathbf{F}^M - \mathbf{F}^0 = [V_1{}^M - V_1{}^0 \quad V_2{}^M - V_2{}^0 \quad V_3{}^M - V_3{}^0]^T \tag{71}$$

and

$$\mathbf{x} = [\Delta I_1{}^b \quad \Delta I_2{}^b \quad \Delta I_3{}^b \quad \Delta I_4{}^b \quad \Delta I_5{}^b]^T \tag{72}$$

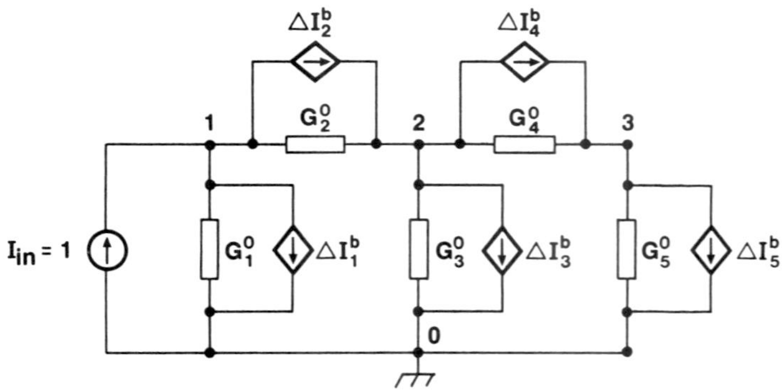

Figure 14.3 Equivalent current sources representing the effect of changes in G_i, $i = 1, 2, \ldots, 5$, for the circuit of Figure 14.2. $\Delta I_i^b = \Delta G_i V_i^b$, where V_i^b is the voltage across the ith element.

where ΔI_i^b, $i = 1, 2, \ldots, 5$ are the equivalent current sources representing ΔG_i, $i = 1, 2, \ldots, 5$, shown in Figure 14.3. The nominal responses $\mathbf{F}^0 = [V_1^0 \quad V_2^0 \quad V_3^0]^T$ can be calculated as $\mathbf{F}^0 = [5/8 \quad 2/8 \quad 1/8]^T$.

Case 1: We assume that no elements have much greater deviation from nominal than others. Table 14.1 shows the results of diagnosis using the l_1 and l_2 techniques and the quadratic programming method. It is demonstrated that the least-squares method gives a more reasonable solution, while the other two methods have mistakenly detected, e.g., G_4 as nonfaulty while this element actually changed 30% for CUT #1. However, the l_2 optimization method may also fail to give correct results; see CUT #3, where the G_2 and the G_5 are not detected as out of tolerance.

Case 2: We assume that only a few elements are faulty and that they have much greater deviation from nominal than the rest of the elements, which are within the specified tolerance of ±5%. Table 14.2 shows the results of diagnosis using the three optimization techniques presented. It can be seen that both the l_1 and quadratic techniques give much sharper results than the l_2 technique. In many cases, both l_1 and the quadratic optimization produce the same solution. In some cases, as shown for CUT #2 and CUT #3 in Table 14.2, one method yields a better solution than the other.

For the quadratic programming technique, we used $\delta = 10^{-6}$ and $\beta = 10^{10}$. The QPSOL FORTRAN package for quadratic programming [28] was utilized to perform step 3 in Section 5 with a limit on the number of iterations for each quadratic programming as 3.

Table 14.1 Results of Diagnosis Using Optimization Techniques for the Circuit of Figure 14.2, Case 1

			Detected $\Delta G_i/G_i^0\%$, $i = 1, 2, \ldots, 5$		
CUT	Measurement $\mathbf{V}^M$	Actual $\Delta G_i/G_i^0\%$ $i = 1, 2, \ldots, 5$	l_2 optimization	Quadratic programming	l_1 optimization
#1	0.5730	4.4	4.36	14.02	13.23
	0.2326	18.0	18.07	1.80	3.14
	0.1186	9.0	7.61	0.00	0.00
		30.0	33.04	0.00	4.00
		25.0	27.93	−3.85	0.00
#2	0.6437	−2.0	−2.38	0.00	0.00
	0.2241	−12.0	−11.41	−15.07	−15.07
	0.1145	6.0	5.28	7.92	7.92
		20.0	23.73	4.35	4.35
		15.0	18.58	0.00	0.00
#3	0.6266	3.0	−0.42	0.00	0.00
	0.2412	−8.0	−2.44	−3.12	−3.12
	0.1307	−3.4	1.96	0.60	0.60
		10.0	17.69	18.28	18.28
		−7.0	−0.50	0.00	0.00

Table 14.2 Results of Diagnosis Using Optimization Techniques for the Circuit of Figure 14.2, Case 2

CUT	Measurement $\mathbf{V}^M$	Actual $\Delta G_i/G_i^o\%$ $i = 1, 2, \ldots, 5$	Detected $\Delta G_i/G_i^o\%$, $i = 1, 2, \ldots, 5$: l_2 optimization	Quadratic programming	l_1 optimization
#1	0.5000	0.0	16.98	0.00	0.00
	0.3333	200.0	149.06	200.00	200.00
	0.1667	0.0	−8.49	0.00	0.00
		0.0	−33.96	0.00	0.00
		0.0	−33.96	0.00	0.00
#2	0.5933	2.0	1.95	1.77	5.77
	0.2207	6.0	6.08	6.36	0.00
	0.1755	−3.0	9.68	0.00	0.00
		300.0	238.72	288.35	235.89
		3.0	−12.78	0.00	−13.51
#3	0.2688	200.0	63.71	199.62	199.04
	0.1304	40.0	304.67	40.73	41.87
	0.0660	−3.0	93.19	0.00	0.00
		4.5	378.57	0.00	2.45
		2.0	367.12	−2.39	0.00

9.2 Diagnosis of a 28-Node Circuit

Kellermann [63] experimented with the nonlinear optimization problem of (9) with $p = 1$, on a 28-node circuit shown in Figure 14.4. The nominal values of the elements $G_i = 1.0$ and tolerances $\varepsilon_i = \pm 0.05$, $i = 1, 2, \ldots, 52$. All outside nodes are assumed to be accessible for measurements. The actual circuit includes four faults where elements G_{41}, G_{44}, G_{45}, and G_{48} have -50% deviation from nominal. All other element values are within their tolerances. The diagnosis was performed successfully with only one excitation. Resulting deviations for G_{41}, G_{44}, G_{45}, and G_{48} are -46, -54, -45, and -53%,

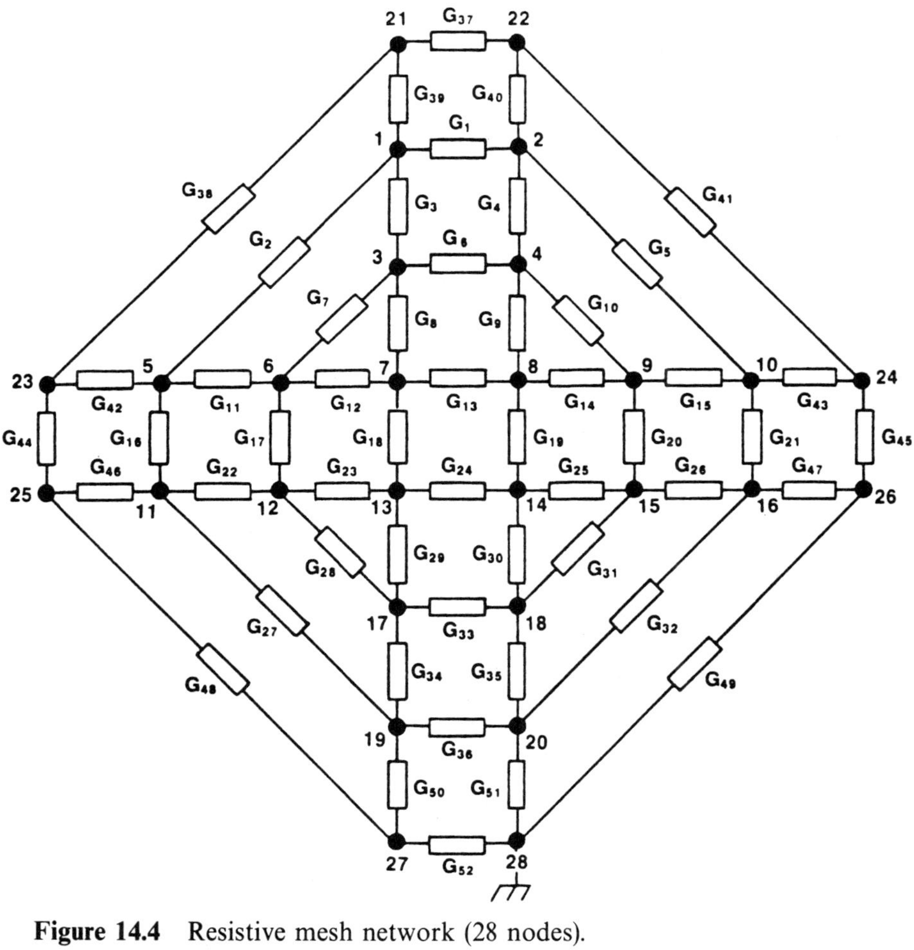

Figure 14.4 Resistive mesh network (28 nodes).

respectively. Deviations for other elements are mostly zero except for a few small nonzero values.

9.3 GaAs FET Modeling: Multicircuit Approach

This example is due to Bandler et al. [51]. They used the equivalent circuit at normal operating bias (including the carrier), as illustrated in Figure 14.5, and created artificial measurements using TOUCHSTONE [64]. Two sets of *S*-parameter (scattering) measurements were created, one set using the parameters reported by Curtice and Camisa [52] (operating bias $V_{ds} = 8.0$ V, $V_{gs} = -2.0$ V, and $I_{ds} = 128.0$ mA) and the other by changing the values of C_1, C_2, L_g, and L_d to simulate the effect of taking different reference planes for the carriers. Both sets of data are shown in Figure 14.6, where the *S*-parameters of the two circuits are plotted on a Smith chart. Although the maximum number of possible variables, namely 32 (16 for each circuit), were allowed for in the optimization, the intrinsic parameters were found to be the same between the two circuits, and, as expected, C_1, C_2, L_g, and L_d changed from circuit 1 to 2. Table 14.3 summarizes the parameter values obtained. The problem involved 128 nonlinear functions (real and imaginary parts of four *S*-parameters, at eight frequencies, for two circuits), 16 linear functions, and 32 variables.

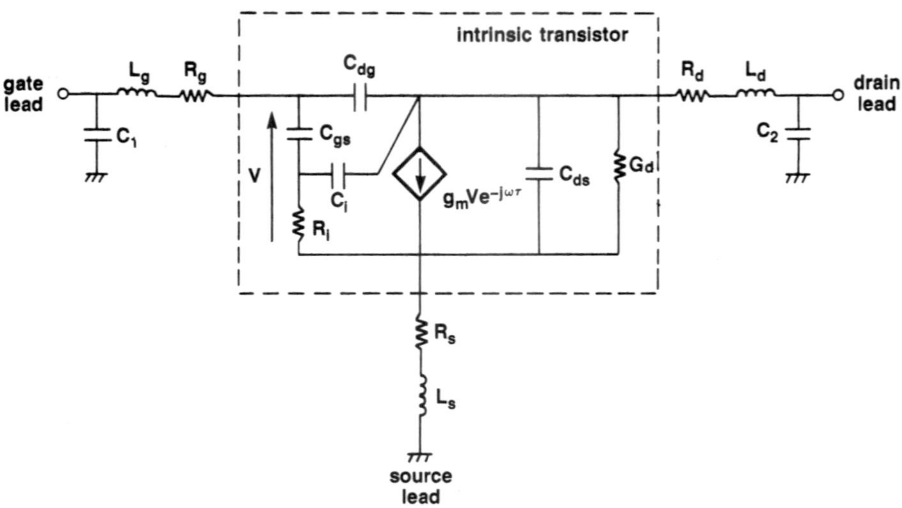

Figure 14.5 Equivalent circuit of carrier-mounted FET (device model B1824-20C).

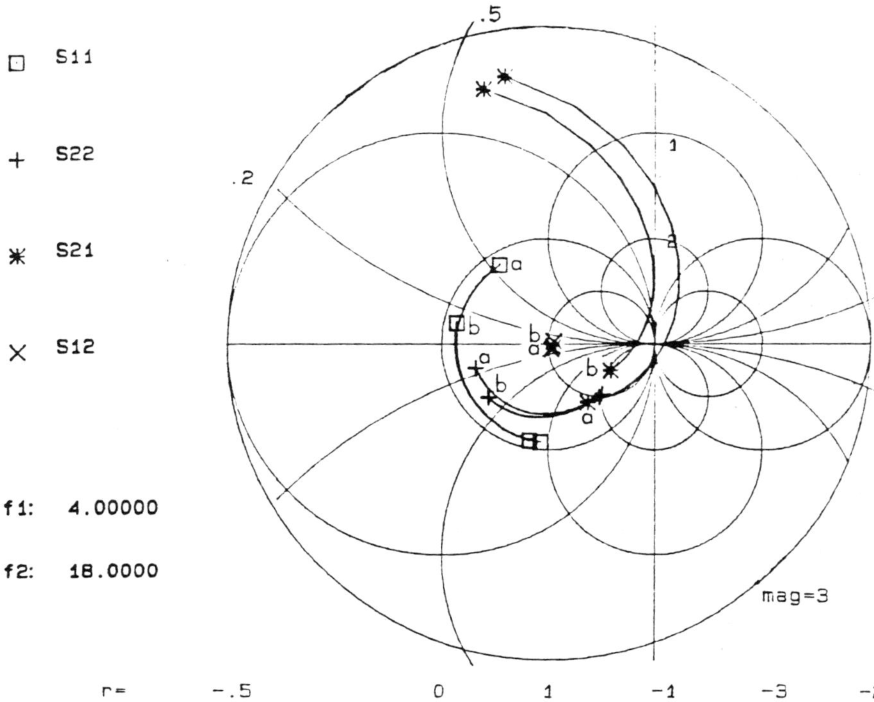

Figure 14.6 Smith chart display of scattering parameters S_{11}, S_{22}, S_{12}, and S_{21} for the carrier-mounted FET, before and after adjustments on parameters. Points a and b mark the high-frequency end of the original and perturbed network responses, respectively.

9.4 A High-Pass Filter Example for Postproduction Tuning

The high-pass notch filter circuit shown in Figure 14.7 was used by Bandler and Salama to demonstrate postproduction tuning algorithms [55]. The circuit example was originally employed by Alajajian [60]. R_3, R_5, R_6, and R_7 are tunable parameters. The nominal and actual element values are given in Table 14.4.

To use the functional tuning approach of (61), Bandler and Salama defined f_i as the absolute value of V_{out} from its nominal, that is, using (57) with $F(\phi, \omega) = V_{out}(\phi, \omega)$ and $F^d(\omega) = V_{out}(\phi^0, \omega)$. Twenty frequencies on the interval 410–505 Hz were used. The limits in (61b) are $\rho_{Uj} = -\rho_{Lj} = 0.02$. After 11 iterations, the tuned responses very closely approached the nominal responses, as shown in Figure 14.8a. After tuning, the values for tunable parameters $[R_3 \quad R_5 \quad R_6 \quad R_7] = [201.952 \quad 2.115 \quad 13.061 \quad 0.973]$.

Table 14.3 Results for the GaAs FET Example

Parameter	Original circuit	Perturbed circuit
C_1 (pF)	0.0440	0.0200[a]
C_2 (pF)	0.0389	0.0200[a]
C_{dg} (pF)	0.0416	0.0416
C_{gs} (pF)	0.6869	0.6869
C_{ds} (pF)	0.1900	0.1900
C_i (pF)	0.0100	0.0100
R_g (Ω)	0.5490	0.5490
R_d (Ω)	1.3670	1.3670
R_s (Ω)	1.0480	1.0480
R_i (Ω)	1.0842	1.0842
G_d^{-1} (kΩ)	0.3761	0.3763
L_g (nH)	0.3158	0.1500[a]
L_d (nH)	0.2515	0.1499[a]
L_s (nH)	0.0105	0.0105
g_m (S)	0.0423	0.0423
τ (ps)	7.4035	7.4035

[a]Significant change in parameter value.

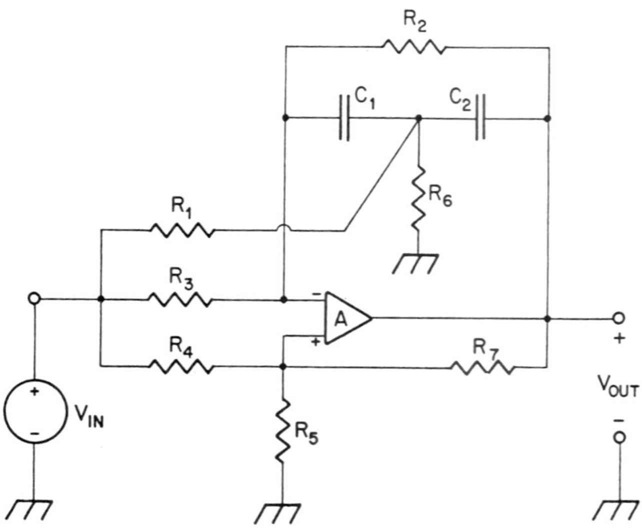

Figure 14.7 The high-pass notch filter circuit.

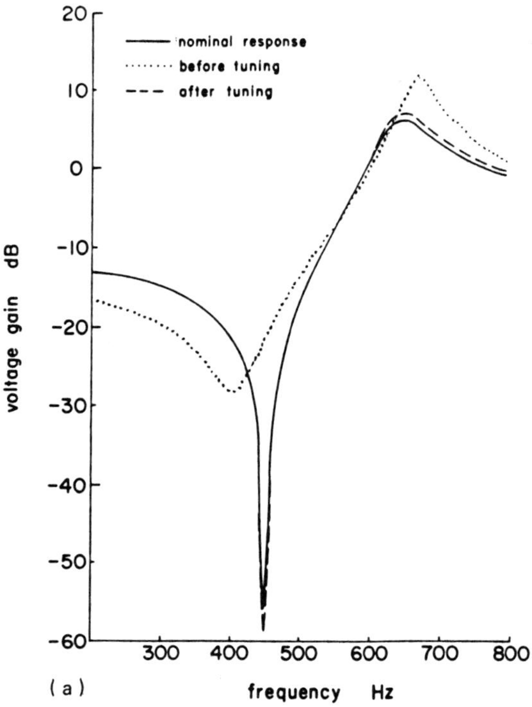

Figure 14.8 Responses for tuning of the high-pass notch filter. (a) Functional tuning. (b) Deterministic tuning.

Table 14.4 Element Values for the High-Pass Filter of Figure 14.7

Element	Nominal value	Actual value	Percentage deviation
R_1 (kΩ)	13.260	13.260	0.0
R_2 (kΩ)	93.0	93.0	0.0
R_3 (kΩ)	214.0	192.6	−10.0
R_4 (kΩ)	2.0	2.0	0.0
R_5 (kΩ)	2.0	1.8	−10.0
R_6 (kΩ)	12.467	11.221	−10.0
R_7 (kΩ)	10.00	9.00	−10.0
C_1 (μF)	0.01	0.00973	−2.07
C_2 (μF)	0.01	0.00965	−3.35
A	10,000.0	10,000.0	0.0

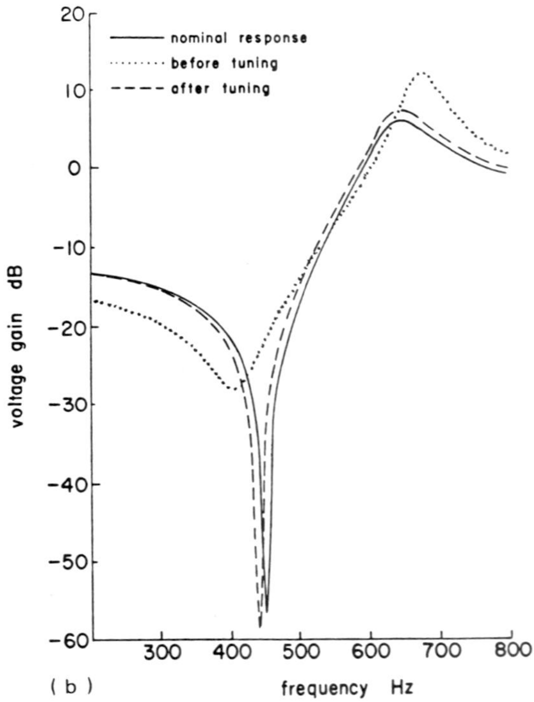

(b)

The deterministic approach of (62)–(65) was performed with $\mathbf{F} = [F_1 \quad F_2 \quad \cdots \quad F_5]^T$, where the F_i are coefficients in the transfer function of the filter $\Gamma = (s^2 + F_1 s + F_2)^{-1}(F_3 s^2 + F_4 s + F_5)$. **B** of (64) was taken as diag$\{4, 0.04, 4, 10^{12}, 0.0625\}$ and $\beta_j = 0.001$. The response associated with the tuning is shown in Figure 14.8b. After tuning, the values for tunable parameters $[R_3 \quad R_5 \quad R_6 \quad R_7]$ are $[184.487 \quad 2.241 \quad 13.747 \quad 0.9993]$.

10 DISCUSSION

Close links and similarities exist between optimization techniques for modeling, diagnosis, and tuning. In this section, relevant common aspects are discussed.

10.1 Sensitivity Matrix

Suppose $\mathbf{f}(\boldsymbol{\phi})$ is defined by (46) for modeling and diagnosis and by (55) or (57) for design and tuning. Let $\boldsymbol{\phi}^0$ be the design nominal. Define the $n \times m$

sensitivity matrix as

$$\mathbf{S}(\boldsymbol{\phi}) \triangleq \operatorname{diag}\{\boldsymbol{\phi}^0\} \frac{\partial \mathbf{f}^T(\boldsymbol{\phi})}{\partial \boldsymbol{\phi}} \operatorname{diag}\{\mathbf{f}(\boldsymbol{\phi}^0)\}^{-1} \tag{73}$$

$\boldsymbol{\phi}^*$ is said to be a regular point [65] of $\mathbf{S}(\boldsymbol{\phi})$ if there exists an open neighborhood of $\boldsymbol{\phi}^*$ in which $\mathbf{S}(\boldsymbol{\phi})$ has constant rank. Parameter identification (or modeling) is usually performed with the assumption that the actual parameter $\boldsymbol{\phi}^a$ is at a regular point and $\text{Rank}[\mathbf{S}(\boldsymbol{\phi}^a)] = n$. Otherwise, if $\text{Rank}[\mathbf{S}(\boldsymbol{\phi}^a)] < n$, that is, the measurement is not sufficient, we should either use the diagnosis technique introduced in Sections 3 to 6 or seek possible additional measurements by creating any or a combination of (1) more accessible nodes for excitation and/or measurement, (2) more frequency points, (3) other types of responses (e.g., voltage and current), and (4) additional circuits obtained by perturbing a few parameters in the CUT. Research has been performed on the selection of excitation and measurement ports and frequencies [42] as well as the multitype response and multicircuit concepts, e.g., [51].

In tuning problems, it is desired that the submatrix containing the first n_t rows of $\mathbf{S}$ (assuming that only the first n_t elements in $[\phi_1 \quad \phi_2 \quad \cdots \quad \phi_n]^T$ are tunable) has a rank which should be as high as the rank of $\mathbf{S}$. Such rank comparison implicates the degree of difficulty to achieve the desired response by tuning ϕ_i, $i = 1, 2, \ldots, n_t$, only.

By checking the $\mathbf{S}$ matrix, possible decomposition can be carried out, sequentially optimizing subsets of responses versus variables that are sensitively related [10].

10.2 Large-Change Sensitivity

The embedding of large-change sensitivity calculations in an optimization procedure, where only a small subset of circuit parameters are updated each iteration, can greatly increase the efficiency. The application of Householder's formula in fault diagnosis was reported [66–68]. Such application can reduce reevaluation of $\mathbf{F}(\boldsymbol{\phi})$ from the order of n to r, r being a rank measure of the subcircuit to be updated. r is less than or equal to the number of parameters in the subcircuit [33, 69].

10.3 Convergence

For problems using the l_1 and minimax optimization method of Hald and Madsen [17, 18, 23–26], superlinear or quadratic convergence is guaranteed. The convergence for Merrill's quadratic approach was reported to be about two or three iterations. For a decomposed problem, sequential optimization may diverge if the subproblems are not well defined or not reasonably ordered. Therefore, it may be desirable to have the system less decomposed as the solution is being approached. Usually, an optimization converges only to a local minimum unless the objective and the constraints satisfy certain conditions. Global optimization methods are being studied [70].

10.4 Possible Difficulties and Disadvantages

Poor or unacceptable results in computer-aided circuit optimization are felt to be most likely due to bad preparation of the problem, lack of understanding of the hazards that can be encountered, and the wrong choice of algorithm [5]. Compared with other techniques for modeling, diagnosis, and tuning (if applicable), optimization techniques often require more computer time and storage. The choice of starting point is often a demanding task for satisfactory solution and fast convergence.

11 CONCLUSION

We have presented basic principles of optimization techniques for modeling, diagnosis, and tuning. Emphasis is centered on the problem formulation and related properties rather than mathematical sophistication of optimization procedures and detailed circuit aspects of MDT. Further research can be directed toward effective modeling techniques to improve the validity of identified parameters. The use and organization of decomposition need further investigation. The desired outcome is an automatic procedure capable of identifying circuit parameters and making decisions concerning physical adjustments based on monitored response and identified parameters.

ACKNOWLEDGEMENTS

The authors thank Dr. T. Ozawa, editor of this book, for his invitation of this contribution. The authors benefited from the work of Dr. A. E. Salama of Cairo University, Giza, Egypt. Fruitful interactions, particularly on the modeling problem, with Dr. S. Daijavad, now at IBM T. J. Watson Research Center, Yorktown Heights, N.Y., and Dr. S. H. Chen, now with Optimization Systems Associates Inc., Dundas, Ontario, Canada, are gratefully appreciated.

REFERENCES

1. G. C. Temes and D. A. Calahan, Computer-aided network optimization: The state-of-the-art, *Proc. IEEE*, vol. 55, pp. 1832–1863, 1967.
2. G. C. Temes, Optimization methods in circuit design, in *Computer Oriented Circuit Design*, F. F. Kuo and W. G. Magnuson, Jr., eds., Prentice-Hall, Englewood Cliffs, N.J., 1969.

3. A. D. Waren, L. S. Lasdon, and D. F. Suchman, Optimization in engineering design, *Proc. IEEE*, vol. 55, pp. 1885–1897, 1967.
4. J. W. Bandler, Optimization methods for computer-aided design, *IEEE Trans. Microwave Theory Tech.*, vol. MTT-17, pp. 533–552, 1969.
5. J. W. Bandler, Computer-aided circuit optimization, in *Modern Filter Theory and Design*, G. C. Temes and S. K. Mitra, eds., Interscience, New York, 1973.
6. J. W. Bandler and M. R. M. Rizk, Optimization of electrical circuits, *Mathematical Programming Study on Engineering Optimization*, vol. 11, pp. 1–64, 1979.
7. S. W. Director, Survey of circuit oriented optimization techniques, *IEEE Trans. Circuit Theory*, vol. CT-18, pp. 3–10, 1971.
8. C. Charalambous, A unified review of optimization, *IEEE Trans. Microwave Theory Tech.*, vol. MTT-22, pp. 289–300, 1974.
9. R. K. Brayton, G. D. Hachtel, and A. L. Sangiovanni-Vincentelli, A survey of optimization techniques for integrated-circuit design, *Proc. IEEE*, vol. 69, pp. 1334–1362, 1981.
10. J. W. Bandler and Q. J. Zhang, An automatic decomposition approach to optimization of large microwave systems, *IEEE Trans. Microwave Theory Tech.*, vol. MTT-35, December 1987.
11. D. G. Luenberger, *Linear and Nonlinear Programming*, 2nd ed., Addison-Wesley, Reading, Mass., 1984.
12. A. Emmett, Karmarkar's algorithm: A threat to simplex?, *IEEE Spectrum*, vol. 22, no. 12, pp. 54–55, Dec. 1985.
13. N. Karmarkar, A new polynomial-time algorithm for linear programming, *Combinatorica*, vol. 4, pp. 373–395, 1984.
14. G. C. Temes and D. Y. F. Zai, Least *p*th approximation, *IEEE Trans. Circuit Theory*, vol. CT-16, pp. 235–237, 1969.
15. J. W. Bandler and C. Charalambous, Theory of generalized least pth approximation, *IEEE Trans. Circuit Theory*, vol. CT-19, pp. 287–289, 1972.
16. J. W. Bandler and C. Charalambous, Practical least pth optimization of networks, *IEEE Trans. Microwave Theory Tech.*, vol. MTT-20, pp. 834–840, 1972.
17. J. Hald and K. Madsen, Combined LP and quasi-Newton methods for nonlinear l_1 optimization, *SIAM J. Numer. Anal.*, vol. 22, pp. 68–80, 1985.
18. J. Hald, A 2-stage algorithm for nonlinear l_1 optimization, Institute for Numerical Analysis, Technical University of Denmark, Lyngby, Rep. No. NI-81-03, 1981.
19. J. E. Dennis, Jr., Non-linear least squares and equations, in *The State of the Art in Numerical Analysis*, D. Jacobs, ed., Academic Press, New York, 1977.

20. D. W. Marquardt, An algorithm for least-squares estimation of nonlinear parameters, *SIAM J. Appl. Math.*, vol. 11, pp. 431–441, 1963.
21. M. Z. Nashed, ed., *Generalized Inverses and Applications*, Academic Press, New York, 1976.
22. C. R. Rao and S. K. Mitra, *Generalized Inverse of Matrices and Its Applications*, Wiley, New York, 1971.
23. J. Hald and K. Madsen, Combined LP and quasi-Newton methods for minimax optimization, *Math. Program.*, vol. 20, pp. 49–62, 1981.
24. J. W. Bandler and W. M. Zuberek, MMLC—a Fortran package for linearly constrained minimax optimization, Department of Electrical and Computer Engineering, McMaster Univ., Hamilton, Canada, Rep. SOS-82-5-U2, 1983.
25. J. W. Bandler, W. Kellermann and K. Madsen, A nonlinear l_1 optimization algorithm for design, modelling and diagnosis of networks, *IEEE Trans. Circuits Syst.*, vol. CAS-34, pp. 174–181, 1987.
26. J. W. Bandler, W. Kellermann, and K. Madsen, A superlinearly convergent minimax algorithm for microwave circuit design, *IEEE Trans. Microwave Theory Tech.*, vol. MTT-33, pp. 1519–1530, 1985.
27. P. E. Gill and W. Murray, Linearly-constrained problems including linear and quadratic programming, in *The State of the Art in Numerical Analysis*, D. Jacobs, ed., Academic Press, New York, 1977.
28. P. E. Gill, W. Murray, M. A. Saunders, and M. H. Wright, User's guide for QPSOL: A Fortran package for quadratic programming, Systems Optimization Laboratory, Department of Operations Research, Stanford Univ., Stanford, Calif., Tech. Rep. SOL 84-6, 1984.
29. G. D. Hachtel, T. R. Scott, and R. P. Zug, An interactive linear programming approach to model parameter fitting and worst-case circuit design, *IEEE Trans. Circuits Syst.*, vol. CAS-27, pp. 871–881, 1980.
30. S. W. Director and R. A. Rohrer, The generalized adjoint network and network sensitivities, *IEEE Trans. Circuit Theory*, vol. CT-16, pp. 318–323, 1969.
31. S. W. Director and R. A. Rohrer, Automated network design—the frequency domain case, *IEEE Trans. Circuit Theory*, vol. CT-16, pp. 330–337, 1969.
32. F. H. Branin, Jr., Network sensitivity and noise analysis simplified, *IEEE Trans. Circuit Theory*, vol. CT-20, pp. 285–288, 1973.
33. J. W. Bandler and Q. J. Zhang, Large change sensitivity analysis in linear systems using generalized Householder formulas, *Int. J. Circuit Theory Appl.*, vol. 14, pp. 89–101, 1986.
34. J. W. Bandler, S. Daijavad, and Q. J. Zhang, Computer aided design of branched cascaded networks, *Proc. IEEE Int. Symp. Circuits Syst.*, Kyoto, Japan, pp. 1579–1582, 1985.

35. C. G. Broyden, A class of methods for solving nonlinear simultaneous equations, *Math. Comput.*, vol. 19, pp. 577–593, 1965.
36. J. W. Bandler, S. H. Chen, S. Daijavad and K. Madsen, Efficient optimization with integrated gradient approximations, *IEEE Trans. Microwave Theory Tech.*, vol. MTT-36, February 1988.
37. R. DeCarlo and R. Saeks, *Interconnected Dynamical Systems*, Marcel Dekker, New York, 1981.
38. M. N. Ransom and R. Saeks, The connection function—theory and application, *Int. J. Circuit Theory Appl.*, vol. 3, pp. 5–21, 1975.
39. M. N. Ransom and R. Saeks, Fault isolation with insufficient measurements, *IEEE Trans. Circuit Theory*, vol. CT-20, pp. 416–417, 1973.
40. J. W. Bandler, R. M. Biernacki, and A. E. Salama, A linear programming approach to fault location in analog circuits, *Proc. IEEE Int. Symp. Circuits Syst.*, Chicago, pp. 256–260, 1981.
41. J. W. Bandler, R. M. Biernacki, A. E. Salama, and J. A. Starzyk, Fault isolation in linear analog circuits using the l_1 norm, *Proc. IEEE Int. Symp. Circuits Syst.*, Rome, pp. 1140–1143, 1982.
42. J. W. Bandler and A. E. Salama, Fault diagnosis of analog circuits, *Proc. IEEE*, vol. 73, pp. 1279–1325, 1985.
43. A. E. Salama, Fault analysis and parameter tuning in analog circuits, Ph.D. Thesis, McMaster Univ., Hamilton, Canada, 1983.
44. J. W. Bandler and A. E. Salama, Recent advances in fault location of analog networks, *Proc. IEEE Int. Symp. Circuits Syst.*, Montreal, pp. 660–663, 1984.
45. K. H. Leung and R. Spence, Multiparameter large change sensitivity analysis and systematic exploration, *IEEE Trans. Circuits Syst.*, vol. CAS-22, pp. 796–804, 1975.
46. H. M. Merrill, Failure diagnosis using quadratic programming, *IEEE Trans. Reliability*, vol. R-22, pp. 207–213, 1973.
47. I. Barrodale and F. D. K. Roberts, An efficient algorithm for discrete l_1 linear approximation with linear constraints, *SIAM J. Numer. Anal.*, vol. 15, pp. 603–611, 1978.
48. R. K. Brayton and R. Spence, *Sensitivity and Optimization*, Elsevier, Amsterdam, 1980.
49. C. Tsironis and R. Meierer, Microwave wide-band model of GaAs dual gate MESFET's, *IEEE Trans. Microwave Theory Tech.*, vol. MTT-30, pp. 243–251, 1982.
50. H. Kondoh, An accurate FET modelling from measured S-parameters, *IEEE Int. Microwave Symp. Dig.* (Baltimore, Md.), pp. 377–380, 1986.
51. J. W. Bandler, S. H. Chen and S. Daijavad, Microwave device modelling using efficient l_1 optimization: a novel approach, *IEEE Trans. Microwave Theory Tech.*, vol. MTT-34, pp. 1282–1293, 1986.

52. W. R. Curtice and R. L. Camisa, Self-consistent GaAs FET models for amplifier design and device diagnostics, *IEEE Trans. Microwave Theory Tech.*, vol. MTT-32, pp. 1573–1578, 1984.
53. J. W. Bandler, P. C. Liu, and H. Tromp, A nonlinear programming approach to optimal design centering, tolerancing and tuning, *IEEE Trans. Circuits Syst.*, vol. CAS-23, pp. 155–165, 1976.
54. E. Polak and A. Sangiovanni-Vincentelli, Theoretical and computational aspects of the optimal design centering, tolerancing and tuning problem, *IEEE Trans. Circuits Syst.*, vol. CAS-26, pp. 795–813, 1979.
55. J. W. Bandler and A. E. Salama, Postproduction tuning employing network sensitivities, *Proc. European Conf. Circuit Theory and Design*, The Hague, Netherlands, pp. 704–709, 1981.
56. K. Antreich, E. Gleissner, and G. Müller, Computer aided tuning of electrical circuits, *Nachrichtentech. Z.*, vol. 28, no. 6, pp. 200–206, 1975.
57. R. L. Adams and V. K. Manaktala, An optimization algorithm suitable for computer-assisted network tuning, *Proc. IEEE Int. Symp. Circuits Syst.*, Newton, Mass., pp. 210–212, 1975.
58. J. W. Bandler and A. E. Salama, Functional approach to microwave postproduction tuning, *IEEE Trans. Microwave Theory Tech.*, vol. MTT-33, pp. 302–310, 1985.
59. P. V. Lopresti, Optimum design of linear tuning algorithms, *IEEE Trans. Circuits Syst.*, vol. CAS-24, pp. 144–151, 1977.
60. C. J. Alajajian, A new algorithm for the tuning of analog filters, Ph.D. Thesis, Univ. of Illinois, Urbana-Champaign, 1979.
61. C. J. Alajajian, T. N. Trick, and E. I. El-Masry, On the design of an efficient tuning algorithm, *Proc. IEEE Int. Symp. Circuits Syst.*, Houston, Texas, pp. 807–811, 1980.
62. D. E. Hocevar and T. N. Trick, Automatic tuning algorithms for active filters, *IEEE Trans. Circuits Syst.*, vol. CAS-29, pp. 448–458, 1982.
63. W. Kellermann, Advances in optimization of circuits and systems using recent minimax and l_1 algorithms, Ph.D. Thesis, McMaster Univ. Hamilton, Canada, 1986.
64. TOUCHSTONE, EEsof Inc., Westlake Village, Calif., 1985.
65. R. Saeks, A. Sangiovanni-Vincentelli, and V. Visvanathan, Diagnosability of nonlinear circuits and systems—part II: Dynamical systems, *IEEE Trans. Circuits Syst.*, vol. CAS-28, pp. 1103–1108, 1981.
66. A. T. Johnson, Jr., Efficient fault analysis in linear analog circuits, *IEEE Trans. Circuits Syst.*, vol. CAS-26, pp. 475–484, 1979.
67. H. S. M. Chen and R. Saeks, A search algorithm for the solution of the multifrequency fault diagnosis equations, *IEEE Trans. Circuits Syst.*, vol. CAS-26, pp. 589–594, 1979.

68. G. C. Temes, Efficient methods of fault simulation, *Proc. 20th Midwest Symp. Circuits Syst.*, Lubbock, Texas, pp. 191–194, 1977.
69. S. B. Haley and K. W. Current, Response change in linearized circuits and systems: Computational algorithms and applications, *Proc. IEEE*, vol. 73, pp. 5–24, 1985.
70. A. Groch, L. M. Vidigal, and S. W. Director, A new global optimization method for electronic circuit design, *IEEE Trans. Circuits Syst.*, vol. CAS-32, pp. 160–170, 1985.

Index

Adjoint network, 385
Algebraic method, 206, 231–232
Ambiguity set, 256, 331, 345
  intersection of, 347
Assume-and-check method, 255
ASTAP, 65, 118
Augmented network, 109
Autonomous circuit, 195

Back substitution, 50
Backward difference formula, 172
Base push-out, 23
Base widening effect, 23
Base-width modulation, 18, 23
Bigenerator, 209, 219
Bilinear function, 212
Block Gauss-Jacobi WR algorithm, 120
Block-Gauss-Seidel WR algorithm, 121
Body factor, 6
Boltzmann distribution, 2
Bordered block diagonal (BBD) matrix, 37
Boundary plane, 68–69
Boundary-value problem, 170, 174
Branch tearing, 43
Broyden formula, 385

Catastrophic failure (*see* Hard failure)
CCM (*see* Component connection model)
Chain path graph, 220
Closed system, 207–209
Coates graph, 271, 273, 274
Common tree, 221, 249, 275, 276
Compact square function, 88
Complementarity
  linear, 74
Complementary pivot method, 338
Complementary problem, 74–79, 337

Component connection model
(CCM), 300-304, 389
Computer-aided design, 233
Collocation, 188
Continuity
of piecewise linear mapping, 67
matrix notation for, 70
Controlled source, 140, 220, 241
Convergence, 120, 410
rate of, 174
Conversion matrix, 191
Corner, 287
Cramer's rule, 207
Crout algorithm, 46
Current graph (I-graph), 144, 220,
243, 275

Dang model, 31-32
Decomposition
graph, 229
hierarchical, 211, 229
nodal, 367
relaxation, 94, 105-110
structural, 94, 100-105
temporal, 94, 105, 119
Decomposition approach (technique)
for circuit simulation, 93-115
for diagnosis, 365-380
for modeling, 395
Decoupling vector, 121
Deficiency, 252
Diagnosability (*see also* Testability),
241-264, 311-313
t-, 370
Diagnosis equation, 267, 268, 291,
305, 307, 309, 315
Diakoptics, 37
DIANA, 119
Digital circuit, 207, 232
Discrete Fourier transform, 211, 214
inverse α-dimensional, 211
Distributed circuit, 207, 233
Dynamic system, 77

Early effect, 18
Early voltage, 19, 20
Ebers-Moll model, 2, 13, 14-17, 18
Eigenvalue method
nodal analysis, 206
state variable, 206
Eigenvalue problem, 208
Electrical connectivity, 256
Emitter efficiency, 21
Euler (method)
explicit, 172, 187
implicit, 173, 187
Expansion method, 170, 186-195

Fault analysis (diagnosis), 219, 385
Fault diagnosis equation (*see* Diagnosis equation)
Fault dictionary (directory), 219,
325-363
integer-code, 351
Fault isolation (location, localization), 255, 265, 277, 344, 373,
374, 378
Fault model, 242
Fault region, 277, 279, 373
Fault verification, 366
Faulty element evaluation, 281-290
Feussner's principle, 230
FFT (*see* Fourier transform)
Field-dependent mobility, 8
Finite-difference method, 170, 183-
185, 201
Flat-band voltage, 6
Flow graph (*see also* Coates graph),
133, 271
Fluid model, 2, 4
Formula manipulation language, 234
Forward substitution, 50
Fourier transform, 157, 210
discrete (DFT), 211, 214
fast (FFT), 210
finite, 210
multidimensional, 211

[Fourier transform]
one-dimensional, 212
Frequency domain solution
of SC networks, 154–160, 166
Full signal (FS), 156
Function-space method, 187

Galerkin method, 188
Generalized common tree, 221
Generalized eigenvalue problem, 208
Generalized least *p*th function, 383
Generalized matrix inversion, 383, 390
Gradient approach, 385
nongradient, 385
Gradual-case approximation, 5
Group delay, 164, 166
Gummel algorithm, 26
Gummel-Poon model, 1, 13, 17–18, 22, 23

Hard failure (fault), 242, 327, 390
Harmonic balance, 189, 200, 201
Hierarchical analysis, 229
Hierarchical decomposition, 211, 229
Hierarchical structure, 90
Hysteresis, 83

I-graph (*see* Current graph)
Implicit integration rule, 78
IMSL, 314
Indefinite admittance matrix, 230
Initial-value problem, 172
Injection node, 287, 288
Integer-code fault dictionary, 351
Integer labeling method, 76
Interpolation, 210, 213, 218, 231
Isolating gate, 103
Iteration factor of WR algorithm, 125
Iterative method, 206

Jacobian, 39, 42, 88, 174, 308
harmonic, 191

Katzenelson algorithm, 94–99
KCL test, 369, 370, 374
k-connection, 272
Knee current, 20

Laplace expansion, 208
Least-squares method, 188, 390
Lemke's algorithm, 76–77, 337
Linear complementary problem (LCP) (*see* Complementary problem)
Linear network, 207
Linear programming, 382, 392
Linking current, 15, 16
LINPACK, 314, 317
Lipschitz-continuous function (mapping), 122, 174
L-matrix, 75
Logic gate model, 86
Loop set
spanning, 224
LU (L/U) decomposition, 46–50, 89
partitioned, 49

MACRO, 119
MACSYMA, 234
Mason's gain formula, 219, 224
MATH, 234
Matrix partition method, 211
Maximally common trees (MCT), 249
Metal-oxide-semiconductor field effect transistor (MOSFET), 1, 5–13, 28, 66, 82
Modeling, 381, 393–396, 405, 410
of transistors, 1–36
Model interconnection, 79
Monotone convergence, 123
MOS (*see* Metal-oxide-semiconductor field effect transistor)

MOTIS, 119
Multicircuit approach, 395, 405
Multifrequency fault diagnosis (testing), 290–295, 299
Multiple excitation, 262, 282
Multiport constraint equation, 339
Multirate effect, 131

Narrow-channel effect, 1, 5, 8, 11
 inverse, 1, 11
Newton-Raphson method (algorithm, iteration), 65, 66, 67, 173, 178, 308–310, 313
Nodal analysis eigenvalue method, 206
Nodal decomposition, 367
Nodal equation, 267
Nodal formulation, 39
Node fault, 256, 265
Node fault diagnosis, 267, 271, 284
 algebraic condition for, 267
 topological condition for, 271
Node fault testability
 f-, 269, 271
Node tearing, 43, 94
Noncanceling term evaluation, 219, 226–228
Nonlinear programming, 382
Norator, 209, 219, 220, 241
Nullator, 219, 220, 241
Numerical interpolation method, 206, 210–219

Operational amplifier (OPAMP), 143, 147
Optimization
 of network performance, 205
 least *p*th, 383
 technique, 382–416
Oscillation condition, 208
Oscillator, 195

Pao-Sah model, 31, 33–34
Parameter extraction method, 206, 231
Parameter identification, 410
Partial derivative method, 212
Particle method, 2
Partition (partitioning)
 of vectors, 39
 of networks (circuits), 106, 125
 overlapped, 130
Partitioned network, 100
Piecewise linear analysis, 65–92
Piecewise linear circuit simulator, 67
Piecewise linear mapping, 71, 81
Piecewise linear function, 94
Piecewise linear resistive network, 336
Pivot, 73, 77
 zero, 74
Pivoting process, 72
P-matrix, 74
Poisson formula, 155, 158
Pole zero calculation, 206
Positive definite (PD) matrix, 74
Principal partition, 249
Projection method, 187

QPSOL, 401
Quadratic form of tableau, 309
Quadratic minimization, 75
Quadratic programming, 384, 391

Rank one update, 90
Rational matrices, 206
 inversion of, 213
REDUCE, 234
RELAX, 119
Relaxation (decomposition), 94, 105–110
Renumbering for sparsity, 56

Samanskii method, 174
Samples and held signal, 156
Semianalytical method, 187

Sensitivity analysis (evaluation), 161, 166, 206, 233
  large change, 219, 339, 410
Sensitivity function, 207
Sensitivity matrix, 409–410
Shooting method, 170, 176–183, 196–200, 201
  parallel (multiple), 181–183
Short-channel effect, 1, 5, 8
  correction factor for, 8
Signal flow graph method, 206, 219–229
Simulation, 118, 304
  parallel, 131–136
Simulation-after-test, 325
Simulation-before-test, 325
Simulator (simulation program), 32 65–67, 79, 88, 118–119
SLATE, 119
Soft failure (fault), 242, 326
Solvability
  measure of, 291, 292, 295
Sorting scheme, 208
Space-charge region recombination, 18
SPICE, 1, 65, 118, 119
SPLICE, 119
Square wave generator, 85
SSVDC, 317
State variable eigenvalue method, 206
Strictly copositive (SCP) matrix, 74
Strictly semimonotone matrix (SSM), 75
Strong inversion state, 6
Sum of squared deviation (SSD), 334
Symbolic network function, 211
  fully, 211
  partially, 211
Switch, 140, 338
Switched-capacitor (SC) network, 139–167, 207, 233
Switching period, 142
Switching phase, 140

Tableau (equation), 304, 305–307, 309
Tearing, 37, 119
  node, 43, 94
  branch, 43
Testability (*see also* diagnosability)
  f-node, 269, 271
  topological condition for, 271
Test frequency, 312
Test frequency bounds, 312–313
Threshold voltage, 5, 6, 8
Time domain solution of SC networks, 153–154, 166
Topological algorithm for fault region, 279
Topological formula, 230
Topological method, 208, 229–231
TOUCHSTONE, 405
Transfer function, 207
Transposed system, 163
Trapezoidal rule, 78
Tree enumeration method, 206, 229–230
Tuning, 381, 396–399, 410
  preproduction, 396
  postproduction, 397–399, 406
  sequential, 399
Two graphs (two-graph method), 143, 230, 243, 275

Unity gain buffer, 144

Variational method, 187
Vector labeling algorithm, 76
Voltage graph (*V*-graph), 144, 220, 243, 275

Waveform relaxation, 66, 117–138
Well posedness, 311
Windowing technique, 131

Z-transform, 154